2/10/16
$145.00

The War on Drugs in Sport

This book is an innovative and compelling work that develops a modified moral panic model illustrated by the drugs in sport debate. Drawing on Max Weber's work on moral authority and legitimacy, McDermott argues that doping scandals create a crisis of legitimacy for sport governing bodies and other elite groups. This crisis leads to a moral panic, where the issue at stake for elite groups is perceptions of their organizational legitimacy. The book highlights the role of the media as a site where claims to legitimacy are made, and contested, contributing to the social construction of a moral panic. The book explores the way regulatory responses, in this case anti-doping policies in sport, reflect the interests of elite groups and the impact of those responses on individuals, or "folk devils." *The War on Drugs in Sport* makes a key contribution to moral panic theory by adapting Goode and Ben-Yehuda's moral panic model to capture the diversity of interests and complex relationships between elite groups. The difference between this book and others in the field is its application of a new theoretical perspective, supported by well-researched empirical evidence.

Vanessa McDermott is a Research Fellow at RMIT University in Melbourne, Australia.

Routledge Research in Sport, Culture and Society

The War on Drugs in Sport
Moral Panics and
Organizational Legitimacy

Vanessa McDermott

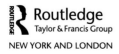

Routledge
Taylor & Francis Group

NEW YORK AND LONDON

First published 2016
by Routledge
711 Third Avenue, New York, NY 10017

and by Routledge
2 Park Square, Milton Park, Abingdon, Oxon OX14 4RN

Routledge is an imprint of the Taylor & Francis Group, an informa business

© 2016 Taylor & Francis

The right of Vanessa McDermott to be identified as author of this work has been asserted in accordance with sections 77 and 78 of the Copyright, Designs and Patents Act 1988.

Library of Congress Cataloging-in-Publication Data
CIP data has been applied for.

ISBN: 978-1-138-81201-7 (hbk)
ISBN: 978-1-315-74905-1 (ebk)

Typeset in Sabon
by Apex CoVantage, LLC

Printed and bound in the United States of America by Publishers Graphics, LLC on sustainably sourced paper.

To Bernie, Bethany, Jacob and Emily

Contents

Abbreviations

AAA	Australian Athletes' Alliance
ABS	Australian Bureau of Statistics
ACC	Australian Crime Commission
ADC	Anti-Doping Code
ADF	Australian Drug Foundation
ADRV/s	Anti-Doping Rule Violation/s
AFL	Australian Football League
AFLPA	Australian Football League Players Association
AIS	Australian Institute of Sport
AOC	Australian Olympic Committee
ASADA	Australian Sports Anti-Doping Agency
ASC	Australian Sports Commission
ASDA	Australian Sports Drug Agency
CAS	Court of Arbitration for Sport
CoE	Council of Europe
DHEA	Dehydroepiandrosterone
EPO	Erythropoietin
FIBA	International Basketball Federation
FIFA	Fédération Internationale de Football Association
FIMS	Fédération Internationale Médicine-Sportive
FINA	Fédération Internationale de Natation
GDP	Gross Domestic Product
GDR	German Democratic Republic
GGOs	Global Governance Organizations
HGH	Human Growth Hormone
IAAF	International Amateur Athletic Federation
IDP	Illicit Drugs Policy
IHF	International Hockey Federation
IICGADS	International Intergovernmental Consultative Group on Anti-Doping in Sport
ISTI	International Standard for Testing and Investigations
IOC	International Olympic Committee

MLB	Major League Baseball
NADA/s	National Anti-Doping Agency/ies
NADO	National Anti-Doping Organization
NDARC	National Drug and Alcohol Research Centre
NDC	National Deviancy Conference
NFL	National Football League (United States)
NHL	National Hockey League
NOC/s	National Olympic Committee/s
NRL	National Rugby League
NSO/s	National Sporting Organizations
OMADA	Olympic Movement Anti-Doping Agency
OMADC	Olympic Movement Anti-Doping Code
PCR	Polymerase Chain Reaction testing
PED/s	Performance Enhancing Drugs
RTP	Registered Testing Pool
SDCM	Sport Drug Control Model
SGBs	Sport Governing Bodies
TSPG	Targeted Sports Participation Growth program
UCI	Union Cycliste Internationale
UIPMB	Union Internationale de Pentathlon Moderne et Biathlon
UNESCO	United Nations Educational, Scientific and Cultural Organization
USADA	United States Anti-Doping Authority
USOC	United States Olympic Committee
USSR	Union of Soviet Socialist Republics
WADA	World Anti-Doping Agency
WADC	World Anti-Doping Code
WHO	World Health Organization

Acknowledgments

The origins of this book can be traced to the southwest coast of 1960s England and Stanley Cohen's analysis of media, police and community responses to a clash of youth subcultures. Learning of these events when I was an undergraduate, the extraordinary reaction and construction of the deviant 'folk devil' resonated with my deeply held convictions around equality and social inclusion. More specifically, Cohen's (1972) analysis and Goode and Ben-Yehuda's (1994) later elaboration of the moral panic concept highlighted the way that powerful groups can manipulate debates and that this has sometimes extreme and undoubtedly unequal and marginalizing consequences for individuals. Together with C. Wright Mills's (1973) "sociological imagination," a moral panic analysis of the "prism" of our social surroundings not only illuminates the different interests at play, but also reveals that there is always room for resistance and change. The moral panic concept provides a powerful tool with which to ask critical questions and create spaces within which to challenge dominant accounts with alternative narratives.

Considering the debate around performance-enhancing drugs in sport provides a valuable opportunity to ask questions that challenge often taken-for-granted aspects of modern sport. Sport is constructed as not only reflecting, but also epitomizing the values that characterize 'healthy' societies. Not only that, sport is constructed as the vehicle for the creation of the 'ideal' human. This is not least because of the so-called natural physical prowess of elite athletes (a notion that is open to much debate in the context of modern medicalized sport) but also because, as the World Anti-Doping Agency (WADA) describe it, at its essence sport is the "celebration of the human spirit, body and mind" based on an ethical foundation that includes values such as "fair play," "respect for rules and laws," "dedication and commitment," "honesty," and "character" (WADA 2015). These are clearly important values, not only in sport, but also in our everyday social interactions with one another.

The problem, however, is that privileging sport as a 'special case' on the basis of values such as these creates a situation that enables issues of exclusion and inequality, such as those around gender, race or social mobility, to be hidden. These types of constructions conceal the fact that while there are opportunities for inclusion, these remain spread unevenly. As Spaaij, Farquharson and Marjoribanks (2015, 400) write, this means that sport is "ultimately a site for social reproduction of hierarchy and social stratification" (e.g., see also Hargie, Mitchell and Somerville 2015; Wheaton 2015). More specifically for this book, these constructions not only create boundaries of inclusion and exclusion, which have come to include anti-drugs regulation and ideas of the 'clean' athlete, but also mean that those boundaries must be policed in order to protect the community. In other words, an appropriate "policing agent" (Erikson 1966), such as WADA, is required in order to protect sport as a site where important societal values are located, linked to broader community well-being.

Placing values-based constructions of sport as the rationale underpinning anti-doping regulation means that athletes take center stage as the exemplars, or ambassadors, of this 'ideal type' sporting community. As such they experience the consequences of boundary maintaining rules and regulations, including anti-doping regulation, firsthand. From a moral panic perspective, athletes are primed as potential 'folk devils' because successful anti-doping regulation requires a subject against which such regulation is implemented. However, this also makes it more difficult to ask questions concerning what might be at stake for those 'policing agents' and other organizational stakeholders in modern sport in terms of maintaining a 'clean' sporting community. This brings us back to the value of a moral panic analysis, which helps to identify what interests might be at stake for elite groups in the construction of a moral panic.

Approaching the doping debate using the legitimacy-inspired modified moral panic model presented in this book means that the analysis then is not limited to why some athletes dope and ways to address such behavior. These are important issues. However, as I describe in this book, a more nuanced analysis, which brings social structures, such as the media, sporting organizations and anti-doping authorities, into the analysis enables us to ask questions concerning the impact of doping on these groups and their regulatory responses to that. There are important aspects to consider because anti-doping regulation has specific and real consequences for athletes, not all of which can be considered as living up to the ideals of equality and other values articulated in descriptions of sport (Henne 2015).

This book, which grew out of my doctoral research work, would not have been possible without assistance and support from many people. I appreciate the Australian Postgraduate Award funded by the Department of Innovation, Industry, Science and Research that enabled me to undertake this project. The Australian National University provided resources including office space and funding for fieldwork and conferences that made this project possible. I especially value the intellectual generosity, and especially their introduction to the sociological imagination as well as the moral panic concept, from Andrew Hopkins, Kevin White and others at The Australian National University throughout my undergraduate career and, later, as colleagues. Without their dedicated and committed approach to sharing knowledge, this journey would never have begun. Thank you to Jan Hayes, for your thoughtful comments on drafts and the time and space to write as well as helping me to stay on track and focused.

Of course, this project would not have been possible without the support of my family. Thank you to my daughters, Bethany and Emily, for not quite understanding what I was actually doing but never doubting I could 'do it.' Throughout this process, I have been privileged to watch you grow into strong and empowered women, thinking critically and reflectively upon the social world and your place in it. Finally, I would like to thank the two people without whom this project would not have been possible. To my husband, Bernie Hogan, I cannot put into words how much I value and appreciate your love and support throughout this long process. You found me when I was lost, sad and lonely and made me feel not only safe and loved, but helped me give voice to the arguments in this book. I also cannot express adequately my appreciation for the support from Dr. Alastair Greig at The Australian National University. There is no doubt that without Alastair's guidance, encouragement and generosity of time in reading and re-reading drafts this project would not have reached completion.

REFERENCES

Cohen, S. 1972. *Folk Devils and Moral Panics: The Creation of the Mods and Rockers*. London: MacGibbon and Kee.

Erikson, K. T. 1966. *Wayward Puritans: A Study in the Sociology of Deviance*. New York: John Wiley and Sons, Inc.

Goode, E., and Ben-Yehuda, N. 1994. *Moral Panics: The Social Construction of Deviance*. Cambridge, Massachusetts: Blackwell Publishers.

Hargie, O., Mitchell, D. H., and Somerville, I. 2015. " 'People have a Knack of Making you Feel Excluded if they Catch on to your Difference': Transgender Experiences of Exclusion in Sport." *International Review for Sociology of Sport*. doi: 10.1177/1012690215583283.

Henne, K. 2015. *Testing for Athlete Citizenship: Regulating Doping and Sex in Sport*. New Brunswick, NJ: Rutgers University Press.

Mills, C. W. 1973. *The Sociological Imagination*. Middlesex, England: Penguin Books.

Spaaij, R., Farquharson, K., and Marjoribanks, T. 2015. "Sport and Social Inequalities." *Social Compass* 9 (5): 400–411.

WADA (World Anti-Doping Agency). 2015. "World Anti-Doping Code 2015." https://wada-main-prod.s3.amazonaws.com/resources/files/wada-2015-world-anti-doping-code.pdf. Accessed 3 September 2014.

Wheaton, B. 2015. "Assessing the Sociology of Sport: On Action Sport and the Politics of Identity." *International Review for Sociology of Sport* 50 (4): 634–639.

Permissions Acknowledgments

Some portions of the Introduction appeared in McDermott, V. 2013. "Adding Legitimacy to the Moral Panic Toolkit." *Critical Criminology Newsletter*, 21:3.

Excerpts from the following paper appear in the Introduction and in Chapter 1: McDermott, V. 2014. "Legitimacy and Consensus in Moral Panic Theory," The annual conference of The Australian Sociological Association, "Challenging Identities, Institutions and Communities," 24–27 November 2014, University of South Australia, Adelaide (https://www.tasa.org.au/wp-content/uploads/2014/12/McDermott.pdf).

Excerpts from the following paper appear in Chapter 4: McDermott, V. 2012. "Legitimating the Fight against Drugs in Sport: The Australian Government and the Australian Football League," The annual conference of The Australian Sociological Association 2012, "Emerging and Enduring Inequalities," The University of Queensland, 26–29 November 2012. (http://www.tasa.org.au/uploads/2012/11/McDermott-Vanessa.pdf)

Excerpts from the following paper appear in the Introduction, Chapter 2 and the Conclusion: Schneider, A. 2000. "Olympic Reform, Are We There Yet?" Paper presented at the *Bridging Three Centuries*, Fifth International Symposium for Olympic Research, The University of Western Ontario, London, Ontario, Canada, September 2000.

Introduction

The moral panic concept, and its associated 'folk devils,' has become one of the most significant contributions to criminology and sociology in the twentieth century. First presented by Jock Young (1971), it was Stanley Cohen's (1972) *Folk Devils and Moral Panics: The Creation of the Mods and Rockers* that popularized the concept (Behlmer 2003; Garland 2008). The origins of moral panic theory can be traced to the intellectual context of the New Deviancy Conference (NDC) at the University of York in 1968. Young and Cohen were founding members of the NDC,[1] which formed at a time when traditional sociological perspectives were challenged and studies of deviance became a central concern in sociology (Plummer 2013; Young 2009). As part of a larger body of work that emerged during this period, Cohen's ideas and research significantly altered the way that criminologists and sociologists—and over time the media and in popular culture—conceptualize social phenomena (Ben-Yehuda 2009; Goode 2012; Innes 2005).

The popularity of the moral panic concept has also had problematic effects. According to Young (2009, 4–5), the concept's insights can be lost due to a "tendency to pluck the concept out of its intellectual context" and apply it to a "rather listless" range of events. More critical assessments suggest that its popularity reflects the concept's lack of theoretical, definitional and evidential integrity (Thompson and Greek 2012). Criticisms of Cohen's original model have nevertheless yielded theoretical innovations that, while emphasizing different elements or adding to the original model, have enhanced its analytical power in ways that are also attuned to societal developments since Cohen's earlier writings (for example, see Hier 2008; Rohloff and Wright 2010).

In this book I highlight the concept's ability to shed light on contemporary issues by presenting a modified moral panic model applied to the debate around performance-enhancing drugs (PEDs) in elite sport as a case study. In doing so, I follow in the constructionist tradition, drawing on and modifying the moral panic model presented by Eriche Goode and Nachman Ben-Yehuda (2009). I respond to a concern posited by Ben-Yehuda (2009, 2):

But what happens to moral panics in multicultural societies where morality itself is constantly contested and negotiated? Consensus about morality in such societies is not a simple or taken-for-granted issue and, therefore, the entire issue of launching moral panics within more general processes of moral entrepreneurship, legislation, policing and regulation has had to be reconceptualized.

In response to this question, I argue that for some moral panics in societies where consensus is contested and negotiated amongst and between diverse social actors, situating a Weberian-inspired consideration of legitimacy within a moral panic framework adds to its explanatory power. Adding legitimacy to a moral panic framework is valuable because it places the focus on the "multifaceted relationships among diverse social agents, fragmented media, representation, and reality" in a moral panic (Hier 2008, 174). Cohen (2002, xxv) had also hinted at the role of legitimacy and moral authority in moral panic theory. He noted that the construction of risk refers to more than assessment or management of risk but "takes a moral turn" that includes evaluations of the "character and moral integrity of the claims-makers. Do they have a right to say this? Is their expertise merely another form of moral enterprise?" Claims of legitimacy and moral authority can contribute to the construction of a moral panic, making them central elements to consider critically.

I apply a legitimacy-inspired moral panic theory to the debate around the use of PEDs or doping in elite sport. The argument here is that doping events can be conceptualized as creating a crisis of legitimacy for sport governing bodies (SGBs), challenging their authority to govern and control their particular sporting community. To avert such a crisis and restore perceptions of legitimacy, doping is constructed as a moral panic involving PED-using 'folk devils' (Cohen 2002). From this perspective, doping is presented as a specific problem of particular concern (Beamish 2009) that threatens community well-being (Goode and Ben-Yehuda 2009), in this case that of the sporting community. This approach contrasts with the current dominant approach to drugs in sport, which tends to focus on changing athletes' behavior or identifying individual personality traits, behaviors and risk factors that may influence the attitudes and motivations of athletes. However, less analysis is conducted of what might be at stake for organizational actors in the doping debate.

The value of investigating the debate over PEDs as an example of a socially constructed moral panic is that it requires "studying those who impute deviance as much as studying the deviants" (Freidson 1970, 215–216). What is at issue is not the objective status of the condition, in this case PED use in sport, but the claims of stakeholders that the condition represents a social problem (Blumer 1971; McCorkle and Miethe 1998). The area of interest here is the nature of stakeholder interactions and "who participates in them, what is at stake, whose definitions prevail and who is affected by them and how" (Ericson, Baranek and Chan 1987, 7). Applying such an approach to PEDs moves the focus away from the athlete-user and incorporates into the analysis broader social structures, such as the media and sporting bodies. As Dingelstad et al. (1996, 1830) note in their discussion of the social construction of drug debates:

> The prime explanatory variable is "interests" . . . groups that stand to gain or lose from a particular way of understanding the world, including corporations, governments, professions . . . through the social constructionist approach: something becomes a social problem when relevant actors define it to be one.

The legitimacy-inspired moral panic model presented in this book helps to identify what interests might be at stake for elite groups in the construction of a moral panic. More specifically, it expands the analysis beyond the somewhat limited observation that economic imperatives or issues of social control motivate elite groups. Rather, situating legitimacy within a moral panic framework demonstrates that elite interests, including the ability to pursue a commercial agenda and maintain control of their particular community, rests on perceptions that their authority is legitimate and valid. In other words, legitimacy is the cornerstone upon which rests the ability of elites to successfully achieve other goals.

I consider which interest groups, or stakeholders, might benefit from constructing doping as a moral panic, involving PED-using 'folk devils' and what these groups stand to lose from continued media reports of doping. Throughout this book, I present evidence to demonstrate that what is at stake for elite SGBs are perceptions of their organizational legitimacy to control their sporting communities. This contributes to the social construction of doping as deviant behavior, with PED-using 'folk devils.' Identification of a group or individual responsible for the problematic behavior is central to a moral panic, as it provides a focus for collective action in the form of an institution-specific regulatory response. The significance of this in the context of PEDs is that it provides opportunities for some elite SGBs to restore their legitimacy by implementing and supporting measures of social control, such as the World Anti-Doping Agency (WADA), as the appropriate and necessary institutional solution to address the problematic behavior. From that perspective, implementing strict anti-doping measures is an opportunity for sporting organizations to enhance their authority by positioning themselves as 'doing the right thing' in protecting the integrity of the sporting community. This is important because such an approach has specific and real consequences for athletes and others who are the subjects of such regulation.

Illustrating this point, a recent work that draws on Howard Becker's (1963) ideas is that of Kathryn Henne (2015, 2) who argues that there are "vested interests in the regulation of athletes' bodies, as they [athletes] communicate values attributed to sport." Thus, she explains, the evolution of anti-doping regulation constitutes an institutionalized 'moral crusade' conducted by 'moral entrepreneurs.' One, of many, consequences that emerge is an embodied form of "athlete citizenship" based on athletes' conformity, or not, with anti-doping policies as testing protocols are 'inscribed' on their bodies. Henne's analysis enables a consideration of broader social inequalities, particularly those associated with color, gender and geographical location (e.g., athletes from the global South) that are inherent in modern elite sport. Similarly to this book, Henne's work contrasts with the dominant approach to anti-doping by not only bringing the influence of broader social issues into the discussion, but also by reminding us of the impact of ideologically driven anti-doping campaigns on individuals' lives. While this is a valuable contribution to the debate around anti-doping and anti-doping regulation, in this book I emphasize that a legitimacy-inspired moral panic lens highlights the way that dominant groups' concern with maintaining the legitimacy and authority to control their particular sporting communities influences anti-doping regulation.

Before discussing the value of applying legitimacy-inspired moral panic framework to consider doping as a moral panic, I next outline events that sparked a legitimation crisis for the International Olympic Committee (IOC) and that affected SGBs globally. The IOC's response to doping is important because the organization has positioned itself as the vanguard of regulation and control of drugs in sport (Boyes 2001). As such, its efforts to identify and sanction 'drug cheats' have significant implications for perceptions of the legitimacy of the IOC as well as other organizations responsible for sports governance.

DOPING, LEGITIMACY AND THE INTERNATIONAL OLYMPIC COMMITTEE

The debate over doping is not a recent development and has long centered on the activities of the IOC and its role as the dominant organization in control of Olympic competition. The importance of legitimacy for the IOC's leadership is evident in arguments emphasizing the ideological values attached to the Olympic Games (Boyes 2001; Schneider 2000). These issues are summarized by Schneider (2000, 225), who notes that:

> . . . the world public identifies Olympic values of excellence, dedication, fair play, and international peace as key ingredients of the Olympic Games. The Olympic Games command the sponsorship they do because the public supports the Games. The Olympic rings connote a higher set of ethics and values and this is what the public support is based on . . . if the public comes to see Olympic values mocked by the practices of the IOC, then the sponsorship value of the Olympic Games will diminish.

Preservation of Olympic ideals is therefore not just the right thing to do, but it is also the best way of preserving the financial success of the Games.

Schneider here points to the significance of meeting community expectations, or public support, in order to maintain positive perceptions of organizational legitimacy. Further, while emphasizing values of excellence, dedication and fair play, the actions of the IOC as "guardians of the Olympic Movement" are located in a broader social context influenced by political and commercial imperatives (Chapter 2, this volume). In this contested socioeconomic space, ensuring that governance frameworks are transparent is necessary in order for the IOC to maintain public support and positive perceptions of its legitimacy and moral authority (Schneider 2000). This includes anti-doping efforts because, as Schneider (2000, 228) writes, doping threatens the Olympic Movement especially if public perceptions are that "Olympic sport is systemically tainted, that no one has the power or the will to do anything about it . . . the outcome will be a worldwide disaffection that will send the moral (and commercial) value of the Games into terminal decline." Thus, active engagement with anti-doping initiatives is integral to the IOC's ability to maintain public and commercial support for the Olympics.

History has demonstrated that failure to protect the values encapsulated by the Olympic Movement can have significant consequences for the legitimacy of the IOC, which I discuss in more detail than I do here in Chapter 2. In the context of doping, although taking steps to address this issue much earlier, several events in 1998 and 1999 adversely affected the IOC's legitimacy and moral authority. These events were the 1998 Tour de France doping scandal, statements by IOC President Samaranch in the Spanish newspaper *El Mundo* and the 1999 Salt Lake City Olympic bribery scandal (MacAloon 2001). I discuss these events in detail in Chapter 2; however, a brief summary follows.

The 1998 Tour de France, *El Mundo* and Salt Lake City

The 1998 Tour de France doping scandal unfolded as French customs officers intercepted Festina cycling team masseur Willy Voet with large amounts of erythropoietin (EPO) and human growth hormone (HGH). Voet's arrest led to police investigations of Tour de France teams and medical personnel (MacAloon 2001; Voet 2001; Waddington 2000). These events challenged the legitimacy and authority of the anti-doping efforts of elite SGBs as magistrates and police took over anti-doping activism (Hoberman 2001; MacAloon 2001). Exacerbating concerns over the IOC's legitimacy resulting from the doping 'busts' by the French authorities in the Tour were Samaranch's comments, reported in the Spanish newspaper *El Mundo*. Samaranch suggested reductions in the list of banned substances and a redefinition of doping. For many, these recommendations implied a decline in the IOC's moral commitment to addressing doping, with significant consequences for their moral authority and legitimacy. MacAloon (2001, 216) writes that "surrender and abandonment of the field, especially under some self-serving rationalization, would remove any claim an organization had to moral standing as a true social movement in sport." IOC members sought to counter any negative impact on perceptions of the IOC's legitimacy by claiming that Samaranch's comments were simply "a personal opinion" and did not affect the integrity of the organization as a whole (MacAloon 2001, 214).

To demonstrate their commitment to anti-doping, the IOC convened the 1999 Lausanne World Conference on Doping in Sport. However, further challenging the position of the IOC as leaders in sport management and administration were accusations of bribery and corruption facing two IOC officials regarding the Salt Lake City bid to host the 2002 Winter Olympics (Crowther 2002). The 1999 Conference was called prior to, but held after, the Salt Lake City bribery scandal, which broke in December 1998. Nevertheless, the bribery scandal contributed to perceptions that the IOC lacked effective leadership and authority (Hoberman 2001; Schneider 2000). At the opening of the Lausanne conference, General Barry R. McCaffrey, director of drug policy in the United States government under the Clinton administration, stated: "Let me sadly but respectfully note that recent examples of alleged corruption, lack of accountability, and failure of leadership have challenged the legitimacy of this institution. These events have tarnished the credibility of the movement" (cited in Rosen 2008, 112).

A direct outcome of the conference was the creation of WADA as an IOC initiative supported by a range of other global actors, including sporting federations and governments as well as public and private bodies (Mendoza 2002, see also WADA 2009). WADA is central to any examination of the anti-doping debate, as this organization emerged in direct response to accusations that the IOC's leadership failed to implement an effective anti-doping system that maintained order and stability in sport (Hoberman 2001). Of interest for this book is the extent to which WADA, as a problem-specific organizational response to doping, provides an example of an institutionalized moral panic driven by elite SGBs' efforts to restore perceptions of their legitimacy.

The World Anti-Doping Agency

A principal task facing WADA is international harmonization of SGBs' anti-doping efforts with a universally binding list of banned substances and a framework of sanctions as well as research and education. To achieve these goals, WADA established the World Anti-Doping Code (WADC) in 2003 (WADA 2008; Chapter 3, this volume). However, the relationship between WADA and SGBs is not necessarily harmonious, with some SGBs reluctant to pass the necessary authority to external regulatory organizations. For example, the Fédération Internationale de Football Association

(FIFA) argued that neither the IOC nor WADA has the right to dictate the terms of disciplinary action or doping sanctions in their sport (Dvorak et al. 2006). This would suggest that an obstacle facing WADA is the desire of SGBs to retain the authority to control their particular sporting communities. I examine the response of SGBs, their interaction with WADA and the extent to which this can be seen in terms of issues of governance and control in Chapter 4, using an Australian sporting organization as a case study.

Shifting ideas regarding sport, or the transformation from playful activity for its own sake to a more extrinsically oriented view, plays a central role in the debate around PEDs. Eitzen and Frey (1991, 508) describe play as "an activity where entry and exit are free and voluntary, rules are emergent and temporary . . . utility of action is irrelevant and the result is uncertain." The transformation from play to modern sport can be associated with other processes of social change, such as industrialization, capitalism, the advance of liberal democracy and mass communications (Horne 2006). This transformation has also been described as the secularization, commodification, rationalization, bureaucratization, quantification, commercialization and spectacularization of sport (Brohm 1978; Eitzen and Frey 1991; Guttmann 1988; Hemphill 1992; Page 1973; Whannel 2005). The more instrumental, performance oriented goals of modern sport illustrate the 'scientization' of sport, which emphasizes "strategies, technical improvement, nutritional and psychological interventions, or any technique to manipulate or engineer the athlete to perform better" (Eitzen and Frey 1991, 509). In this modern industrial sporting complex, and in contrast to play, sport is "hardly voluntary":

> Rules are formal, generalizable and enforced by formal regulatory bodies; the outcome is serious for individuals and organizations not actually participating in the physical activity, and winning (the outcome) is more important than participation (the process). (Eitzen and Frey 1991, 508)

The area of interest for this book is the role of the IOC, and later WADA, as "formal regulatory bodies" seeking to maintain support for their authority to determine and enforce anti-doping rules. The Salt Lake City bribery scandal as well as ongoing doping scandals contributed to a perception that the leadership of the IOC was in crisis (Schneider 2000). In this context, WADA transformed institutional authority regarding anti-doping regulation that, using the WADC, increasingly controls athletes' behavior (Chapter 3, this volume). Like Miah (2002), rather than viewing the creation of WADA as a 'clean break' from the IOC's authoritative position, I argue that the creation of WADA can be seen as a means by which elite SGBs, including the IOC, restore perceptions of legitimacy based on the introduction of specific measures to control doping as a particular problem (Beamish 2009) in sport.

Nevertheless, despite the creation of WADA and the WADC, media reports of doping incidents continue. This raises questions over the ability of WADA to create an anti-doping culture, which has implications for its legitimacy and moral authority. From this perspective, WADA must demonstrate that, rather than raising questions concerning their legitimacy, doping scandals justify their existence as the necessary institutional response to PED-using 'folk devils' (see also Hawdon 2001; Zatz 1987). One consequence of this is that, to bolster their legitimacy and demonstrate their commitment and ability to catch 'cheats,' WADA, but also SGBs' anti-doping authorities and governments introduce increasingly stringent measures to monitor, control and modify athlete behavior. From a moral panic perspective, these types of responses can be described as a process of 'escalation,' 'diffusion' or 'widening-the-net' (Cohen 2002; Goode and Ben-Yehuda 1994b) where new measures of social control are activated or existing measures strengthened. However, before discussing these elements of a moral panic, I next establish the context for the claims of this book by briefly outlining the significance of legitimacy in modern social life, with a particular focus on sport governance.

LEGITIMACY, MORAL AUTHORITY AND SPORTS GOVERNING BODIES

Legitimacy is a foundational sociological concern. Max Weber (1969) noted the interconnected nature of legitimacy and moral authority in the organization of modern social life. He stressed the importance of legitimacy for legally formed and procedurally regulated types of authority characteristic of modern societies. The legitimacy of groups in positions of power, Weber (1969, 214) explained, rests on "the probability that to a relevant degree the appropriate attitudes will exist, and the corresponding practical conduct ensue." Jürgen Habermas (1976) also emphasized the importance of legitimacy, arguing that for any authority to be viewed as legitimate, certain conditions must be fulfilled. These conditions are "that (a) the normative order must be established positively, and (b) those legally associated must believe in its legality, that is, in the formally correct procedure for the creation and application of laws" (Habermas 1976, 98). In other words, legitimacy refers to the extent to which an organization is seen to be "duly constituted and to have valid authority in a relevant area" (Donovan et al. 2002, 276). Any system of authority aiming to maintain social order requires that members of the community perceive claims to legitimacy to be valid (Weber 1969). This is important because belief in the validity of such claims confirms the moral authority of claim-makers to determine appropriate attitudes and conduct for the group.

Morality is also important, as it orients social actions that mark community boundaries based on a set of social criteria, or rules, which evaluate behavior as acceptable, and permissible, for the group or community (Ben-Yehuda 1986). In modern societies, explains Ben-Yehuda, moral boundaries and evaluations of behavior undergo constant processes of negotiation and renegotiation by social groups. In this context, enforcement practices, regulatory frameworks or procedural mechanisms are concerned with moral principles and justifications, questions of right and wrong, and must be open to public scrutiny to be seen as legitimate (Battin et al. 2008; Bok 1989). This means that claims to legitimacy and moral authority cannot be taken for granted, even when manipulated by elite groups, which can include organizations responsible for sport governance, including anti-doping regulation.

The diversity of stakeholders in modern life, including in sport, means that there are different notions of how legitimacy operates in particular communities. As Pakulski (1986, 37) points out, legitimacy is a dynamic analytical concept that is not necessarily clear or easily applied:

> Legitimacy appears to be relative, gradational, dynamic and 'multi-dimensional.' The same rulers may be accepted as legitimate by some, and rejected as usurpers by others. . . . Bases of legitimacy may change and they may be analyzed on such 'dimensions' as credibility, prestige and deference and in such aspects as economic decisions, political activities, propaganda, etc.

In the context of governmental activity, legitimacy includes a subjective component influenced by the quality of governance and delivery of expected outcomes (Connor 2009; Pierre and Røiseland 2011; Rothstein 2009). Modern sport governance, with elite groups such as FIFA and the IOC enjoying monopoly positions with their legitimacy rarely questioned, complicates the development of a legitimacy based explanatory model for SGBs (Connor and Kirby 2011). Nevertheless, SGBs must also address the subjective or 'Janus faced' nature of legitimacy "in that it must be both asked for and received (or denied)" (Connor and Kirby 2011, 8). Bette and Schimank (2001, 52–53) suggest that in the commercial context of modern sport, continued doping scandals carry the potential to give elite sports a 'bad reputation':

> . . . without the interest of the audience, neither mass media nor economic or political sponsors are interested in elite sports. . . . For them, only the interest of the public is of importance which manifests itself as viewing figures, circulations, publicity value. . . . It is these environmental actors and the audience who pays to get into the stadiums where the money comes from. Sport associations need these resources to reproduce themselves and to grow . . . the doping problem could result in a crisis of legitimacy which seriously harms elite sports and its associations.

There is currently little evidence to suggest that audiences are turning away from sport due to continued doping scandals. Nevertheless, to ensure continued commercial gains from audience support, not to mention perceptions of organizational legitimacy, SGBs actively demonstrate a commitment to anti-doping. The growth in the number of sporting 'choices' also means that maintaining the image of sport as drug-free is increasingly important for SGBs to build participation rates and develop their sport.

Organizations governing sport are responsible for the governance and regulation of their particular sport. As a result, they are uniquely situated to create an anti-doping culture centered on compliance with a regulatory framework that defines the boundaries of the sporting community (Donovan et al. 2002; Girginov 2006). According to the Vice-Chair of the Jamaican Anti-Doping Committee, SGBs are mandated to oversee the terms of conditions for participation and the "taking of a drug to enhance performance is entirely inconsistent with the kind of achievement sporting federations are required to advance" (Vasciannie 2006, *Jamaica Gleaner*). Successfully fulfilling this mandate requires that SGBs maintain stakeholder support for their legitimacy and moral authority to establish and monitor the boundaries of their sporting community. This includes from members of the sporting community, the media, athletes and the public(s).

The current anti-doping approach focuses on changing individual behavior and enforcing compliance with agreed moral boundaries, which is PED-free sporting participation, through deterrence-based testing programs, sanctions and education (Donovan et al. 2002). These procedural elements are premised on the intrinsic value of sport, described as the "spirit of sport," which is the "essence of Olympism" and includes a moral values-based foundation of: "ethics, fair play and honesty, health, excellence in performance, character and education, fun and joy, teamwork, dedication and commitment, respect for rules and laws, respect for self and other Participants, courage, community and solidarity" (WADA 2015, 14). Placing these values at the core of the anti-doping campaign creates a normative order based on a set of moral criteria that marks community boundaries and evaluates doping as undesirable behavior fundamentally contrary to the spirit of sport. For example, Peter Ueberroth, former Chairman of the US Olympic Committee, described doping as a "cancer" that not only undermines the credibility of sporting performances, compromises athletes' health and "unfairly tilts the playing field in favor of those that cheat," but also "tears at the fabric of what makes sport unique and important to our society" (cited in AP 2006). However, claims to legitimacy cannot be taken for granted, as social actors, including sporting communities, constantly renegotiate community boundaries and moral evaluations of behavior. Consequently, WADA as well as SGBs that are bound by the WADC must actively work to maintain support for this values-based normative order and for their claims to the moral authority and legitimacy to implement and enforce anti-doping rules.

Nonetheless, throughout the world, SGBs have been criticized for failing to deal effectively with doping, with some commentators claiming that these organizations no longer enjoy the legitimacy and moral authority to create an anti-doping culture (Hoberman 2001; MacAloon 2001). For example, UK Athletics was accused of undermining the fight against doping following the appointment of Linford Christie as mentor to Britain's sprinters (Agencies 2006; *BBC Sport* 2006). Christie, who won the 100 meters gold medal at the 1992 Barcelona Olympics, tested positive for nandrolone in 1999 and was banned for two years (Agencies 2006). Prior to the 2012 London Olympics, media reports described UK Athletics' invitation of Vesteinn Hafsteinsson, who tested positive for nandrolone at the 1984 Los Angeles Olympics, to a coaching clinic for British track and field athletes as "the worst possible example" (Brookes 2011, *Mail Online*). The world swimming organization, the Fédération Internationale de Natation (FINA), has been criticized for failing "to make even the most tentative gesture to keep drugs from our sport" (Leonard 2001, 229). According to a media report, irrespective of the efforts of "administrators, drug testers and anti-doping bodies . . . the doping crisis is undermining any legitimacy that sport still holds" (AP 2006).

Such media reports have the potential to influence a withdrawal of support for SGBs and contribute to a crisis of legitimacy for those organizations. At the same time, however, media reports can also restore flagging support by providing opportunities for SGBs to promote a specific institutional response to doping. As much of the debate takes place in the media and as media reports can influence public perceptions (in this case ideas of the legitimacy of SGBs' anti-doping efforts), consideration of the media's role in the social construction of a moral panic is a central element in this examination. I next outline the role of legitimacy within a moral panic framework applied to the debate surrounding PEDs.

MORAL PANICS AND LEGITIMACY: THE CASE OF PERFORMANCE-ENHANCING DRUGS IN SPORT

Weber's concept of legitimacy can enhance understandings of efforts by elite groups to maintain authority in some moral panics. Considering legitimacy is useful because it analytically captures power relationships between organizations and the way these shape debates. Although privileged, elite groups cannot take for granted claims to the moral authority or legitimacy in order to 'pull the strings.' Rather, these groups must, at least to a certain extent, actively work to generate and maintain support for the legitimacy of an institutional response to a *specific* problem that is of *particular* concern, which is a central feature of a moral panic (Beamish 2009). Further, the diversity of stakeholders in modern life means that there are different notions of how legitimacy operates in particular communities. I noted earlier in this Introduction that legitimacy is multi-dimensional in nature (Pakulski 1986). Examining legitimacy in the context of a moral panic provides an opportunity to consider its multi-dimensional character and the associated implication that "it will operate differently in different contexts, and how it works may depend on the nature of the problems for which it is the purported solution" (Suchman 1995, 573).

Similarly, as Goode and Ben-Yehuda (2009, 247) point out, moral panics do not necessarily follow formal, specific stages consisting of a "beginning, middle and a predictable end." Rather, moral panics may produce different effects and take different forms leading to different outcomes under specific circumstances. Placing legitimacy at the core of a moral panic analysis also addresses some criticisms of both Cohen's original model and later adaptations, such as Goode and Ben-Yehuda (1994a, 2009). In particular, the subjective aspect of legitimacy highlights how dominant groups work to generate and maintain support for their claims to authority, which are contested by a range of other stakeholder groups. In contrast to societal control, imposed from the top-down, authority and legitimacy must be negotiated. This constructs audiences as active participants, as legitimacy must be granted.

The inclusion of legitimacy in a moral panic model also addresses the different ways in which the media's role in a moral panic has been theorized. The British version of moral panic theory is exemplified by the work of Hall et al. (1978) and their analysis of mugging in 1970s Britain. They argued that the law and order campaign in response to mugging (as a moral panic) "had the overwhelming single consequence of legitimating the recourse to the law, to constraint and statutory power, as the main, indeed the only, effective means left of defending hegemony" (Hall et al. 1978, 278). This approach emphasizes the influential role of the media who, rather than presenting objective accounts, are "cued in" to specific news topics by those in authoritative positions (Hall et al. 1978, 57). Some moral panic theorists have criticized claims that elite groups orchestrate a moral panic as underplaying the active role of other social agents (Goode and Ben-Yehuda 2009). Others have argued that such an approach fails to "account for occasions on which the media may take the initiative in *challenging* the so-called primary definers and forcing them to respond" (Schlesinger 1990, 67, cited in Critcher 2002, 529; emphasis in original).

The media do, however, play a key role in generating, or maintaining, public concern in a moral panic, particularly on issues with which audiences have limited or no direct experience (Gonzenbach 1992). Media reports identify 'troublemakers' using morality-focused individualized language to contrast 'demon criminals' with 'responsible authorities' (Ericson et al. 1987; 1991). This also reassures audiences that there are institutional solutions presented in media reports (Wagner-Pacifici 1986). Identifying the deviant group and responsible agents prepared to take action to solve the problem brings even small digressions from the norm into the public eye, enabling calls for greater regulation and control. This process 'normalizes' expressions of hostility toward 'folk devils,' stresses the importance of official agents of social control and informs audiences about the community's moral constraints and values (Lull and Hinerman 1997; Sanders 1990).

Nevertheless, it would be a misrepresentation to generalize audiences as passive consumers or recipients of information. Rather, audiences filter messages through social networks and knowledge frameworks and are influenced by their own interests, which may not coincide with those of dominant groups, including the media (Goode and Ben-Yehuda 2009; Reiner 2007). This is significant in terms of building legitimacy, as a failure to persuade audiences can lead to perceptions that these groups are "incompetent, impractical or illegitimate" (Throgmorton 1991, 154). Consequently, while perhaps often supporting the claim-making activities of dominant groups, the media are sites where claims to legitimacy and moral authority are both made and contested. Thus, the media are not simply conduits for the discourse of elite groups but can play a role in directing and influencing narratives around particular social issues, driven by their own organizational needs—including legitimacy.

Including legitimacy in a moral panic analysis shifts the focus from a temporary event, a crisis, to focus on consequences over time. Moral panics build on a fear that the well-being and fundamental values of society are under threat from a certain category of deviant individuals. This requires that 'something must be done' by those in positions of authority or power (Cohen 2002). Similar to traditional moral panic theory, the 'folk devil' continues to provide a focus for regulation and collective action. However, rather than a 'panic,' the issue becomes how to regulate against ongoing forms of problematic behavior or persons rendered as problematic. This attempts to move beyond assumptions that moral panics are "exceptional rather than ordinary forms of action" (Hier 2008, 171). Instead of a concern with the 'origins' or 'tipping point' that might be the focus of conventional moral panic analyses, the emergent issues are the "implications of volatile moralization for the development of different regulatory approaches" (Hier et al. 2011, 263). One consequence of this is that it enables dominant groups to introduce more stringent measures to regulate the deviant group.

Goode and Ben-Yehuda (2009, 35) describe this as "strengthening the social control apparatus" and include the introduction of more stringent measures to control the so-called deviant group. Cohen (2002, 66–67) describes this process as "diffusion," in which a number of other agents of social control, such as policing bodies, are drawn into the control system. Hall et al. (1978) describe the same process as a "spiral of signification" in which each "new twist" increases concern and anxiety (see also Garland 2008). To deal with new or increasing perceived threats, connections between and among enforcement agencies are either activated or strengthened, (Cohen 2002). Goode and Ben-Yehuda (1994b, 156) describe this as operating under the "widening-the-net principle."

Irrespective of this, the construction of a moral panic is contested ground. Competitive media arenas, with multiple claims and issues vying for attention, mean that not all moral panics become institutionalized parts of the social environment (Best 1990, 1999; Hilgartner and Bosk 1988). Cohen (2002, 1) acknowledged this, writing that while some moral panics have little impact, others have more "serious and long-lasting repercussions and might produce such changes as those in legal and social policy or even in the way society conceives of itself." The forms of moral panic of interest here are those that lead to institutional responses or enforcement mechanisms, which can include the introduction of legislative measures to control the deviant individuals and their behavior (Goode and Ben-Yehuda 1994b). These forms of moral panic are important for organizational claims to legitimacy because they signal to the 'threatening agents' that the community is prepared for the imminent danger. Implementing regulatory or enforcement mechanisms tells the community that "steps are being taken against the threat" (Goode and Ben-Yehuda 2009, 138). This also brings legitimacy into the moral panic framework, highlighting the complexities of power operating in these spaces. The significance of a problem-specific institutional response is that it enables dominant groups to respond to challenges and reassert their power and values, or claims to authority and legitimacy, through a regulatory framework (Gusfield 1963; Schneider 1985).

These contested episodes actually constitutively contribute to wider systems of moral regulation (Hier et al. 2011) and these processes tend to 'evolve' over time. This is because, despite imposing regulatory measures, the 'danger' from the particular behavior or group remains. Thus, the strengthening of existing regulatory and control measures or introduction of new mechanisms is justified in order to prevent the contamination spreading to other parts of society. Consequently, some moral panics leave a significant legacy that contributes to social change and acts as a historical antecedent for later moral panics (Goode and Ben-Yehuda 2009; Killingbeck 2006). Analytically attending to legitimacy highlights ways in which these processes also provide opportunities for elite groups to position themselves as 'doing the right thing'—as leaders in law and order campaigns or protecting the health or integrity of a community. In doing so, however, the evaluative and subjective nature of legitimacy means that dominant groups cannot take their claims to moral authority for granted. To maintain support, dominant groups must engage in ongoing work to generate consensus, from the public and other stakeholders, that the particular behavior or issue in question continues to threaten social order and warrants a strong institutional response.

The model proposed by Cohen (1972) and elaborated upon by Goode and Ben-Yehuda (1994a, 2009) provides an important conceptual framework. The value of this approach is that it enables us to broaden the analysis to consider the role of other social actors and institutions. It provides tools with which to answer questions such as:

Why is a social problem 'discovered' in one period rather than another? What steps are taken, and by whom, to remedy a given condition? Why . . . take steps to remedy this condition but not that, even more harmful, one? Who wins, and who loses, if a given condition is recognized as a social problem? (Goode and Ben-Yehuda 1994b, 152)

A modified moral panic model that includes a Weberian-inspired consideration of legitimacy helps us identify, as Gusfield (1981, 5) noted decades ago, which institutional actors are responsible for "doing something" about the problematic behavior. As well as identifying stakeholders and the influence of these actors on the construction of PED use as deviant behavior, it is essential to examine what such a course means to those groups. As Erikson (1966, 11) points out:

When a community calls the deviant individual to account, it is making a statement about the nature and placement of its boundaries. . . . Members of a community inform one another about the placement of their boundaries by participating in the confrontations which occur when persons who venture out to the edges of the group are met by policing agents . . . they demonstrate . . . where the line is drawn between behavior that belongs in the special universe of the group and behavior that does not.

These types of interactions link members together and, by marking the border between right and wrong, draw the normative contours of a community (Becker 1963; Cromer 1978; Erikson 1966). In this book, I investigate the role of the media and elite SGBs as stakeholders, or claim-makers, in the anti-doping debate and the establishment of a problem-specific 'policing agent' to monitor the boundaries of the sporting community. In other words, some moral panics contribute to social change by creating "ongoing, long-lasting organizational structures" to deal with behavior defined by dominant groups, including the media and other elites, as problematic and threatening social stability (Goode and Ben-Yehuda 2009, 247). Of interest here is the extent to which the doping debate illustrates an institutionalized moral panic underpinned by elite groups' concern to restore or enhance perceptions of their legitimacy leading to a problem-specific organization, namely WADA. Also of interest is the way that WADA reflects elite SGBs' efforts to restore their legitimacy in the face of continued media coverage of doping.

CONCLUSION

The complex nature of contemporary social debates, such as that over drugs in sport, includes a diverse range of stakeholders making and contesting claims to legitimacy. This requires a theoretical framework that takes into account the power relationships between these groups as well as their different interests and objectives. Situating legitimacy within a moral panic framework provides a useful mechanism with which to accomplish this task. Social groups negotiate community boundaries based on moral evaluations of acceptable behavior. Consequently, claim-makers cannot take legitimacy for granted and must actively seek and maintain community support for any claims to authority. This is illustrated using the debate around doping in elite sport. The argument in this book is that in the context of a crisis of legitimacy for SGBs, socially constructing doping as an institutionalized moral panic with PED-using folk devils helps SGBs keep a firmer hold on the power and rewards associated with modern sport. The approach presented contrasts with most current methods used to discuss PEDs, which remain focused on changing individual behavior (Chapter 1, this volume).

CHAPTER STRUCTURE

In this book, I use a Weberian consideration of legitimacy complemented by a moral panic framework to demonstrate that the debate over doping can be conceptualized as a moral panic, involving PED-using 'folk devils.' More specifically, the doping debate illustrates an institutionalized moral panic, with a problem-specific organization (namely WADA) and a regulatory framework (namely the WADC or WADC-aligned policies) to maintain boundaries between the law-abiding 'us' and the deviant PED-using 'other' (Goode and Ben-Yehuda 2009). Underpinning this construction and much of the anti-doping debate are SGBs' efforts to maintain the moral authority and legitimacy to govern and control their particular sporting community. I present evidence for these claims in six chapters.

In Chapter 1, I establish the rationale for the theoretical approach used in this book, which is a modified moral panic model with legitimacy at its core. A large proportion of research and academic literature discussing PEDs in sport remains focused at the level of the athlete-user. Approaching the doping debate using the modified moral panic model presented here means that the analysis then is not limited to why some athletes dope and ways to address such behavior. While these are important issues, the approach presented here brings broader social structures into the analysis, such as the media, sporting organizations and anti-doping authorities. This enables us to ask questions concerning the impact of doping on these groups and their regulatory responses to that. These are important aspects to consider because, as Henne (2015) notes, they lead to specific and real consequences for athletes.

I commence with several socio-historical case studies to illustrate that contested claims to legitimacy are an important part of the doping debate. In Chapter 2, I present the first of three case studies, which includes an outline of the socio-historical context around changing attitudes to substance use in sport and the doping debate. The focus in Chapter 2 is on the IOC and the way that challenges to the legitimacy of the IOC had implications for other SGBs due to criticism of the IOC's leadership role in anti-doping efforts. That leads to a discussion in Chapter 3 of the creation of WADA, the second case study, as a direct result of perceptions that the IOC had failed to maintain order and stability in the sporting community. There I discuss WADA as a means to reinstate SGBs' legitimacy and consider doping as an institutionalized moral panic. In this context, WADA transformed institutional authority in sports management, including anti-doping regulations that, using the WADC, increasingly control athletes' behavior. I also point to organizational tensions in the sporting community as WADA endeavors to implement a globally harmonized anti-doping framework. Modifications to the WADC bring other individuals and groups, which include SGBs and governments, more explicitly under WADA's authority, which raises issues of governance and control between organizational actors.

I examine these issues in Chapter 4 using an Australian SGB, namely the Australian Football League (AFL), as the third and final case study. The AFL administers one of Australia's largest football[2] codes and, following the creation of WADA, faced considerable pressure from the Australian federal government to reform their anti-drugs in sport policies (see McDermott 2012; Stewart 2006, 2007a). I illustrate the way that claim-makers bring diverse objectives to the doping debate, which influences the policy and regulatory frameworks that are applied to the issue. A review of media coverage of doping in Chapter 5 demonstrates that the debate can be conceptualized as a moral panic with PED-using folk devils. This emphasizes that, while not all issues become moral panics, the media can generate concern over an issue and influence the responses of social actors, such as governments and law enforcement agencies (Goode and Ben-Yehuda 2009). The media are not only the means by which moral panics are articulated by dominant groups, but can also be the "spark or . . . beating heart" of a moral panic (Goode and Ben-Yehuda 2009, 90). However, Goode and Ben-Yehuda further explain, while not all "threats" presented by the media "catch fire with the public," nevertheless, "singling out threats, generating alarm, and directing attention to folk devils are among the media's most important functions." Dominant groups use the media to 'frame' issues, such as doping, as problematic and present appropriate institutional solutions, namely WADA. At the same time, claims to legitimacy do not go uncontested and media forums provide opportunities for other stakeholders, such as other SGBs and athletes, to challenge WADA's claims to legitimacy and moral authority.

In Chapter 6, I present qualitative interview data from members of the Australian grassroots sporting community in order to gauge public perceptions of the legitimacy of WADA and the WADC, as applied by Australian sporting organizations. The interviews I discuss formed part of my doctoral research and were conducted in 2007. The relevance of investigating public perceptions of the current anti-doping framework lies in their role as a key sporting stakeholder and one that is important for the commercial success of SGBs. This adds another level of analysis that contrasts with considerations of legitimacy from an organizational perspective and highlights its multi-dimensional nature. The concluding chapter draws together the evidence presented throughout the book and outlines the implications and inferences that emerge. These chapters do not allow me to make any claims that Australian, or any other elite SGBs, WADA or the IOC are experiencing a crisis of legitimacy. Rather, they highlight areas in which these organizations could take action to improve public perceptions of their commitment to anti-doping and, consequently, perceptions of their legitimacy.

NOTES

1 NDC founding members included Paul Rock, Kit Carson, David Downes, Ian Taylor and Mary McIntosh (Plummer 2013).
2 The term football can be used to describe an array of games, such as soccer, American football, Australian football, Gaelic football, rugby union and rugby league (Stewart 2007b). In using the term Australian football, I refer to the game that is administered by the AFL and which is variously described as Australian Rules, AFL or simply "footy" (Stewart 2007b, 5). In using the descriptor Australian football, I follow the lead of the AFL website, which consistently refers to "Australian football" (Nicholson 2006, 1).

REFERENCES

Agencies. 2006. "Gold Medal Tainted by Drugs." *The Age*, 8 August 2006. http://www.theage.com.au/news/sport/gold-medal-tainted-by-drugs/2006/08/07/1154802822652.html. Accessed 8 August 2006.

AP (Associated Press). 2006. "Sports Losing the Battle Against Doping Image and Credibility Taking a Hit." *The Winnipeg Sun*, 31 July 2006. http://winnipegsun.com/Sports/OtherSports/2006/07/31/1711477-sun.html. Accessed 1 August 2006.

Battin, M. P., Luna, E., Lipman, A. G., Gahlinger, P.M., Rollins, D. E., Roberts, J. C., and Booher, T. L. 2008. *Drugs and Justice: Seeking a Consistent, Coherent, Comprehensive View*. Oxford: Oxford University Press.

BBC Sport. 2006. "Radcliffe Attacks Christie Role." *BBC Sport*, 13 August 2006. http://news.bbc.co.uk/sport2/hi/athletics/4788157.stm. Accessed 7 April 2011.

Beamish, R. 2009. "Steroids, Symbolism and Morality: The Construction of a Social Problem and Its Unintended Consequences." In *Elite Sport, Doping and Public Health*, edited by Moller, V., McNamee, M. and Dimeo, P., 55–73. Odense: University of Southern Denmark.

Becker, H. S. 1963. *Outsiders*. New York: Free Press.

Behlmer, G. K. 2003. "Grave Doubts: Victorian Medicine, Moral Panic, and the Signs of Death." *The Journal of British Studies* 42 (2): 206–235.

Ben-Yehuda, N. 1986. "The Sociology of Moral Panics: Toward a New Synthesis." *Sociological Quarterly* 27 (4): 495–513.

———. 2009. "Moral Panics—36 Years On." *British Journal of Criminology* 49: 1–3.

Best, J. 1990. *Threatened Children: Rhetoric and Concern about Child-Victims.* Chicago: University Press of Chicago.

———. 1999. *Random Violence: How We Talk about New Crimes and New Victims.* Berkeley: University of California Press.

Bette, K., and Schimank, U. 2001. "Coping with Doping: Sport Associations Under Organisational Stress." In *Proceedings from the Workshop Research on Doping in Sport,* 51–69. Oslo: The Research Council of Norway.

Blumer, H. 1971. "Social Problems As Collective Behavior." *Social Problems* 18 (3): 298–306.

Bok, S. 1989. *Lying Moral Choice in Public and Private Life.* New York: Vintage Books.

Boyes, S. 2001. "The International Olympic Committee, Transnational Doping Policy and Globalisation." In *Drugs and Doping in Sport Socio-Legal Perspectives,* edited by O'Leary, J., 167–179. London: Cavendish Publishing.

Brohm, Jean-Marie. 1978. *Sport: A Prison of Measured Time.* London: Ink Links.

Brookes, J. 2011. "UK Athletics Sanction Drugs Cheat to Help Coach British Medal Hopeful Okoye." *Mail Online,* 31 July 2011. http://www.dailymail.co.uk/sport/othersports/article-2020585/UK-Athletics-sanction-drugs-cheat-help-coach-young-British-medal-hopeful-Okoye.html?ito=feeds-newsxml. Accessed 1 August 2011.

Cohen, S. 1972. *Folk Devils and Moral Panics: The Creation of the Mods and Rockers.* London: MacGibbon and Kee.

———. 2002. *Folk devils and moral panics: the creation of the Mods and Rockers* 3rd ed. Abingdon, Oxon, New York: Routledge.

Connor, J. 2009. "Legitimacy and Decline: The Role of the Australian Democrats." In *Forum of Federations' Political Parties and Civil Society Roundtable.* Australian Parliament House, Canberra. http://www.forumfed.org/en/events/event.php?id=457, accessed 9 September 2010.

Connor, J., and A. Kirby. 2011. "Sport and Global Governance: Foul Play Rewarded with Legitimacy." The annual conference of the International Sociological Association, Global Governance: Political Authority in Transition, Montreal, Quebec, Canada, 16–19 March, 2011. http://www.isanet.org/Conferences/Montreal-2011, accessed 9 September 2011.

Critcher, C. 2002. "Media, Government and Moral Panic: The Politics of Paedophilia in Britain 2000–1." *Journalism Studies* 3 (4): 521–535.

Cromer, G. 1978. "Character Assassination in the Press." In *Deviance and Mass Media,* edited by Winick, C., 241–255. Beverley Hills, CA: Sage Publications.

Crowther, N. 2002. "The Salt Lake City Scandals and the Ancient Olympic Games." *International Journal of the History of Sport* 19 (4): 169–178.

Dingelstad, D., Gosden, R., Martin, B., and Vakas, N. 1996. "The Social Construction of Drug Debates." *Social Science and Medicine* 43 (12): 1829–1838.

Donovan, R.J., Egger, G., Kapernick, V., and Mendoza, J. 2002. "A Conceptual Framework for Achieving Performance Enhancing Drug Compliance in Sport." *Sports Medicine* 32 (4): 269–284.

Dvorak, J., Graf-Baumann, T., D'Hooghe, M., Kirkendall, D., Taennler, H., and Saugy, M. 2006. "FIFA's Approach to Doping in Football." *British Journal of Sports Medicine* 40: 3–12.

Eitzen, D.S., and Frey, J.H. 1991. "Sport and Society." *Annual Review of Sociology* 17: 503–522.

Ericson, R. V, Baranek, P. M., and Chan, J.B.L. 1987. *Visualizing Deviance a Study of News Organisations.* Milton Keynes: Open University Press.

———. 1991. *Representing Order*. Toronto: University of Toronto Press.

Erikson, K. T. 1966. *Wayward Puritans A Study in the Sociology of Deviance*. New York: John Wiley and Sons.

Freidson, E. 1970. *Profession of Medicine: A Study of the Sociology of Applied Knowledge*. Chicago: University of Chicago Press.

Garland, D. 2008. "On the Concept of Moral Panic." *Crime Media Culture* 4 (1): 9–31.

Girginov, V. 2006. "Creating a Corporate Anti-doping Culture: The Role of Bulgarian Sports Governing Bodies." *Sport in Society* 9 (2): 252–268.

Gonzenbach, W. J. 1992. "A Time-Series Analysis of the Drug Issue, 1985–1990: The Press, The President and Public Opinion." *International Journal of Public Opinion* 4 (2): 126–147.

Goode, E. 2012. "The Moral Panic: Dead or Alive?" Presentation at Seminar 1, *Moral Panics Seminar Series*, 23 November, Edinburgh: Edinburgh University.

Goode, E., and Ben-Yehuda, N. 1994a. *Moral Panics: The Social Construction of Deviance*. Cambridge, MA: Blackwell Publishers.

———. 1994b. "Moral Panics: Culture, Politics and Social Construction." *Annual Review of Sociology* 20 (3): 149–171.

———. 2009. *Moral Panics: The Social Construction of Deviance*. Chichester, West Sussex: Wiley-Blackwell Publishing.

Gusfield, J. R. 1963. *Symbolic Crusade, Status Politics and the American Temperance Movement*. Urbana: University of Illinois Press.

———. 1981. *The Culture of Public Problems Drinking-Driving and the Symbolic Order*. Chicago: University of Chicago Press.

Guttmann, A. 1988. *A Whole New Ballgame: An Interpretation of American Sports*. Chapel Hill: University of North Carolina Press.

Habermas, J. 1976. *Legitimation Crisis*. London: Heinemann Educational.

Hall, S., Critcher, C., Jefferson, J., Clarke, J., and Roberts, B. 1978. *Policing the Crisis: Mugging, The State, and Law And Order*. London: The MacMillan Press.

Hawdon, J. E. 2001. "The Role of Presidential Rhetoric in the Creation of a Moral Panic: Reagan, Bush and the War on Drugs." *Deviant Behaviour* 22 (5): 419–445.

Hemphill, D. 1992. "Sport, Political Ideology and Freedom." *Journal of Sport and Social Issues* 16 (1): 15–33.

Henne, K. 2015. *Testing for Athlete Citizenship: Regulating Doping and Sex in Sport*. New Brunswick, NJ: Rutgers University Press.

Hier, S. 2008. "Thinking Beyond Moral Panic: Risk, Responsibility, and the Politics of Moralization." *Theoretical Criminology* 12 (2): 173–190.

Hier, S., Lett, D., Walby, K., and Smith, A. 2011. "Beyond Folk Devil Resistance: Linking Moral Panic and Moral Regulation." *Criminology and Criminal Justice* 11 (3): 259–276.

Hilgartner, S., and Bosk, C. L. 1988. "The Rise and Fall of Social Problems: A Public Arenas Model." *The American Journal of Sociology* 94 (1): 53–78.

Hoberman, J. 2001. "How Drug Testing Fails: The Politics of Doping Control." In *Doping in Elite Sport: The Politics of Drugs in the Olympic Movement*, edited by Wilson, W. and Derse, E., 241–274. Champaign, IL: Human Kinetics.

Horne, J. 2006. *Sport in Consumer Culture*. New York: Palgrave Macmillan.

Innes, M. 2005. "A Short History of the Idea of Moral Panic." *Crime Media Culture* 1 (1): 106–111.

Killingbeck, D. 2006. "The Role of Television News in the Construction of School Violence as a 'Moral Panic'." In *Constructing Crime: Perspectives on Making News and Social Problems*, edited by Potter, G. W. and Kappeler, V. E., 213–228. Long Grove, IL: Waveland Press.

Leonard, J. 2001. "Doping in Elite Swimming: A Case Study of the Modern Era from 1970 Onward." In *Doping in Elite Sport: The Politics of Drugs in the*

Olympic Movement, edited by Wilson, J. and Derse, E., 225–239. Champaign, IL: Human Kinetics.

Lull, J., and Hinerman, S. 1997. *Media Scandals: Morality and Desire in the Popular Culture Marketplace*. Cambridge, England: Polity Press.

MacAloon, J. 2001. "Doping and Moral Authority: Sport Organisations Today." In *Doping in Elite Sport: The Politics of Drugs in the Olympic Movement*, edited by Wilson, W. and Derse, E., 205–224. Champaign, IL: Human Kinetics.

McCorkle, R. C., and Miethe, T. D. 1998. "The Political and Organizational Response to Gangs: An Examination of a 'Moral Panic' in Nevada." *Justice Quarterly* 15 (1): 41–64.

McDermott, V. 2012. "Legitimating the Fight against Drugs in Sport: The Australian Government and the Australian Football League." The annual conference of The Australian Sociological Association, *Emerging and Enduring Inequalities*, The University of Queensland, 26–29 November 2012.

Mendoza, J. 2002. "The War on Drugs in Sport: A Perspective from the Front-Line." *Clinical Journal of Sport Medicine* 12: 254–258.

Miah, A. 2002. "Governance, Harmonisation, and Genetics: The World Anti-Doping Agency and Its European Connections." *European Sport Management Quarterly* 2 (4): 350–369.

Nicholson, M. 2006. "Moving the Goalposts: Change and Challenge in a Competitive Football Market." In *Football Fever: Moving the Goalposts*, edited by Nicholson, M., Stewart, B. and Hess, R., 1–10. Hawthorne, VIC: Maribyrnong Press.

Page, C. H. 1973. "The World of Sport and Its Study." In *Sport and Society: An Anthology*, edited by Talamini, J. and Page, C. H., 1–40. Boston: Brown Little.

Pakulski, J. 1986. "Legitimacy and Mass Compliance: Reflections on Max Weber and Soviet-Type Societies." *British Journal of Political Science* 16 (1) (Jan. 1986): 35–56.

Pierre, J., and A. Røiseland. 2011. "Democratic Legitimacy by Performance? Exploring a Research Field." 6th ECPR General Conference, University of Iceland, Reykjavik, 25–27 August, 2011, http://ecpr.eu/filestore/paperproposal/5607187b-73a7-4084-afd7-79d66e32f45c.pdf.

Plummer, K. 2013. "Inspirations: The National Deviancy Conference." http://kenplummer.com/2013/02/08/inspirations-the-national-deviancy-conference/, accessed 16 June 2013.

Reiner, R. 2007. "Media-Made Criminality: The Representation of Crime in the Mass Media." In *The Oxford Handbook of Criminology*, edited by Maguire, M., Morgan, R. and Reiner, R., 302–337. Oxford, England: Oxford University Press.

Rohloff, A., and Wright, S. 2010. "Moral Panic and Social Theory: Beyond the Heuristic." *Current Sociology* 58 (3): 403–419.

Rosen, D. M. 2008. *Dope: A History of Performance Enhancement in Sports from the Nineteenth Century to Today*. Westport, CT: Praeger.

Rothstein, B. 2009. "Creating Political Legitimacy: Electoral Democracy Versus Quality of Government." *American Behavioral Scientist* 53: 311–330.

Sanders, C. R. 1990. "'A Lot of People Like It': The Relationship Between Deviance and Popular Culture." In *Marginal Conventions: Popular Culture, Mass Media and Social Deviance*, edited by Sanders, C. R., 3–13. Bowling Green, Ohio: Bowling Green State University Popular Press.

Schneider, A. 2000. "Olympic Reform, Are We There Yet?" Paper presented at the Bridging Three Centuries, Fifth International Symposium for Olympic Research, University of Western Ontario, London, Ontario, Canada.

Schneider, J. W. 1985. "Social Problems Theory: The Constructionist View." *Annual Review of Sociology* 11: 209–229.

Stewart, B. 2006. "The World Anti-Doping Agency and the Australian Football League: The Irresistible Force Bludgeons the Immoveable Object." In *Football Fever: Moving the Goalposts*, edited by Nicholson, M., Stewart, B. and Hess, R., 107–114. Hawthorne, VIC: Maribyrnong Press.

———. 2007a. "Drugs in Australian Sport: A Brief History." *Sporting Traditions* 23 (2):65–78.

———. 2007b. "The Political Economy of Football: Framing the Analysis." In *The Games Are Not the Same: The Political Economy of Football in Australia*, edited by Stewart, B., 3–22. Carlton, VIC: Melbourne University Press.

Suchman, M.C. 1995. "Managing Legitimacy: Strategic and Institutional Approaches." *The Academy of Management Review* 20 (3): 571–610.

Thompson, B., and Greek, C. 2012. "Mods and Rockers, Drunken Debutants, and Sozzled Students: Moral Panic or the British Silly Season?" *Sage OPEN* 2 (3) (July–September 2012): 1–13. doi: 10.1177/2158244012455177.

Throgmorton, J.A. 1991. "The Rhetorics of Policy Analysis." *Policy Sciences* 24 (2) (May 1991): 153–179.

Vasciannie, S. 2006. "As Fast As a Drug." *Jamaica Gleaner*, 7 August 2006. http://www.jamaica-gleaner.com/gleaner/20060807/cleisure/cleisure2.html. Accessed 7 August 2006.

Voet, W. 2001. *Breaking the Chain Drugs and Cycling: the True Story*. London: Yellow Jersey Press.

WADA (World Anti-Doping Agency). 2008 (July). "What Is the Code—Introduction." World Anti-Doping Agency. http://www.wada-ama.org/en/dynamic. ch2?pageCategory.id=267. Accessed 14 July 2008.

———. 2009 (January). "WADA History." http://www.wada-ama.org/en/dynamic. ch2?pageCategory.id=311. Accessed 30 January 2009.

———. 2015. "World Anti-Doping Code 2015." https://wada-main-prod. s3.amazonaws.com/resources/files/wada-2015-world-anti-doping-code.pdf. Accessed 3 September 2014.

Waddington, I. 2000. *Sport, Health and Drugs a Critical Sociological Perspective*. London: E and FN Spon.

Wagner-Pacifici, R.E. 1986. *The Moro Morality Play: Terrorism as Social Drama*. Chicago: University of Chicago Press.

Weber, M. 1969. *Economy and Society*. 2 vols. Berkeley: University of California Press.

Whannel, G. 2005. "The Five Rings and the Small Screen: Television, Sponsorship, and New Media in the Olympic Movement." In *Global Olympics : Historical and Sociological Studies of the Modern Games*, edited by Young, K. and Wamsley, K.B., 161–177. Amsterdam: Elsevier JAI.

Young, J. 1971. "The Role of the Police as Amplifiers of Deviance, Negotiators of Reality and Translators of Fantasy." In *Images of Deviance*, edited by Cohen, S., 27–61. Harmondsworth: Penguin.

———. 2009. "Moral Panic Its Origins in Resistance, Ressentiment and the Translation of Fantasy into Reality." *British Journal of Criminology* 49: 4–16.

Zatz, M.S. 1987. "Chicano Youth Gangs and Crime: The Creation of a Moral Panic." *Contemporary Crises* 11 (2): 129–158.

1 Locating Legitimacy and Moral Panics

A legitimacy-inspired moral panic framework provides a valuable analytical framework that can be applied to a contemporary social issue. I illustrate this claim by considering the doping debate as an institutionalized moral panic. The emphasis here is to use a moral panic lens to consider the way that doping impacts on, and challenges, the legitimacy and moral authority of SGBs in terms of governing and controlling their particular sporting community. I first outline the significance of legitimacy and moral authority in modern social life before moving to summarize the moral panic theoretical framework. I contrast that with the current dominant approach to drugs in sport to highlight that a legitimacy-inspired moral panic framework provides an alternate way to consider the issue.

LEGITIMACY

The work of Weber provides a useful starting point to discuss legitimacy and moral authority in modern social life. Weber was concerned with identifying the basis of legitimacy and moral authority in differing modes of domination and administration, particularly in relation to their universality and stability (Cantelon and McDermott 2001; Thomas 1984; Weber 1969). While primarily considering political institutions (Spencer 1970), Weber also recognized that domination can occur in a range of relationships, such as "a family, a business or economic enterprise, the state or a church" (Thomas 1984, 225). What is important for this book is that Weber (1969) emphasized that the ability of any social system to maintain order reflects the need of any power or group in a position of authority for its claims to legitimacy to be perceived as valid. This is significant, as belief in the validity of such claims confirms the moral authority of claim-makers to determine appropriate attitudes and conduct for the group and the types of rules to maintain stability. As Weber (1969, 214) stated:

> It is by no means true that every case of submissiveness to persons in positions of power is primarily (or even at all) oriented to this belief. . . .

What is important is the fact that in a given case the particular claim to legitimacy is to a significant degree, and according to its type, treated as 'valid' . . . this fact confirms the position of the persons claiming authority and that it helps to determine the choice of means of its exercise.

Weber argued that legitimate authority, using rules to orient behavior and achieve social order and stability is based, in part, on the fact that "it has been established in a manner which is recognized to be legal" (Weber 1954, 130). Weber termed this form of domination "rational" or "legal." From this perspective, claims to legitimacy are based in a "belief in the legality of patterns of normative rules and the right of those elevated to authority under such rules to issue commands" (Weber 1947, 328). The validity of the authority of those in positions of power, Weber (1969, 954) explained:

. . . may be expressed . . . in a system of consciously made rational rules (which may be either agreed upon or imposed from above), which meet with obedience as generally binding norms whenever such obedience is claimed by him whom the rule designates. In that case, every single bearer of powers of command is legitimated by that system of rational norms, and his power is legitimate insofar as it corresponds with the norm.

Compliance based on perceptions of legitimacy requires a framework that combines rules and regulations 'grounded' on prescribed norms because these support the legitimacy of authority and expectations of compliance (Matheson 1987). For Weber, these represent different aspects of the same phenomenon that underpin all ordered human interaction. He classifies these as comprised of two fundamental components: norms and authority (Spencer 1970). Elaborating on the relationship between these, Spencer (1970, 124) writes:

Norms are rules of conduct towards which actors orient their behavior. Ordered interaction is achieved when a high probability exists that a significant number of actors in a given context will orient their behavior to the same norms. The essence of authority is a relationship between two or more actors in which the commands of certain actors are treated as binding by the others. Authority is thus a sphere of legitimate command and where authority exists ordered interaction is also possible.

Legitimacy is essential to the ability of either norms or authority to ensure social order and stability (Spencer 1970). The reference to "actors" emphasizes the subjective element in this process. For Weber (1969, 214), subjectivity could be conceptualized as a function of self-interest, custom or belief in the existence of legitimate order, noting that: "Loyalty may be hypocritically simulated . . . on purely opportunistic grounds, or carried out in practice for reasons of material self-interest. Or people may submit from individual weakness and helplessness because there is no acceptable alternative." However, Weber did not view these considerations as representing sufficiently reliable forms of compliance. Rather, he suggests that irrespective of the motivational foundation, what is important is that the claim to legitimacy is treated as valid (Matheson 1987; Weber 1954). Whether considered from the perspective of individuals' motivations or the legitimacy of authority, both require explanatory frameworks that "legitimate" or "make rightful" the particular behavior (Matheson 1987, 200). As Matheson (1987, 200) notes: "Power-holders have an interest in securing obedience motivated by a belief in legitimacy, for legitimate authority is a less 'costly' form of authority than either coercive or reward-based authority. . . . Legitimate authority obviates the need for surveillance and rewards, since subordinates feel obliged to obey no matter whether there is a 'reward' for compliance or not."

In other words, neither fear of sanctions nor expediency alone will generate perceptions of legitimacy. Rather, it requires subjective acceptance by social actors based either on voluntary agreement or decisions by an authority held to be legitimate (Pakulski 1986). Perceptions of legitimacy leading to compliance require a framework of rules and regulations underpinned by prescribed norms or values (Matheson 1987). Irrespective of their form, the subjective component of these frameworks suggests an element of negotiation (Holton 1987). Rather than a reliance on routine submission or imposition of authority from above, successful governance requires support, or consent, which while voluntary is nevertheless predicated on perceptions of the legitimacy of authority (Pakulski 1986; Spencer 1970). Legitimacy, Suchman (1995, 574) writes, "is a generalized perception or assumption that the actions of an entity are desirable, proper, or appropriate within some socially structured system of norms, values, beliefs, and definitions."

Legitimacy emerges as a dynamic concept that is not necessarily clear or easily applied. Rather it appears to be "multi-dimensional" (Pakulski 1986), which implies that its operation is dependent upon the nature of the problem under discussion (Suchman 1995). The subjective, evaluative component of legitimacy means that dominant groups must actively work to generate and maintain support for their legitimacy and moral authority, including compliance with regulatory frameworks (Pakulski 1986, see also Bernstein 2004; Buchanan and Keohane 2006; Cashore 2002; Grafstein 1981; Hurd 1999, Koppell 2005, 2007). Applying a legitimacy-based explanatory model to SGBs is complicated by the monopoly position of many of these organizations, with their legitimacy rarely questioned (Connor and Kirby 2011). Palmer (2000, 364) describes elite SGBs, such as the IOC, FINA or FIFA, as "powerful organizations which enjoy wealth, celebrity, status and global influence on a scale with few rivals."

One application of legitimacy to the issue of drugs in sport is the work of Donovan et al. (2002) and their development of a Sport Drug Control

Model (SDCM). They suggest that compliance with anti-doping regulations is more likely if those regulations and enforcement agencies are perceived as legitimate. They also note that perceptions of legitimacy are influenced by scientifically accurate testing protocols as well as consistent and equitable application of any sanctions. Research testing the SDCM with elite Australian athletes suggested that legitimacy was less influential than other elements of the model in terms of athletes' appraisals of threats and benefits associated with PED use (Gucciardi, Jalleh and Donovan 2011). A later survey of elite Australian athletes found that athletes' view that anti-doping procedures were fair enhanced their perceptions of organizational legitimacy, which meant that anti-doping compliance was more likely (Jalleh et al. 2014). These findings suggest support for Donovan et al.'s claim that compliance is linked to perceptions that enforcement agencies are legitimate and hold the moral authority to impose such a regulatory framework.

Morality is important sociologically, as it orients social actions that mark community boundaries based on a set of social criteria, or rules, which evaluate "behavior and goals as good or bad, desirable or undesirable" (Ben-Yehuda 1986, 495; Lidz and Walker 1980). In modern complex societies, moral boundaries and evaluations of behavior undergo constant processes of negotiation and renegotiation by social groups and, as a result, legitimacy cannot be taken for granted (Ben-Yehuda 1986). Emphasizing this point, Ericson et al. (1991, 8) write that:

> Moral authority is always subject to consent, and legitimacy is always something that is granted. There is institutional space for choice in consenting to a given moral authority and in granting legitimacy, albeit circumscribed by institutional frames and their imprints on reality and morality.

Frames include stipulating appropriate norms, classifying certain behavior as prohibited as well as sanctions attached to that behavior (Entman 2004). An organization's ability to obtain consent and support for the legitimacy and authority to stipulate 'frames' hinges on two central elements. These are that organizations establish a normative order for their particular community and that rules and regulations are created in a legally correct manner (Habermas 1976). This highlights Weber's (1969) point that compliance requires a framework based on norms or values with decisions perceived as legitimate because they are derived from appropriately formulated and enacted procedures or laws. Further, maintaining legitimacy and moral authority requires organizations to search for and sanction individuals deviating from procedural norms (Ericson et al. 1991). In other words, organizations must make convincing claims that their actions are in accord with existing social norms supported or enforced by appropriate procedural laws. Failure to do so carries the potential for a crisis of legitimacy to emerge.

The notion of crisis is useful as, rather than a total collapse, it helps to conceptualize social change as a transformative process mediated through cultural agency and conflict (Andrews 2000; Holton 1987). For an organizational crisis of legitimacy, this may include accounts (using, for example, socio-historical case studies as presented later in this book) examining how organizations institutionalize conflict and reconstruct relationships experiencing stress (Holton 1987). From this perspective, and in the context of drugs in sport, the 1998 Tour de France doping scandal contributed to a crisis of legitimacy for the IOC. That scandal transformed anti-doping approaches, resulting in the creation of WADA as a new institutional anti-doping response (Chapter 2, this volume). The establishment of WADA transformed interactions between sporting organizations, including strengthening existing relationships and incorporating new actors, such as the state and policing bodies, into the realm of sporting regulation (Rasmussen 2005; Chapter 3, this volume). Organizational interactions bring issues of governance and control into the frame. These relationships are often contentious, with various groups seeking to retain the authority and legitimacy to control their particular sporting community (Chapter 4, this volume).

In such a contested environment, maintaining or restoring social order and stability leads organizations to implement behavior-defining rules and enforcement practices, such as codes of conduct (Stewart, Nicholson and Dickson 2005), that define behavioral boundaries of their sporting community. In Weberian terms these represent "consciously made rational rules" (Weber 1969, 954) as stabilizing mechanisms to regulate the particular organizational community (Ericson et al. 1991; Chapter 3, this volume). Enforcement practices, regulatory frameworks or procedural mechanisms are concerned with moral principles and justifications, questions of right and wrong, and must be open to public scrutiny to be seen as legitimate (Battin et al. 2008; Bok 1989). This emphasizes the point that claims to legitimacy and moral authority cannot be taken for granted, as Wuthnow et al. (1984, 222) emphasize in reference to Habermas's work on legitimation:

> The legitimacy of the modern state no longer rests on tradition or absolute values, but is rooted in conceptions of proper procedures—procedures deemed legitimate if they have been established according to norms of legality and constitutionality and if they conform to certain conceptions of citizenship and representation. They are intended to serve as mechanisms for negotiating policies oriented towards the common good. . . . They are not taken for granted as the way things simply must be, but are consciously subjected to scrutiny to determine if they in fact produce desired consequences.

Although directed at modern state governance, Habermas's analysis can be extended to organizations as procedure or "obsessive attention to detail is the defining characteristic of legitimacy in modern bureaucratic life"

(Ericson et al. 1987, 356). The area of interest for this book is the location of control, power and authority in the modern sporting environment.

Heightening this importance of legitimacy are the significant financial rewards associated with the modern industrial sporting complex. Sport has become a global industry with a significant economic impact in terms of revenue generation. This has implications for sporting organizations, media organizations, private corporations as well as state bodies. For example, in the 2004–05 financial year the income generated in Australia by organizations involved in sport and recreation was AUD$8,820.5 million. This added a total industry value of AUD$2,349.6 million, the equivalent of 0.3 percent of Australia's Gross Domestic Product (GDP) for 2004–05 (ABS 2006). As Connor (2009) notes, estimates revealed that in 2000 sport added GB£9.8 billion to the British economy and employed around 400,000 people, just under two percent of the workforce. Financial benefits from sport include contracts with individual athletes, clubs, venues and leagues creating sponsorship as a multi-billion dollar global industry (Andrews and Jackson 2001). Commercial sponsorship of sport is not new. Rather, Tomlinson (2005, 39) explains, the difference in the modern sporting context is the "scale of commercial involvement," with sponsorship that targets "whole sports, not just individuals; establishing exclusive rights for set periods, not just one-offs."

Added to this are lucrative new markets created by a globalized media (see also Amis 2005; Harvey and Law 2005). Houlihan (2002) writes that since the 1960s there has been an increasingly interdependent relationship between sport and media organizations. Sporting events are televised to huge audiences, providing broadcasters with a valuable mechanism with which to tap into consumer markets. For example, NBC and its parent company General Electric reached an agreement with the IOC for the 2010 Vancouver Winter and the 2012 London Olympics worth a total of US$2.201 billion (Whannel 2005). To secure broadcasting rights for the 2000 to 2008 Olympics (Summer and Winter), the European Broadcasting Union agreed to a deal worth $1.442 billion (Houlihan 2002). The significant monetary returns associated with global sport illustrate the risks to SGBs, as well as media organizations, of any loss of legitimacy.

So far in this chapter I have discussed the point that organizations' legitimacy and moral authority rest upon their application and enforcement of 'proper procedures' (Habermas 1976; Weber 1969; Wuthnow et al. 1984). These claims to legitimacy cannot be taken for granted but include the subjective, evaluative component of the social audience (Suchman 1995). In other words, observers' perceptions of legitimacy are influenced by organizational responses to particular issues or events (Chapter 6, this volume). As Suchman (1995, 574) notes, legitimacy is socially constructed in "that it reflects a congruence between the behaviors of the legitimated entity and the shared (or assumed shared) beliefs of some social group." A failure by elite SGBs to generate and maintain support potentially creates a crisis of legitimacy. This may particularly be the case when faced with situations placing them under stress, such as continued media coverage of doping. Next, I summarize the moral panic theoretical framework underpinning the claim that media reports of doping potentially create a crisis of legitimacy, contributing to the construction of doping as a moral panic.

MORAL PANICS AND FOLK DEVILS—CRITERIA FOR ANALYSIS

Cohen (1972) suggested that moral panics emerge "every now and then" when conventional morality is challenged or during times of rapid social change. More recent moral panic literature notes that "almost anything can spark off a panic and the trigger can range from something as serious as children killing another child (the murder, in 1993, of James Bulger) to an incident of school bullying" (Thompson 1998, 2; see also McRobbie and Thornton 1995). Moral panics build on a fear that the well-being and fundamental values of society are under threat from a certain category of deviant individuals. This requires that 'something must be done' by those in positions of authority or power (Baerveldt et al. 1998; Cohen 1972). A consequence of this is that it is used to justify dominant groups' introduction of more stringent measures to regulate the deviant group, including "tougher or renewed rules, more intense public hostility and condemnation, more laws, longer sentences, more police, more arrests, and more prison cells" (Goode and Ben-Yehuda 2009, 35). This can be examined from a Weberian foundation, which points out that:

> . . . it is conceivable that such controls can actually be established, that the ends for and the ways of its exercise become articulated in reglementations [regulations], that special agencies are created for its exercise and special appellate agencies for the resolution of questions of doubt, and that, finally, the controls are constantly made more strict. In such a case this kind of domination might become quite like the authoritative domination of a bureaucratic state agency over its subordinates, and the subordination would assume the character of a relationship of obedience to authority. (Weber 1969, 944)

As well as highlighting the role of legitimacy and moral authority, this Weberian approach emphasizes that power relationships are part of the debate.

Also of interest in a moral panic is the key role of the media in generating ideas about the extent and seriousness of the threat. Using melodramatic vocabulary and language, described by Cohen (1972) as the moral panic 'inventory,' the media create disproportional perceptions of danger by exaggerating the focus of attention and the seriousness of the event (Fritz and Altheide 1987; Hawdon 2001). Cohen's (1972) analysis of media reports of the 1960s Mods and Rockers moral panic revealed consistent use of language such as "riot," "orgy of destruction," "battle" and "attack." These accounts distorted and exaggerated the number of young people involved, the amount of damage inflicted and the social impact of the events (Goode and Ben-Yehuda 2006; McRobbie and Thornton 1995). Cohen (1967, 125–126) refers to the consequence of this process as "community sensitization" when, once identified, even "extremely small deviations from the norm became noticed, commented on, judged, and reacted to" (Goode and Ben-Yehuda 2009, 22). The significance of the moral panic inventory is that it provides legitimacy to claims that seek to persuade the public that threats to social order from moral deviants are real (Victor 1998).

This highlights the subjective component of legitimacy as well as the media's influence in shaping public perceptions and focusing attention on particular issues. Audiences incorporate media definitions and language to frame ideas about problems and social issues and, as a result, media reports have considerable influence over the types of issues that become part of public discourse (Welch et al. 2000). Media-defined categories selected as newsworthy are those often primarily concerned with deviance (Altheide 1997; Pritchard and Hughes 1997). This performs an important normative function by marking the boundaries of a community and reinforcing shared identities (Erikson 1966; Tucher 1994). Using authoritative voices, metaphoric language, pictures and headlines, media reports present a 'common-sense' understanding of deviance juxtaposed against the desired state of affairs to emphasize the importance of social order and build consensus about the way things should be (Ericson et al. 1987, 1991; Parenti 1986).

Emphasizing that ideological and political imperatives underpin media reports, by calling attention to social issues, the media maintain an issue as politically important. The significance of this is that it influences audiences' attitudes and increases acceptance of more "repressive, tough on crime policy proposals" (Pritchard and Hughes 1997, 49). The issue of illicit drug use in the broader social context illustrates this point. Media reports use dramatic examples, such as random acts of drug violence and language supporting law enforcement "crackdowns." This type of reportage enables dominant groups to frame the issue as "another war on drugs" requiring more "law and order," such as increased sentences and zero tolerance (Chermak 1997, 712). This has particular relevance for this book and the role of the media in legitimating WADA as a "special agency" using the WADC to regulate athletes with controls that are "constantly made more strict" (Weber 1969, 944).

However, as well as identifying issues as social problems, the media open up opportunities to demand reform, change and progress using selected key organizational spokespersons as "socially accredited experts" to define the problem and its solution (Becker 1967, 241; Cohen 1972; Ericson et al. 1987). This enables organizations to situate themselves as the 'natural' choice to maintain or restore order and is important for organizational legitimacy. However, to be successful, organizations must construct and "sell" the problem as well as its solution (Boxill and Unnithan 1995, 74; Ericson et al. 1987, 1991). Any failure to persuade an audience has the potential to create perceptions of incompetency or damage claims to legitimacy (Throgmorton 1991). This process is evident in the drugs in sport debate. WADA takes advantage of its authoritative position to use media reports to present doping as problematic and the WADC as the necessary response (Chapter 5, this volume). Demonstrating that claims to legitimacy cannot be taken for granted, other stakeholder groups, such as elite SGBs, use the media to contest WADA's claims to legitimacy (Chapter 4, this volume).

There are also implications here for the legitimacy of media organizations. A successful moral panic requires that media attention touches a "responsive chord" in the general public (Goode and Ben-Yehuda 2006, 25). However, audiences are not "zombies . . . brainwashed over the airwaves" (Goode and Ben-Yehuda 2009, 90) but are influenced by their own interests, which may not coincide with those of dominant groups (Goode and Ben-Yehuda 1994b). Audiences bring their own predispositions and interpretations to reading and viewing 'news,' which influence the meanings they attach to information and perceptions of media credibility (Reiner 2007). Consequently, media organizations seek to maintain their own legitimacy and accept information consistent with their own organizational needs (Chermak 1997; Farnen 1990; Sacco 1995; Schneider 1985). While prepared to trade some integrity in exchange for information, Parenti (1986, 239) notes that:

> . . . there are occasions when the trade-off comes at too high a price. . . . Were it to follow the government (or corporate) line on all such matters the press would cast doubt on its own credibility as a news organization and as a neutral, objective social institution. So the media go along on most stories, but not all the time and sometimes not all the way.

The relative autonomy of the media creates a contested space where journalists 'break the scandals' to which organizations respond using 'spin-doctors' and 'tailor-made' accounts to present their version of events. At the same time, the media's position as powerful agents of social control enables them to criticize and challenge these accounts (e.g., see McKay, Hutchins, and Mikosza 2000). Further, claims that an issue is problematic must compete with numerous other social-problem claims. Best (1990, 15) defines the media as a "social problems marketplace" composed of "particular public arenas" (Hilgartner and Bosk 1988; see also McRobbie and Thornton 1995). The problem for claim-makers is that the number of problems that each 'arena' can handle at one time is limited by structural factors such as space and time (Hilgartner and Bosk 1988). In this contested environment, not all definitions can win out (Best 1999; Fritz and Altheide 1987). This is significant in terms of building legitimacy, Rommetvedt (2005, 757) writes; claim-makers that "argue convincingly that their viewpoints and suggestions promote the public good have better chances of obtaining general acceptance or of acquiring support from the necessary number and kinds of partners."

This picture is complicated by the emergence and availability of relatively cheap forms of 'new media' that enable 'folk devils' to 'fight back' (McRobbie 1994). In some contemporary moral panics, the changing nature of 'experts' includes "extremely articulate . . . skilled representatives from pressure groups and voluntary organizations . . . who now do the job of defending the folk devils" (McRobbie 1994:111). The emergence of 'new media,' such as Twitter or Facebook, carry the potential to open up debates over social issues by bringing a diverse range of voices and influences to challenge dominant political discourses (see Ghareeb 2000; Kwak et al. 2010; McRobbie 1994; Reiner 2007; Schlesinger and Tumber 1994; Seib 2008). However, Reiner (2007) notes that, despite this, past experiences suggest that "the dice are loaded in favor of dominant interests—even if they have to struggle harder for their hegemony." A key point for this book is that the reciprocal nature of the relationship between the media and significant claim-makers remains a central element. Privileged access to the media provides claim-makers, such as elite SGBs, with opportunities to enhance their legitimacy by identifying problems, PED-using athletes, for example, that threaten order and stability. More importantly, media access enables claim-makers, such as WADA, to position themselves as providers of solutions to those problems (Schneider 1985). These are primary characteristics underpinning claim-makers' activities in a moral panic, which Beamish (2009, 56–57) summarizes:

> First they must successfully publicize the behavior deemed as problematic. Second . . . they must also convince others that certain people or behaviors are dangerous, irresponsible, contagious, or undermine the welfare of the community . . . there does not have to be a genuine basis for the claim—all the claims-makers need to do is convince others that this is the case . . . third . . . claims-makers want to convince people that there is not simply a general problem, there is a *specific* problem which is of *particular* concern. (emphasis in original)

This moral panic model provides a useful mechanism with which to consider the claims of dominant actors, and what might be at stake for those groups, in debates over contemporary social issues. However, the popularity of the moral panic concept and a tendency to apply it to "listless" events (Young 2009, 4–5) raises questions around whether it is possible to identify an issue as a moral panic. Building on Cohen's (1972) moral panic model is the work of Goode and Ben-Yehuda (1994a, 2009), who list five criteria in the identification of a moral panic. These are consensus, concern, hostility, disproportionality and volatility. Commencing with consensus, the next section outlines these criteria and modifications that I apply to consider the debate around drugs in sport as a moral panic.

Consensus

Cohen (2002, xi) noted that a successful moral panic required agreement that the "beliefs or action being denounced were not insulated entities ('it's not only this') but integral parts of the society or else could (and would) be unless 'something was done' [sic]." Goode and Ben-Yehuda (2009) also note that social agreement that deviant individuals and their behavior threaten the social order is a central element of a moral panic. However, this obscures the point that moral panics are varied in nature, some stimulate concern only amongst some groups or elements in the community, while others mobilize a majority of citizens (Goode and Ben-Yehuda 1994b). While consensus is important, the character, causes or consequences of the problem are subject to dispute as well as collective negotiation (Garland 2008). For some contemporary moral panics, such as drugs in sport, consensus fails to adequately account for the contested relationships between dominant social actors.

Consensus-Making

To more effectively capture the negotiated nature of consensus evident in the identification of an issue as a social problem, including contested claims to legitimacy, I modify Goode and Ben-Yehuda's (2009) criterion of consensus to '*consensus-making*.' Claims to legitimacy occur in competitive arenas comprised of a range of stakeholder groups with diverse and conflicting interests and not all will agree on the causes, consequences or measures to solve the threat presented by the issue or group. In this context, consensus-making captures the interactive processes involved in selecting, presenting and maintaining attention and concern over issues as social problems. As social reactions in a moral panic can be more or less consensual or more or less divided (Garland 2008), dominant groups must actively work to build and maintain agreement that the issue threatens social order. This includes convincing claims about the definition, legitimacy and urgency of problems as well as those responsible and the necessary mechanisms to control the deviant behavior (Sacco 1995). As Koppell (2008, 195) writes regarding global governance organizations (GGOs):

> Any rulemaking body that is not accepted by key actors offers minimal benefit to other potential members. . . . Without the acquiescence of key . . . organizations, an international organization will be marginalized. . . . If the GGO's rules are ignored by the most significant market participants, there is little reason for the less powerful to go along . . .

once ignored, the GGO may even lose its substantive legitimacy as it no longer achieves the very goals it was created to pursue.

This highlights the importance of consensus-making activities as rule-making organizations, such as WADA, seek to maintain legitimacy and moral authority. In the case of doping as a moral panic, 'consensus-making' more accurately describes the interactive processes as well as power relationships between groups that are evident in the debate. Dominant stakeholders, such as WADA, elite SGBs, governments and media organizations have diverse interests and use narratives around doping to justify the introduction of regulatory mechanisms to achieve specific outcomes that are relevant to their particular sporting communities (Chapter 4, this volume). The modern sporting context also includes athletes, coaches and the public, amongst others, as stakeholders with an interest in anti-doping initiatives (Chapter 6, this volume). Consequently, consensus-making more accurately reflects the multi-dimensional and contested nature of elite SGBs' efforts to generate and maintain support for the legitimacy of particular anti-doping responses, such as WADA.

Cohen's (2002) model emphasized that moral panics require a dimension of community concern that a particular issue threatens social order and agreement that 'something must be done' to maintain social stability. This brings us to the next elements of Goode and Ben-Yehuda's (2009) moral panic criteria, which are concern and hostility.

Concern and Hostility

Goode and Ben-Yehuda (2006, 24–25) describe concern and hostility as the "raw material" with "latent potential" for a public reaction to a given issue from which a moral panic emerges. Concern over an issue can be expressed through a range of channels, such as public opinion polls as well as proposed legislation (Baerveldt et al. 1998). Other avenues include public commentary voiced in letters to the editor and comments in online forums, blogs or other forms of social media. Closely associated with increased concern is the identification of a group or 'folk devil' as responsible for the threatening behavior, creating and perpetuating divisions between 'us' (respectable society) and 'them' (outsiders) (Goode and Ben-Yehuda 1994a). A successful moral panic, writes Cohen (2002, 45), requires the "generation of diffuse normative concerns" with the creation of 'folk devils' reliant on "their stereotypical portrayal as atypical actors against a background that is overtypical." Defining a common enemy, a 'folk devil,' narrows the focus and provides an object against which collective action can be taken (Hawdon 2001). Media reports play an important role here, with suggestions that part of society is in crisis or that the deviant behavior directly attacks fundamental values heightening public concern (Gonzenbach 1992; Johnson et al. 1996; Jones, McFalls and Gallagher 1989). According to von Hoffman (1985, 10):

> If a reporter finds two experts, he can turn any event into an upmarket version of the killer-bee story . . . that is what trend stories really are: the announcement that something bad and goose-pimply is slouching toward the reader's hometown and into his very own suburb.

In addition to raising public concern, suggestions that something 'bad and goose-pimply' threatens the audiences' immediate social environment creates opportunities for expressions of hostility toward those perceived as responsible. This is important in the identification or classification of a moral panic, as without a combination of hostility and concern a moral panic will not develop (Goode and Ben-Yehuda 2009).

Identifying the deviant group normalizes expressions of hostility toward 'folk devils.' More specifically, it emphasizes the importance of official agents of social control that are prepared to take action to solve the problem and return social order and stability (Ericson et al. 1987; Lull and Hinerman 1997; Sanders 1990). Folk devils, explain Goode and Ben-Yehuda (2009, 28–29), are "*deviants*," their behavior is "harmful to society; they are selfish and evil; they must be stopped, their actions neutralized. Only an effort of substantial magnitude will permit us to return to normal" (emphasis in original). As part of increasing concern and normalizing hostility toward the deviant group, the media and other stakeholder groups exaggerate the extent of the threat or, as Jones et al. (1989, 4) describe it, "objective molehills have been made into subjective mountains."

Disproportionality

This brings us to Goode and Ben-Yehuda's (2009) moral panic criterion of disproportionality.[1] In the construction of a moral panic, claim-makers imply that considerably more individuals are engaged in the deviant behavior than actually are. Exaggerated facts and figures create a sense that the deviant behavior is eroding the social order (Goode and Ben-Yehuda 2009). This quantifying of a social problem performs an important ideological function. Statistics provide persuasive evidence that measure the extent, or size, of the problem as well as the efficacy of solutions to the problematic issue or behavior (Best 2002). Large numbers imply a correspondingly large social problem and, while often exaggerated, ground intangible impressions in 'facts' (Best 1999; Blumer 1971; Jenkins 1992; Sacco 1995), which support consensus-making activities. However, in some moral panics, such as those that rely on demonstrating that regulatory frameworks are successfully controlling deviant behavior, statistics can create opportunities to enhance, as well as to challenge, organizational claims to legitimacy.

In the drugs in sport debate, low numbers of positive drugs tests are used to bolster SGBs' claims to legitimacy and demonstrate that the anti-doping framework is effective. At the same time, and demonstrating that contested power relationships are part of the debate, low numbers of positive tests can also lead to challenges to SGBs' organizational claims to legitimacy. This is particularly relevant when doping is constructed as an issue that not only threatens sport but also public health more broadly (e.g., see Howman 2012). From that perspective, rather than supporting organizational claims to legitimacy, some stakeholders use small numbers of positive tests to criticize the anti-doping framework of other stakeholders for failing to detect and sanction PED-using athletes (Chapter 4, this volume). Irrespective of the claims or counter-claims of dominant groups in respect to the extent of the problematic behavior or efficacy of particular regulatory solutions, their responses rely on a level of public concern that the issue represents a significant threat to social order. This provides a focus for hostility and stresses the necessity of a strong regulatory response.

Media reports contribute to disproportional claims about social problems through statements exaggerating the extent of a problem typically commanding attention rather than "what actually happened" (Fritz and Altheide 1987, 476). For example, Fritz and Altheide (1987) traced the role of the media in the social construction of the 'missing children issue' in the United States. They found that claims from selected parents, moral entrepreneurs and government agencies regarding the extent of the problem rather than its nature were widely publicized. Some media reports frequently stated that 1.5 million children went missing each year. Other reports noted that most 'missing' children were more likely to be runaways or involved in custodial disputes. Later research showed that stranger abductions accounted for less than one percent of all missing children (Fritz and Altheide 1987; Lofquist 1997). A significant outcome of the concern generated over missing children was a problem-specific institutional response:

> Understanding the 'problem' was secondary to establishing the legitimacy and organization to 'deal with the problem.' The latter was accomplished by establishing the National Center for Missing and Exploited Children. Once the institutionalization of the problem had been accomplished, moral 'expert' entrepreneurs could provide routine news sources for the mass media. (Fritz and Altheide 1987, 478)

The missing children example illustrates a 'spiral effect' as media and dominant groups interact and influence public opinion. Establishing a problem-specific institution contributes to the idea that the problem is ongoing and therefore necessitates institutional control (Goode and Ben-Yehuda 1994b; Thompson 1998). Cohen (2002, 66–67) described the process where other agents of social control, such as policing bodies, are drawn into the system as "diffusion," which Hall et al. (1978) classify as a "spiral of signification." Goode and Ben-Yehuda (1994b, 156) describe the process as "police 'escalate' their law enforcement efforts, 'diffuse' them from precinct to precinct, and 'innovate' new methods of social control; they operate under the 'widening-the-net' principle."

Nevertheless, the construction of a moral panic is contested ground. The discrepancy between the number of potential problems and the public space, or media arenas, available for addressing them creates a fiercely competitive environment. Consequently, despite extensive media coverage, not all moral panics become institutionalized (Best 1990, 1999; Hilgartner and Bosk 1988). The fact that not all moral panics leave a long-term or institutional legacy was acknowledged in Cohen's (2002, 1) model, noting that "sometimes the panic passes over and is forgotten, except in folklore and collective memory." However, in other instances moral panics do leave a lasting impression, perhaps raising fundamental questions around the way society sees itself or contributing to changes in policy responses. It is these types of moral panic that are of interest here, those that lead to institutional enforcement responses, which can include legislative mechanisms that criminalize the behavior and the individuals argued to be responsible (Goode and Ben-Yehuda 1994b). The idea that appropriate action is being taken is important for perceptions of the legitimacy of institutional responses to the threatening behavior.

There is evidence of the moral panic criterion of disproportionality in the doping debate. The representations of dominant groups, such as the media, elite SGBs as well as governments create the idea that doping has reached 'epidemic' proportions, with PED-using 'folk devils' undermining sport as a valuable social institution (Chapter 5, this volume). The significance of the media lies in their tendency to present reality in terms of only 'sensational' news (Bourdieu 1998). This is an essential part of a moral panic, as sensational media coverage creates an exaggerated perception of the danger or threat presented by the particular issue, while limited coverage can reduce the level of concern (Johnson et al. 1996). In the context of the doping debate, reports that a minority of athletes use PEDs are far from 'sensational' or newsworthy, and unlikely to generate support for an institutional response to doping as a specific problem of particular concern (Beamish 2009). This is important because generating and maintaining the idea that doping remains widespread opens opportunities for SGBs, including WADA, to enhance their legitimacy by providing a regulatory solution to eliminate doping as a moral and physical danger threatening sport.

This leads us to Goode and Ben-Yehuda's (2009) final moral panic criterion of volatility, which is significant in terms of maintaining support for the legitimacy of an institutionalized response to a social problem.

Volatility

Moral panics are also described as 'volatile,' denoting a tendency to erupt suddenly and just as suddenly subside, therefore possessing similar attributes to a fad or craze (Goode and Ben-Yehuda 2009). Typically, moral panics are referred to as events that, whether emerging suddenly as a 'new' social problem or the reappearance of a dormant issue, spark a sense of panic or urgency in the search for a solution. The descriptive term 'panic' implies that individuals react to these situations in extraordinary ways, suggesting havoc, disorganization and chaos. Critics have argued that this "under-emphasizes the presence of deliberate and rational actors" and ignores complex processes involving "active, not merely reactive, efforts by social actors" (Cornwell and Linders 2002, 307–313; see also Hunt 1999). The observation throughout this book is that complex processes, involving a range of social actors, constitute moral panics. These groups include the mass media, other organizations as well as the public that both react to and actively create an issue as a moral panic. Nevertheless, the characterization of moral panics as volatile, coupled with their failure to maintain initial levels of concern, contributes to their description as fadlike.

The relevant point for this book is that unlike a fad, some moral panics leave a significant legacy. These events contribute to social change, acting as precedents for later moral panics with informal or institutional legacies (Goode and Ben-Yehuda 2009; Killingbeck 2006). During the 1970s, for instance, heroin addiction in the United States received substantial media and political attention but was of limited initial impact as a volatile moral panic. What was significant were institutional mechanisms that 'paved the way' for subsequent drug panics in the 1980s and 1990s, including the development of a national drug strategy (Chermak 1997; Wright 2000). A problem-specific organizational response is central to an institutionalized moral panic and also brings legitimacy into the moral panic framework. From this perspective, organizations face the potential for concern over deviant behavior to link with community perceptions that existing procedures have failed to deal with a problem threatening order and stability. From a Weberian perspective, these claims no longer meet community expectations or generate community support and, as a result, no longer enjoy perceptions of validity. The significance of a problem-specific institutional response is that it enables dominant groups to respond to challenges and reassert their power and values, or claims to authority and legitimacy, through a regulatory framework (Gusfield 1963; Schneider 1985). As Gusfield (1967, 178) points out:

> The fact of affirmation through acts of law and government expresses the public worth of one set of norms, of one sub-culture vis-à-vis those of others. It demonstrates which cultures have legitimacy and public domination, and which do not. Accordingly it enhances the social status of groups carrying the affirmed culture and degrades groups carrying that which is condemned as deviant.

There is, however, a further problem facing an institutionalized response to a moral panic that also concerns their claims to legitimacy. In her discussion of the moral panic surrounding Chicano youth gangs and crime in the United States city of Phoenix in the 1970s and 1980s, Zatz (1987) emphasizes the dilemma confronting organizations, such as law enforcement agencies, in their quest for public funds. To secure government funding, they must demonstrate the seriousness of the problem while also managing the "delicate balance between demonstrating the success of the new program . . . justifying the money already spent, and showing a continued need for the infusion of additional funds" (Zatz 1987, 131). As an organization funded by the IOC, the sport movement and government (WADA 2010a), which includes public funds, WADA faces a similar pressure. Similarly, SGBs receive funding from external sources, such as commercial sponsorship agreements or government funding for sport development programs, for example. Consequently, SGBs also face pressure to demonstrate that those funds are effectively applied to achieve their intended outcomes. The challenge for WADA and SGBs is to maintain support for anti-doping initiatives that, while effective, nevertheless remain necessary to control doping to ensure sporting stability.

The concept of volatility in a moral panic is also problematic, as the initial momentum of a moral panic tends to wane over time (Goode and Ben-Yehuda 2009). Consequently, claim-makers cannot take for granted that the issue will continue to be seen as problematic or that their response will continue to be seen as legitimate and appropriate. In addition to competing for attention, media focus on issues tends to fade, and as a result public concern also recedes (Goode and Ben-Yehuda 2009). Regarding the debate over PEDs in sport, Houlihan (2009, 49) stresses the importance of the anti-doping policy regime's ability to "embed its concerns and priorities more securely in the sustained interest and commitment of . . . influential policy actors over the medium to long-term." The moral panic criterion of volatility again highlights the media's role in consensus-making activities that draw public attention to and maintain concern over an issue as a social problem. In this book I demonstrate that elite SGBs, while challenged by media reports of doping, also use the media to perpetuate concern that PED use is an ongoing problem, which justifies or legitimates WADA and the introduction of increasingly stringent measures of social control.

This model, proposed by Cohen (1972, 2002) and elaborated upon by Goode and Ben-Yehuda (1994a, 2009), provides an important conceptual framework with which to consider the doping debate. The value of this approach is that it enables us to broaden the analysis beyond the athlete-user to consider the role of other social actors and institutions. The criteria outlined by Goode and Ben-Yehuda also highlights important characteristics of a moral panic. However, they do not provide a mechanism with which to examine why some issues become a moral panic while others do not. Enhancing the analytical ability of the moral panic framework, and to address questions about why not all issues become moral panics, Goode and Ben-Yehuda (2009) provide three moral panic theories.

Social Theory and Moral Panics

Goode and Ben-Yehuda (2009) outline three 'ideal' moral panic theoretical frameworks comprising a) a grassroots model, b) 'middle level' interest-groups and c) an elite-engineered model. These theories provide us with the tools to answer questions around why some issues become moral panics while other, more harmful conditions, do not (Goode and Ben-Yehuda 1994b). More specifically, for the goals of this book and a consideration of organizational legitimacy, the moral panic theories help us answer the question posed by Gusfield (1981, 5): "Who and what institution gains or is given the responsibility for 'doing something' about the issue." Next, I summarize the grassroots theory, followed by the middle level interest-groups theory and conclude with a summary of the elite-engineered moral panic theory, which I modify to an *elites-engineered* theory.

Grassroots Theory

The grassroots perspective stresses popular participation and argues that moral panics are a 'bottom-up' event motivated by activists' and citizens' concerns with morality and ideology (Goode and Ben-Yehuda 1994b). This perspective situates moral panics as a cultural phenomenon driven by a level of "diffuse anxiety or strain" with "more or less spontaneous eruptions of concern on the part of a large number of people" regarding the threatening behavior or issue (Goode and Ben-Yehuda 1994b, 161). A central element of this form of a moral panic is that public concern is based on the deeply felt attitudes and beliefs of a broad sector of society that there is a real and present danger threatening their values, or "even their very existence" (Goode and Ben-Yehuda 1994b, 161).

The grassroots position claims that moral panics often include populist sentiment, driven by public concerns over the ability of powerful groups, such as large corporations, to cause harm to ordinary citizens (Goode and Ben-Yehuda 2009). Public fear and mistrust of corporate power have been described as the "Goliath Effect" (Fine 1985, 65), where harmful situations that happen to naïve consumers are linked to the greed and influence of large corporations. The appeal to populist sentiment evident in some grassroots moral panics may lead to classifying these events as simply urban legends (see also Brunvand 2001). However, Turner (1987) and Carroll (1987) note that these forms of a moral panic should not be dismissed, as they reflect deep-seated anxieties over living in modern societies held by some sectors of the community. For example, Turner (1987, 295) discussed the rumor that the Church's Fried Chicken franchise was owned by the "Ku Klux Klan and that they were putting something in the chicken that would cause sterility in black male customers." Analysis of this case revealed that it remained popular amongst segments of the community because it reflected tensions in race relations and the vulnerability felt by some individuals (Turner 1987).

The strength of the grassroots moral panic is that concern stems from deeply held feelings and is impervious to manipulation "from above" (Goode and Ben-Yehuda 1994b, 163). From this perspective dominant groups, such as the media or politicians, may influence public concerns. However, if a latent and widespread concern does not already exist or if the public is indifferent to an issue, a moral panic will not develop (Goode and Ben-Yehuda 2009). Although arising more or less spontaneously, a successful moral panic requires that concern is "focused, brought to public attention or awareness, given a specific outlet, harnessed to a mechanism of expression" (Goode and Ben-Yehuda 1994b, 167). However, the grassroots theory does not clarify how or why an issue becomes "harnessed to a mechanism of expression," why a moral panic emerges at a particular time or the manner in which local concerns shift to influence broader social views (Goode and Ben-Yehuda 1994b).

Interest-Group Theory

A theory that examines the way that concern is articulated, given direction and moves from the "bottom of society's socioeconomic ladder," or the grassroots, to the "middle of society's status and power hierarchy" is the interest-group theory (Goode and Ben-Yehuda 2009, 52–58; Hawdon 2001; Jensen, Gerber, and Babcock 1991). This theory suggests that moral panics emerge "somewhere in society's middle rungs" (Goode and Ben-Yehuda 1994b, 160–161). Becker (1963, 147–155) defined members of the interest-group typology as "moral entrepreneurs" including "rule creators" who agitate for social change with new and better rules overseen by a new "rule enforcer" (see also Henne 2015). These individuals are motivated by strong humanitarian ideals intended to "help those beneath them achieve a better status" (Becker 1963, 147–148; Gusfield 1955). The interest-group theory is the most widely used perspective and notes that, for some members of this group, the driving force of the moral panic is sincerely held beliefs that a particular issue is of real concern (Goode and Ben-Yehuda 2009). For example, Zatz (1987) notes that the 1970s and 1980s moral panic over Chicano youth gangs in the United States city of Phoenix also reflected the fact that police officers believed that youth crime was a significant issue threatening the community. The interest-group moral panic theory notes that members of this group include influential claim-makers, each with their own interests and agenda (Cohen 1972; Jenkins 1992; Jenkins and Maier-Katkin 1992; Thompson 1998). The superior moral position of these types of interest-groups enhances their ability to focus media attention on and transform the slant of news stories about particular situations (Becker 1963; Goode and Ben-Yehuda 2009; Zajdow 2008). From the perspective of the interest-group model:

> Advancing a moral and ideological cause almost inevitably entails advancing the status and material interests of the group who expresses

or works for them, and advancing the status and material interests of a group or category may simultaneously advance its ideology and morality. (Goode and Ben-Yehuda 2009, 67)

In other words, rather than a moral panic driven by grassroots concerns or by elite groups' efforts to protect their interests, as in the elite-engineered model discussed shortly, the interest-group model argues that material interests and morality are often "part of the same package" (Goode and Ben-Yehuda 2009, 69). As Goode and Ben-Yehuda (2009) note, separating interests and morality is not clear-cut and it may be more useful to see both as operative, with one more influential than the other in the context of particular moral panics.

Elite-Engineered Theory

The final moral panic theory is the 'elite-engineered' model. In contrast to the grassroots and interest-group models, the elite-engineered model argues that elite groups deliberately and consciously create moral panics to divert public attention from 'real' problems, or issues that undermine elite interests. The elite-engineered approach does not suggest that social problems are conjured from thin air but that the focus of attention is out of all proportion to the concrete nature of the threat (Goode and Ben-Yehuda 2009). Underpinning the notion that elite groups have the ability, and power, to engineer a moral panic is the idea that these groups "dominate the media, determine the content of legislation and the direction of law enforcement, and control much of the resources on which action groups and social movements depend" (Goode and Ben-Yehuda 2009, 135). Elites use access to these resources to shape "shared understandings of normality, dangerousness, acceptable behavior, legitimacy, immorality, and the myriad other definitional components of deviance and conventionality" (Sanders 1990, 4). From the perspective of elite-engineered theory rather than spontaneous expressions shaped by "common-sense views," public opinion is molded by "multiple elite interest-defining layers," with the media playing a central role (Goode and Ben-Yehuda 2009, 135–136). Unlike the grassroots and interest-group perspectives, the elite-engineered view takes a top-down social control approach driven by specific concerns of elite groups to protect their—primarily economic—interests rather than defending morality or ideology (Goode and Ben-Yehuda 2009).

The elite-engineered theory enables examination of interactions between dominant groups because, Goode and Ben-Yehuda (2009, 52–53) write, it notes that "elites in one institution frequently and intimately interact with those in another" and "tend to have interests in common, and act to protect those interests." The interaction between dominant groups, in particular the media and other elite groups, provides opportunities for these to influence public opinion. A significant consequence of this is that it enables the establishment of a specific institutional response to an issue constructed by elite groups as a moral panic. Orthodox application of an elite-engineered theory reduces the public to "puppets . . . being pulled . . . by strings manipulated from above, by . . . the ruling elite" (Goode and Ben-Yehuda 2009, 54). For example, Hall et al. (1978) argue that, rather than originating with the masses, a moral panic around mugging in 1970s Britain was engineered by the capitalist class to defend hegemonic positions of power achieved with the unwitting complicity of the media, legislature, police and the courts (Goode and Ben-Yehuda 1994b). Goode and Ben-Yehuda (2009) disagree with this conceptualization, suggesting that it fails to acknowledge the active role of other social agents, such as the public and the media.

In the context of doping as a moral panic, a further problem with the elite-engineered theory is that it suggests that elite groups share a singularity of purpose. This is not to imply that elite groups do not share common goals, such as maintaining their dominant position. However, applying elite-engineered theory to the issue of drugs in sport does not sufficiently account for the diversity of interest-groups or the contested nature of power relationships between these social actors.

Elites-Engineered Moral Panic Theory

In the context of PEDs in sport as a moral panic, I expand the theoretical model to an '*elites-engineered*' approach in order to capture the plurality of elite groups with diverse and competing interests that are active in the doping debate. An elites-engineered moral panic theory brings issues of governance, control and legitimacy into the analysis as factors that may contribute to the classification of doping as deviant behavior. The intensely codified nature of modern global sport includes laws, rules and regulations to address a range of issues. As well as PED use, these include political boycotts, eligibility of athletes, commercialization and jurisdictional disputes between competing SGBs (Nafziger 1992). In these contested spaces, to maintain support for an overarching anti-doping regulatory framework, including perceptions of the legitimacy of such an approach, requires that a diverse range of SGBs consistently apply anti-doping regulations. This is complicated by the structure of the global sporting community, which is constituted by a range of stakeholder groups that bring with them diverse interests and objectives (Kidd et al. 2001). This highlights the multi-dimensional and contested aspect of legitimacy, as multiple claims to legitimacy overlap with one another in the global sporting community.

Situating legitimacy within a moral panic framework provides an effective mechanism with which to identify "groups that stand to gain or lose from a particular way of understanding the world" (Dingelstad et al. 1996, 1830). In the context of drugs in sport as a moral panic, considering legitimacy within an elites-engineered moral panic theory expands the analysis beyond the individual athlete-user to include power relationships between organizations and the way these shape the debate. This approach contrasts with the explanations for PED use in current anti-doping regulatory dis-courses, which are discussed in the next section.

DISCIPLINARY APPROACHES TO PERFORMANCE-ENHANCING DRUG USE

Explanations for the illegitimate use of drugs in sport draw on a number of disciplinary approaches. Sports medicine focuses on the impact of PEDs on athletes' health and strategies to improve performance within medically sound limits. For example, Ashenden (2002) called for the implementation of a 'Hematological Passport' as one strategy to ensure that athletes compete safely (see also Savulescu and Foddy 2011). Pharmacologists develop and improve new testing technology, and policy makers explore legal solutions supported by resources directed toward drug testing programs (Strelan and Boeckmann 2003). The economics literature applies cost-benefit models to explain athletes' decisions to dope as a rational choice analysis of risks and rewards (see Berentsen 2002; Bird and Wagner 1997; Eber 2008; Haugen 2004; Shermer 2008). Psychology identifies individual personality traits, behaviors and risk factors that may influence the attitudes and motivations of athletes. Sports psychology concentrates on the cognitive or behavioral aspects of drug-taking and the development of behavioral frameworks to promote compliance with anti-doping regulations (see Anshel and Russell 1997; Petroczi 2007). The identification of doping risk factors tied to individual personality traits has had practical consequences and is a central theme of WADA's anti-doping research and efforts to ensure the efficacy of doping prevention strategies (e.g., see Backhouse et al. 2007; WADA 2010c).

This prevailing anti-doping research approach tends to ignore broader social factors, including organizational interactions and responses, placing the individual athlete-user outside the influence of the social structures that constitute the modern sporting context. This is problematic; as Armour et al. (2000) point out, "a social being cannot escape society in order to participate in sport, rather society consists of structures and agents who constitute—and reconstitute—sport." More specifically, an individualist perspective limits its potential to effectively inform anti-doping policy, as Stewart and Smith (2008, 282) emphasize:

> It assumes athlete decision making to be a rational weighing of costs and benefits and also presupposes a universal moral force that condemns drug use . . . the behavioral approach implies that social and reference group pressures will discourage drug use when, in fact, we live in an increasingly drug-tolerant society where drugs are viewed as means of improving people's quality of life.

The elevation of anti-doping to the level of an ethical choice, as research focused on changing individual behavior suggests, diverts attention from the influence of broader political and economic structures and the way that the interactions of a variety of interest-groups impact on the debate (Hollands 1984). This critique does not imply that examining attitudes, behavior and motivations of athletes is not important. Indeed, research has shown that understanding athletes' values, beliefs and motives is central to developing effective anti-doping policy (for example, see British Medical Association 2002; Gucciardi et al. 2010; Moston et al. 2015; Mugford et al. 1999). Research conducted by Donovan et al. (2002) considered the role of attitudes toward the current anti-doping framework. That research suggested that deterrence and compliance with anti-doping regulations are more effective if organizations applying such strategies are perceived as legitimate. Drawing on a broad body of literature discussing the development of anti-drug policies—including PEDs—Battin et al. (2008, 23) reinforce this finding. They emphasize that to be successful, a drug management or control policy requires a framework that incorporates justice, consistency, coherence and comprehensiveness:

> A just theory and policy must also be coherent, otherwise it is not really intelligible as either a theory or policy. Coherence requires not only that a theory or policy be consistent, but also that its parts all relate to each other, that they are involved in the same dialogue, and that they are mutually supporting. In other words, a coherent theory or policy hangs together in such a way that its rationale is apparent and easily evaluated. Coherence is desirable for all the reasons consistency is desirable, but developing a coherent drug policy requires a deeper inquiry into the types of rationales that should shape drug policy.

Battin et al. (2008, 23) also argue that the failure of components of drug regulatory systems to "fit together in a mutually supporting whole" reflects a lack of coherency in the overall system. The success of any regulatory system, including anti-doping regulation, is dependent upon acceptance of its underlying goals (Buti and Fridman 1994; e.g, see Chapter 4, this volume). This highlights the importance of subjective perceptions of legitimacy and, in the case of drugs in sport, means that the rationale underpinning the anti-doping regulatory framework must match, reflect or enable the attainment of the goals of that policy.

However, an approach that privileges social structure at the expense of social interaction and perspectives is equally problematic. What is important is acknowledging and investigating structural factors as well as the way that these are interpreted and evaluated by social actors. This includes examining the definitions and meanings that individuals assign to the actions that result as social structures impact on their behavior (Millham et al. 1972). The point here is that a coherent, consistent anti-doping policy framework requires moving beyond the individual athlete-user to a multi-dimensional model that recognizes that athlete behavior is situated in, and influenced by, the structure and culture of the broader sporting context—including inter-actions between elite SGBs and the way they respond to particular issues defined as problematic (Stewart and Smith 2008). These are relevant points, as the ability to regulate athletes' behavior is more complex than the power to impose sanctions.

CONCLUSION

The dominant approach to PEDs remains focused on regulation and control of athletes at the individual level. However, I have noted in this chapter that an approach that privileges either the individual or social structures fails to adequately address the interactive processes at work in the con-struction of a social problem. Such approaches are particularly problematic in terms of legitimacy, which I argue underpins the social construction of doping as a moral panic. Elite groups cannot take for granted claims to the moral authority or legitimacy to 'pull the strings.' Rather, these groups must engage in consensus-making activities to generate and maintain support for the legitimacy of an institutional response to a specific problem that is of particular concern (Beamish 2009). This highlights the subjective nature of legitimacy. Further, members of the public are not passive 'puppets or marionettes' but, as we have seen, filter messages, including those from the mass media, through complex social networks and knowledge frameworks (Goode and Ben-Yehuda 2009).

In this book I apply a modified Goode and Ben-Yehuda (2009) moral panic model to the debate surrounding PEDs that includes a focus on consensus-making in an elites-engineered moral panic theory. Combined with Weber's (1969) concept of legitimacy, I expand the analysis to consider the way that interactions between social institutions, such as the media, WADA and elite SGBs, impact on the doping debate. While some moral panics may have limited initial impact, others can leave a significant insti-tutional legacy (Goode and Ben-Yehuda 1994b). Of particular interest is the extent to which the creation of WADA constitutes an institutionalized response in the construction of PEDs as a moral panic. From this perspec-tive, the actions of WADA and elite SGBs can be interpreted as perpetuating concern over, and institutionalizing, PEDs as a moral panic with the objec-tive of restoring perceptions of the legitimacy of sporting elites. To bolster and support claims to legitimacy, dominant stakeholders, such as WADA, SGBs and governments, introduce increasingly strict regulatory measures to monitor and control athlete behavior.

NOTE

1 Disproportionality includes: grossly exaggerated figures to highlight the extent of the problem; available evidence that suggests that the 'concrete threat' is non-existent; 'tall tales' about non-existent harm are told and believed; increased levels of attention to a specific condition that does not present a greater or lesser threat than another condition; and attention to a given condition exceeds that of a previous or later time, with no increase in the objective seriousness of the issue (Goode and Ben-Yehuda 2009, 44–46).

REFERENCES

ABS (Australian Bureau of Statistics). 2006. *8680.0 — Sports and Physical Recreation Services, Australia, 2004–05*. Canberra: Australian Bureau of Statistics.

Altheide, D. L. 1997. "The News Media, the Problem Frame, and the Production of Fear." *Sociological Quarterly* 38 (4): 647–668.

Amis, J. 2005. "Beyond Sport: Imaging and Re-imaging a Transnational Brand." In *Sport and Corporate Nationalisms*, edited by Andrews, D. L., 143–165. Oxford: Berg.

Andrews, D. L., and Jackson, S. J. 2001. "Introduction—Sport Celebrities Public Culture, and Private Experience." In *Sport Stars—The Cultural Politics of Sporting Celebrity*, edited by Andrews, D. L. and Jackson, S. J., 1–19. London: Routledge.

Andrews, I. 2000. "From a Club to a Corporate Game: The Changing Face of Australian Football 1960–1999." *International Journal of the History of Sport* 17 (2/3): 225–254.

Anshel, M. H., and Russell, K. G. 1997. "Examining Athletes' Attitudes Toward Using Anabolic Steroids and Their Knowledge of the Possible Effects." *Journal of Drug Education* 27 (2): 121–145.

Armour, K., Jones, R., and Kerry, D. 2000. "Sport Sociology 2000." *Sociology of Sport Online*. http://physed.otago.ac.nz/sosol/v1i1/v1i1a7.htm. Accessed 30 May 2010.

Ashenden, M. 2002. "A Strategy to Deter Blood Doping in Sport." *Haematologica* 87 (3): 225–234.

Backhouse, S. H., McKenna, J., Robinson, S., and Atkin, A. 2007. *International Literature Review: Attitudes, Behaviours, Knowledge and Education—Drugs in Sport: Past, Present and Future*. Leeds Metropolitan University: Carnegie Research Institute.

Baerveldt, C., Bunkers, H., de Winter, M., and Kooistra, J. 1998. "Assessing a Moral Panic Relating to Crime and Drugs Policy in the Netherlands: Towards a Testable Theory." *Crime, Law and Social Change* 29 (1): 31–47.

Battin, M. P., Luna, E., Lipman, A. G., Gahlinger, P.M., Rollins, D. E., Roberts, J. C., and Booher, T. L. 2008. *Drugs and Justice: Seeking a Consistent, Coherent, Comprehensive View*. Oxford: Oxford University Press.

Beamish, R. 2009. "Steroids, Symbolism and Morality: The Construction of a Social Problem and Its Unintended Consequences." In *Elite Sport, Doping and Public Health*, edited by Moller, V., McNamee, M. and Dimeo, P., 55–73. Odense: University of Southern Denmark.

Becker, H. S. 1963. *Outsiders*. New York: Free Press.

———. 1967. "Whose Side Are We On?" *Social Problems* 14: 239–247.

Ben-Yehuda, N. 1986. "The Sociology of Moral Panics: Toward a New Synthesis." *Sociological Quarterly* 27 (4): 495–513.

Berentsen, A. 2002. "The Economics of Doping." *European Journal of Political Economy* 18: 109–127.

Bernstein, S. 2004. "IGHC Working Paper Series: The Elusive Basis of Legitimacy in Global Governance: Three Conceptions." In *Autonomy, Democracy, and Legitimacy in an Era of Globalization*, edited by W. D. Coleman. McMaster University, Ontario: Institute on Globalization and the Human Condition. http://www.religiousstudies.mcmaster.ca/institute-on-globalization-and-the-human-condition/documents/IGHC-WPS_04-2_Bernstein.pdf. Accessed 1 March 2012

Best, J. 1990. *Threatened Children: Rhetoric and Concern about Child-Victims.* Chicago: University Press of Chicago.

———. 1999. *Random Violence: How We Talk about New Crimes and New Victims.* Berkeley: University of California Press.

———. 2002. "Monster Hype." *Education Next* Summer 2002: 51–55.

Bird, E. J., and Wagner, G. G. 1997. "Sport As a Common Property Resource—A Solution to the Dilemmas of Doping." *Journal of Conflict Resolution* 41 (6): 749–766.

Blumer, H. 1971. "Social Problems As Collective Behavior." *Social Problems* 18 (3): 298–306.

Bok, S. 1989. *Lying: Moral Choice in Public and Private Life.* New York: Vintage Books.

Bourdieu, P. 1998. *On Television and Journalism.* Translated by Priscilla Packhurst Ferguson. London: Pluto Press.

Boxill, I., and Unnithan, N. P. 1995. "Rhetoric and Policy Realities in Developing Countries: Community Councils in Jamaica, 1972–1980." *Journal of Applied Behavioral Science* 31 (1): 65–79.

British Medical Association. 2002. *Drugs in Sport: The Pressure to Perform* London: BMJ Books.

Brunvand, J. H. 2001. *Encyclopedia of Urban Legends.* Santa Barbara, CA: Oxford.

Buchanan, A., and Keohane, R. O. 2006. "The Legitimacy of Global Governance Institutions." *Ethics & International Affairs* 4: 405–437.

Buti, A., and Fridman, S. 1994. "The Intersection of Law and Policy: Drug Testing in Sport." *Australian Journal of Public Administration* 53 (4): 489–507.

Cantelon, H., and McDermott, L. 2001. "Charisma and the Rational-Legal Organisation: A Case Study of the Avery Brundage-Reginald Honey Correspondence Leading Up to the South African Expulsion from the International Olympic Movement." *OlyMPIKA: The International Journal of Olympic Studies* X: 33–58.

Carroll, M. P. 1987. " 'The Castrated Boy': Another Contribution to the Psychoanalytic Study of Urban Legends." *Folklore* 98 (2): 216–225.

Cashore, B. 2002. "Legitimacy and the Privatization of Environmental Governance: How Non-State Market-Driven (NSMD) Governance Systems Gain Rule-Making Authority." *Governance: An International Journal of Policy, Administration, and Institutions* 15 (4): 503–529.

Chermak, S. 1997. "The Presentation of Drugs in the News Media: The News Sources Involved in the Construction of Social Problems." *Justice Quarterly* 14 (4): 687–718.

Cohen, S. 1967. "Mods, Rockers and the Rest: Community Reactions to Juvenile Delinquency." *The Howard Journal of Criminal Justice* 12 (2): 121–130.

———. 1972. *Folk Devils and Moral Panics: The Creation of the Mods and Rockers.* London: MacGibbon and Kee.

———. *Folk devils and moral panics: the creation of the Mods and Rockers* 3rd ed. Abingdon, Oxon, New York: Routledge.

Connor, J. 2009. "Towards a Sociology of Drugs in Sport." *Sport in Society* 12 (3): 327–343.

Connor, J., and A. Kirby. 2011. "Sport and Global Governance: Foul Play Rewarded with Legitimacy." The annual conference of the International Sociological Association, Global Governance: Political Authority in Transition, Montreal, Quebec, Canada, 16–19 March, 2011. http://www.isanet.org/Conferences/Montreal-2011, accessed 9 September 2011.

Cornwell, B., and Linders, A. 2002. "The Myth of 'Moral Panic': An Alternative Account of LSD Prohibition." *Deviant Behaviour* 23 (4): 307–330.

Dingelstad, D., Gosden, R., Martin, B., and Vakas, N. 1996. "The Social Construction of Drug Debates." *Social Science & Medicine* 43 (12): 1829–1838.

Donovan, R. J., Egger, G., Kapernick, V., and Mendoza, J. 2002. "A Conceptual Framework for Achieving Performance Enhancing Drug Compliance in Sport." *Sports Medicine* 32 (4): 269–284.

Eber, N. 2008. "The Performance-Enhancing Drug Game Reconsidered A Fair Play Approach." *Journal of Sports Economics* 9 (3): 318–327.

Entman, R. M. 2004. *Projections of Power: Framing News, Public Opinion, and U.S. Foreign Policy*. Chicago: University of Chicago Press.

Ericson, R. V, Baranek, P. M., and Chan, J. B. L. 1987. *Visualizing Deviance: A Study of News Organisations*. Milton Keynes: Open University Press.

———. 1991. *Representing Order*. Toronto: University of Toronto Press.

Erikson, K. T. 1966. *Wayward Puritans: A Study in the Sociology of Deviance*. New York: John Wiley and Sons.

Farnen, R. F. 1990. "Decoding the Mass Media and Terrorism Connection: Militant Extremism as Systemic and Symbiotic Processes." In *Marginal Conventions: Popular Culture, Mass Media and Social Deviance*, edited by Sanders, C. R., 98–116. Bowling Green, OH: Bowling Green State University Popular Press.

Fine, G. A. 1985. "The Goliath Effect: Corporte Dominance and Mercantile Legends." *The Journal of American Folklore* 98 (387): 63–84.

Fritz, N. J., and Altheide, D. L. 1987. "The Mass Media and the Social Construction of the Missing Children Problem." *Sociological Quarterly* 28 (4): 473–493.

Garland, D. 2008. "On the Concept of Moral Panic." *Crime Media Culture* 4 (1): 9–31.

Ghareeb, E. 2000. "New Media and the Information Revolution in the Arab World: An Assessment." *Middle East Journal* 54 (3 The Information Revolution): 395–418.

Gonzenbach, W. J. 1992. "A Time-Series Analysis of the Drug Issue, 1985–1990: The Press, The President and Public Opinion." *International Journal of Public Opinion* 4 (2): 126–147.

Goode, E., and Ben-Yehuda, N. 1994a. *Moral Panics: The Social Construction of Deviance*. Cambridge, MA: Blackwell Publishers.

———. 1994b. "Moral Panics: Culture, Politics and Social Construction." *Annual Review of Sociology* 20 (3): 149–171.

———. 2006. "Enter Moral Panics." In *Constructing Crime: Perspectives on Making News and Social Problems*, edited by Potter, G. W. and Kappeler, V. E., 21–28. Long Grove, IL: Waveland Press.

———. 2009. *Moral Panics: The Social Construction of Deviance*. Chichester, West Sussex: Wiley-Blackwell Publishing.

Grafstein, R. 1981. "The Failure of Weber's Conception of Legitimacy: Its Causes and Implications." *The Journal of Politics* 43 (2): 456–472.

Gucciardi, D. F., Jalleh, G., and Donovan, R. 2010. "Does Social Desirability Influence the Relationship Between Doping Attitudes and Doping Susceptibility in Athletes?" *Psychology of Sport and Exercise* 11 (6): 479–486.

———. 2011. "An Examination of the Sport Drug Control Model with Elite Australian athletes." *Journal of Science and Medicine in Sport* 14 (6): 469–476.

Gusfield, J. R. 1955. "Social Structure and Moral Reform: A Study of the Woman's Christian Temperance Union." *American Journal of Sociology* 61 (3): 221–232.

———. 1963. *Symbolic Crusade, Status Politics and the American Temperance Movement*. Urbana: University of Illinois Press.

———. 1967. "Moral Passage: The Symbolic Process in Public Designations of Deviance." *Social Problems* 15: 175–188.

———. 1981. *The Culture of Public Problems Drinking-Driving and the Symbolic Order*. Chicago: University of Chicago Press.

Habermas, J. 1976. *Legitimation Crisis*. London: Heinemann Educational.

Hall, S., Critcher, C., Jefferson, J., Clarke, J., and Roberts, B. 1978. *Policing the Crisis: Mugging, The State, and Law And Order*. London: MacMillan Press.

Harvey, J., and Law, A. 2005. "'Resisting' the Global Media Oligopoly? The Canada Inc. Response." In *Sport and Corporate Nationalisms*, edited by Andrews, D. L., 187–225. Oxford: Berg.

Haugen, K. K. 2004. "The Performance-Enhancing Drug Game." *Journal of Sports Economics* 5 (1): 67–86.

Hawdon, J. E. 2001. "The Role of Presidential Rhetoric in the Creation of a Moral Panic: Reagan, Bush and the War on Drugs." *Deviant Behaviour* 22 (5): 419–445.

Henne, K. 2015. *Testing for Athlete Citizenship: Regulating Doping and Sex in Sport*. New Brunswick, NJ: Rutgers University Press.

Hilgartner, S., and Bosk, C. L. 1988. "The Rise and Fall of Social Problems: A Public Arenas Model." *The American Journal of Sociology* 94 (1): 53–78.

Hollands, R. G. 1984. "The Role of Cultural Studies and Social Criticism in the Sociological Study of Sport." *Quest* 36 (1): 66–79.

Holton, R. J. 1987. "The Idea of Crisis in Modern Society." *The British Journal of Sociology* 38 (4): 502–520.

Houlihan, B. 2002. *Dying to Win*. Strasbourg Cedex: Council of Europe Publishing.

———. 2009. "Doping, Public Health and the Generalisation of Interests." In *Elite Sport, Doping and Public Health*, edited by Moller, V., McNamee, M. and Dimeo, P., 41–54. Odense: University Press of Southern Denmark.

Howman, D. 2012. "Developing New Alliances to Tackle the Increasing Problem of Doping in Sport." In *Doping as a Public Health Issue Symposium*. Stockholm, Sweden: World Anti-Doping Agency.

Hunt, A. 1999. *Governing Morals: A Social History of Moral Regulation*. Cambridge, England: Cambridge University Press.

Hurd, I. 1999. "Legitimacy and Authority in International Politics." *International Organisation* 53 (2): 379–408.

Jalleh, G., Donovan, R., and Jobling, I. 2014. "Predicting Attitude Towards Performance Enhancing Substance Use: A Comprehensive Test of the Sport Drug Control Model with Elite Australian Athletes." *Journal of Science and Medicine in Sport* 17: 574–579.

Jenkins, P. 1992. *Intimate Enemies: Moral Panics in Contemporary Great Britain*. New York: Aldine de Gruyter.

Jenkins, P., and Maier-Katkin, D. 1992. "Satanism: Myth and Reality in a Contemporary Moral Panic." *Crime, Law and Social Change* 17 (1): 53–75.

Jensen, E. L., Gerber, J., and Babcock, G. M. 1991. "The New War on Drugs: Grass Roots Movement or Political Construction?" *Journal of Drug Issues* 21 (3): 641–667.

Johnson, T. J., Wanta, W., Boudreau, T., Blank-Libra, J., Schaffer, K., and Turner, S. 1996. "Influence Dealers: A Path Analysis Model of Agenda Building During Richard Nixon's War on Drugs." *Journalism and Mass Communication Quarterly* 73 (1): 181–194.

Jones, B. J., McFalls, J. A., and Gallagher, B. J. 1989. "Toward a Unified Model for Social Problems." *Journal of the Theory of Social Behavior* 19 (3):337–356.

Kidd, B., Edelman, R., and Brownell, S. 2001. "Comparative Analysis of Doping Scandals: Canada, Russia, and China." In *Doping in Elite Sport: The Politics of Drugs in the Olympic Movement*, edited by Wilson, W. and Derse, E., 153–188. Champgaign, IL: Human Kinetics.

Killingbeck, D. 2006. "The Role of Television News in the Construction of School Violence as a 'Moral Panic.'" In *Constructing Crime: Perspectives on Making News and Social Problems*, edited by Potter, G. W. and Kappeler, V. E., 213–228. Long Grove, IL: Waveland Press.

Koppell, J. 2005. "Pathologies of Accountability: ICANN and the Challenge of 'Multiple Accountabilities Disorder.'" *Public Administration Review* 65 (1): 94–108.

———. 2007. "Structure of Global Governance: Explaining the Organizational Design of Global Rulemaking Institutions." In *Annual Meeting of the International Studies Association*. Chicago, IL.

———. 2008. "Global Governance Organizations: Legitimacy and Authority in Conflict." *Journal of Public Administration Research and Theory* 18 (2): 177–203.

Kwak, H., Lee, C., Park, H., and Moon, S. 2010. "What Is Twitter, a Social Network or a News Media?" In *World Wide Web Conference Committee*. Raleigh, NC.

Lidz, C. W., and Walker, A. L. 1980. *Heroin, Deviance, and Morality*. Beverly Hills, CA: Sage Publications.

Lofquist, W. S. 1997. "Constructing 'Crime': Media Coverage of Individual and Organizational Wrongdoing." *Justice Quarterly* 14 (2): 243–263.

Lull, J., and Hinerman, S. 1997. *Media Scandals: Morality and Desire in the Popular Culture Marketplace*. Cambridge, England: Polity Press.

Matheson, C. 1987. "Weber and the Classification of Forms of Legitimacy." *The British Journal of Sociology* 38 (2): 199–215.

McKay, J., Hutchins, B., and Mikosza, J. 2000. *'Shame and Scandal in the Family': Australian Media Narratives of the IOC/SOCOG Scandal Matrix*. Paper presented at the Bridging Three Centuries—Fifth International Symposium for Olympic Research, University of Western Ontario, London, Ontario, Canada.

McRobbie, A. 1994. "Folk Devils Fight Back." *New Left Review*: 107–116.

McRobbie, A., and Thornton, A. L. 1995. "Rethinking 'Moral Panic' for Multi-Mediated Social Worlds." *British Journal of Sociology* 46 (4): 559–574.

Millham, S., Bullock, R., and Cherrett, P. F. 1972. "Social Control in Organizations." *The British Journal of Sociology* 23 (4): 406–421.

Moston, S. E., Engelberg, T., and Skinner, J. 2015. "Perceived Incidence of Drug Use in Australian Sport: A Survey of Athletes and Coaches." *Sport in Society: Cultures, Commerce, Media, Politics* 18 (1): 91–105.

Mugford, S., Mugford, J., and Donnelly, D. 1999. *Social Research Project: Athletes' motivations for using or not using performance enhancing drugs*. Canberra.: Australian Sports Drug Agency.

Nafziger, J. A. R. 1992. "International Sports Law: A Reply of Characteristics and Trends." *American Journal of International Law* 86 (3): 489–518.

Pakulski, J. 1986. "Legitimacy and Mass Compliance: Reflections on Max Weber and Soviet-Type Societies." *British Journal of Political Science* 16 (1): 35–56.

Palmer, C. 2000. "Spin Doctors and Sportsbrokers." *International Review for Sociology of Sport* 35 (3): 364–377.

Parenti, M. 1986. *Inventing Reality*. New York: St. Martin's Press.

Petroczi, A. 2007. "Attitudes and Doping: A Structural Equation Analysis of the Relationship Between Athletes' Attitudes, Sport Orientation and Doping Behaviour." *Substance Abuse Treatment, Prevention, and Policy* 2: 34.

Pritchard, D., and Hughes, K. D. 1997. "Patterns of Deviance in Crime News." *Journal of Communication* 47 (3): 49–67.

Rasmussen, K. 2005. "The Quest for the Imaginary Evil: A Critique of Anti-Doping." *Sport in History* 25 (3): 515–535.

Reiner, R. 2007. "Media-Made Criminality: The Representation of Crime in the Mass Media." In *The Oxford Handbook of Criminology*, edited by Maguire, M., Morgan, R. and Reiner, R., 302–337. Oxford: Oxford University Press.

Rommetvedt, H. 2005. "Norway: Resources Count, But Votes Decide? From Neo-Corporatist Representation to Neo-Pluralist Parliamentarism." *West European Politics* 28 (4): 740–763.

Sacco, V. F. 1995. "Media Constructions of Crime." *Annals of the American Academy of Political & Social Science* 539: 141–154.

Sanders, C. R. 1990. " 'A Lot of People Like It': The Relationship Between Deviance and Popular Culture." In *Marginal Conventions: Popular Culture, Mass Media and Social Deviance*, edited by Sanders, C. R., 3–13. Bowling Green, OH: Bowling Green State University Popular Press.

Savulescu, J., and Foddy, B. 2011. "Le Tour and Failure of Zero Tolerance: Time to Relax Doping Controls." In *Enhancing Human Capacities*, edited by Savulescu, J., Meulen, R. H. J. ter and Kahane, G., 304–312. Chichester, West Sussex: Wiley-Blackwell.

Schlesinger, P., and Tumber, H. 1994. *Reporting Crime: The Media Politics of Criminal Justice*. Oxford: Clarendon Press.

Schneider, J. W. 1985. "Social Problems Theory: The Constructionist View." *Annual Review of Sociology* 11: 209–229.

Seib, P. 2008. *The Al Jazeera Effect: How the New Global Media Are Reshaping World Politics*. Washington, DC: Potomac Books.

Shermer, M. 2008. "The Doping Dilemma." *Scientific American*, 31 March 2008. http://www.sciam.com/article.cfm?id=the-doping-dilemma.   Accessed   9 April 2008.

Spencer, M. E. 1970. "Weber on Legitimate Norms and Authority." *The British Journal of Sociology* 21 (2): 123–134.

Stewart, B., Nicholson, M., and Dickson, G. 2005. "The Australian Football Leagues' Recent Progress: A Study in Cartel Conduct and Monopoly Power." *Sport Management Review* (Melbourne, Aust) 8 (2): 95–117.

Stewart, B., and Smith, A. C. T. 2008. "Drug Use in Sport Implications for Public Policy." *Journal of Sport and Social Issues* 32 (3): 278–298.

Strelan, P., and Boeckmann, R. J. 2003. "A New Model for Understanding Performance Enhancing Drug Use by Elite Athletes." *Journal of Applied Sport Psychology* 15: 176–183.

Suchman, M. C. 1995. "Managing Legitimacy: Strategic and Institutional Approaches." *The Academy of Management Review* 20 (3): 571–610.

Thomas, J. J. R. 1984. "Weber and Direct Democracy." *The British Journal of Sociology* 35 (2): 216–240.

Thompson, K. 1998. *Moral Panics*. London: Routledge.

Throgmorton, J. A. 1991. "The Rhetorics of Policy Analysis." *Policy Sciences* 24 (2): 153–179.

Tomlinson, A. 2005. "The Making of the Global Sports Economy: ISL, Adidas and the Rise of the Corporate Player in World Sport." In *Sport and Corporate Nationalisms*, edited by Andrews, D. L., 35–65. Oxford: Berg.

Tucher, A. 1994. *Froth and Scum: Truth, Beauty, Goodness, and the Ax Murder in America's First Mass Medium*. Chapel Hill: University of North Carolina Press.

Turner, P. A. 1987. "Church's Fried Chicken and the Klan: A Rhetorical Analysis of Rumor on the Black Community." *Western Folklore* 4: 294–306.

Victor, J. S. 1998. "Moral Panics and the Social Construction of Deviant Behavior: A Theory and Application to the Case of Ritual Child Abuse." *Sociological Perspectives* 41 (3): 541–565.

von Hoffman, N. 1985. "The Press: Pack of Fools. Killer Bees, Missing Kids, and Other Phoney Stories." *The New Republic* 3681: 9–11.

WADA (World Anti-Doping Agency). 2010a. "About WADA." World Anti-Doping Agency. http://www.wada-ama.org/en/About-WADA/. Accessed 12 August 2010.

———. 2010b. "WADA—Education & Awareness, Social Science Research." World Anti-Doping Agency. http://www.wada-ama.org/en/Education-Awareness/Social-Science/. Accessed 11 April 2010.

———. 2010c. "WADA—Education & Awareness, Social Science Research, Funded Research Projects." World Anti-Doping Agency. http://www.wada-ama.org/en/Education-Awareness/Social-Science/Funded-Projects/. Accessed 11 April 2010.

Weber, M. 1947. *The Theory of Social and Economic Organisation*. New York: Free Press.

———. 1954. *Max Weber on Law in Economy and Society*. Cambridge: Harvard University Press.

———. 1969. *Economy and Society*. 2 vols. Berkeley: University of California Press.

Welch, M., Weber, L., and Edwards, W. 2000. " 'All the News That's Fit to Print': A Content Analysis of the Correctional Debate in the *New York Times*." *The Prison Journal* 80 (3): 245–264.

Whannel, G. 2005. "The Five Rings and the Small Screen: Television, Sponsorship, and New Media in the Olympic Movement." In *Global Olympics: Historical and Sociological Studies of the Modern Games*, edited by Young, K. and Wamsley, K. B., 161–177. Amsterdam: Elsevier JAI.

Wright, R. 2000. " 'I'd Sell You Suicide': Pop Music and Moral Panic in the Age of Marilyn Manson." *Popular Music* 19 (3): 365–385.

Wuthnow, R., Hunter, J., Bergesen, A., and Kurzweil, E. 1984. *Cultural Analysis*. London: Routledge.

Young, J. 2009. "Moral Panic: Its Origins in Resistance, Ressentiment and the Translation of Fantasy into Reality." *British Journal of Criminology* 49: 4–16.

Zajdow, G. 2008. "Moral Panics: The Old and the New." *Deviant Behaviour* 29 (7): 640–664.

Zatz, M. S. 1987. "Chicano Youth Gangs and Crime: The Creation of a Moral Panic." *Contemporary Crises* 11 (2): 129–158.

2 Historical Overview
The International Olympic Committee, Legitimacy and Doping

A modified moral panic model, based on the work of Goode and Ben-Yehuda (2009) and incorporating Weber's (1969) concept of legitimacy, usefully illuminates debates around contemporary social issues. This is because it expands the analysis to consider the way that interactions between organizational actors, such as sporting organizations, impact on debates around social issues, in this case the drugs in sport debate. In this chapter I focus on the role of legitimacy in the doping debate, using the International Olympic Committee (IOC) as a socio-historical case study. There has been in-depth analysis and discussion of the changes to sport and the political and social context surrounding the IOC (e.g., see Brown 2005; Guttmann 1984, 1992, 2004; Hill 1992; Hoberman 1986; Houlihan 1994; MacAloon 1981, 1984, 2006; Riordan 1993, amongst others). I draw on that literature here to outline changing attitudes toward drug use in sport, the IOC's response to PEDs and implications for their legitimacy leading to the creation of the World Anti-Doping Agency (WADA). This positions the doping debate in the socio-historical context within which it is situated.

In the next section I briefly discuss the historical basis for the moral authority and legitimacy of the IOC, including the manner in which attitudes toward drugs in sport in the twentieth century affected the IOC's legitimacy in the context of anti-doping regulation. The complexity of factors that influenced the introduction of anti-doping policies has been extensively canvassed (e.g., see Dimeo 2007, 2009; Henne 2015; Hoberman 1992, 2005; Houlihan 2002; Møller 2005; Wrynn 2004). My focus is on key events to consider their relationship to perceptions of the IOC's legitimacy and the events that contributed to the creation of WADA (Chapter 3, this volume).

THE IOC AND LEGITIMACY

Claims that the IOC is in a crisis or lacks legitimacy are not recent developments and not limited to the issue of PEDs. Hoberman (1986, 5) explains that "political scandals" have "tarnished" the Olympic Games, noting that "there is inherent in global sport, and in the Olympic movement in particular, a moral vacuum from which political crisis derive." Some examples of issues that confronted the IOC include political tension between China and Taiwan, the 'two Koreas,' the Tlatelolco (1968 Mexico Olympics) and Black September (1972 Munich Olympics) massacres as well as the expulsion and re-admittance of South Africa (Berg 2008; Houlihan 2005; Riordan 1993; Torres and Dyreson 2005). However, the IOC has long held onto idealized notions of its role as promoter of social order and cohesion. This can be traced to Baron Pierre de Coubertin's 1894 revival of the ancient Olympics. Coubertin founded the modern Olympics on values associated with the ideals of amateurism, with participation linked to "love of sport and play" (Allison 1993; Hill 1993).

A Weberian lens can also be applied to the early sporting context. From this perspective, amateur athletes competed based on shared values over the "love of the activity and its intrinsic moral and physical benefits" and voluntarily agreed to the authority of athletic associations as 'guardians' of the amateur order (MacAloon 1981, 301 n229; 2006). Legitimacy based on a framework of rational, consciously crafted rules is also evident in the early Olympic Movement. Influencing Coubertin in his Olympic revival was the shift toward codified rules and regulations to order social life, including sport, which took place during the Industrial Revolution. Described as a process of "sportization," that period linked codified sporting contests with the introduction of more formalized rules and norms to govern social behavior (Boyes 2001, 171). Implementation of codified rules and regulations, or codes of conduct, required institutional foundations, such as the early IOC, which, in addition to being intended as a vehicle for social change, performed an educational role and championed moral values underpinning the Olympic Movement through the *Olympic Charter* (Schneider 2000). Schneider (2000, 225) explains that de Coubertin's "grand vision" for Olympic sport as a force for social change included "the personal and moral development of young people and that a great international sporting festival could bring the world together in peace and celebration . . . the IOC, through the *Olympic Charter*, still expresses these noble sentiments."

The ideals of Olympic sport and its function as a moral and educational tool to steer social change are clearly evident in the *Olympic Charter*. Emphasizing this point, Schneider (2000, 225) describes the Olympic Movement as a "public trust . . . established to promote the ideals of Olympism." However, as guardians of the Olympic Movement and the ideals of Olympism, the IOC's legitimacy rests on their accountability to stakeholders. In the modern sporting context, stakeholders include the public, athletes, governments and commercial interests (Schneider 2000). Accountability has implications for the IOC's legitimacy and requires transparency on their part, with activities including policy initiatives open to public scrutiny. These elements are also important for the legitimacy of anti-drug policies (Battin et al. 2008; Buti and Fridman 1994; Chapter 1, this volume). Before discussing those issues, I next outline the socio-historical context surrounding drug use in sport and broader social factors influencing attitudes toward doping and the changing nature of modern sport.

OVERVIEW—DRUG USE IN SPORT

Drug and substance use in sport have a long history. Over time, a range of groups, including early Olympians, Roman gladiators, the ancient Greeks and South American Indians, used stimulants such as herbal mixtures, wild mushrooms and plant seeds to improve performance, overcome fatigue and injury and increase endurance (Birchard 2000; Buti and Fridman 2001; Woodland 1980; Yesalis and Bahrke 2005). There is no evidence describing such substance use as doping or deviant behavior. Ordway and Rofe (1998, 16) note that "no moral distinction was made between a heavyweight wrestler choosing to eat fatty meat and a Roman gladiator using non-dietary substances to enhance bravery and aggression." Historical evidence traces the origin of doping to an eighteenth century drink known as 'dop,' a type of South African brandy of walnut extract, xanthines and alcohol used to improve endurance in ceremonial dances. Over time the term came to refer to other stimulating drinks (WADA 2006). The sporting connection to doping appears in the nineteenth century with a narcotic potion described as dop used to influence the outcome of bets by reducing racehorses' and greyhounds' winning chances (Donohoe and Johnson 1986; Verroken 2005; Voy 1991). Anti-doping policies and testing began in horseracing at the turn of the twentieth century driven by concerns that the practice was unfair to gamblers (Stokvis 2003; Verroken 2000; Yesalis and Cowart 1998). This is not to suggest that human athletes did not use substances to enhance performance. However, as the historical evidence shows, these practices were not labeled as contrary to sporting ideals.

Evidence from the nineteenth century reveals that growth in scientific and physiological knowledge as well as the changing nature of modern sport influenced athletes' use of a range of substances. Increasing professionalization of sport and developments in sporting technology, such as the bicycle, contributed to widespread substance use. Events such as velodrome races, where "men pushed themselves and their machines to the limit" (Hoberman 1992, 129), six day cycle races and pedestrian marathons (Yesalis and Bahrke 2005), as well as a growing public interest in quantified records (Guttmann 2004), contributed to the commonplace use of a range of substances. These included ether soaked sugar cubes, strychnine tablets, brandy and cocaine, caffeine, alcohol, nitroglycerin, digitalis, opium and heroin (Cashmore 1990; Donohoe and Johnson 1986; Houlihan 2002; Kennedy 2000; Yesalis and Bahrke 2005). Extreme sporting events, which required "almost superhuman strength to survive" (Møller 2009, 14), meant that substances were tools used to accomplish a difficult task. This also meant that sport provided an ideal forum for scientific investigation, focused on measuring and exploring the effects of substances on human physiology. Warnings focused on dangers to athletes' health and not on substance use as deviant behavior undermining the integrity of sport (Hoberman 1992).

Nineteenth century training models focused on "tapping the hereditary potential" of athletes "rather than artificially manipulating the organism itself" (Beamish and Ritchie 2005, 416). With the exception of some trainers who guarded their "doping recipes" (Yesalis and Bahrke 2005, 443), there were no efforts at concealment to avoid sanction (Hoberman 1992). There are claims that substance use led to athletes' deaths (Donohoe and Johnson 1986; Ordway and Rofe 1998; Sheil 1998; Verroken and Mottram 2005). However, ethical or moral considerations that these practices threatened the integrity of sport or the legitimacy of newly forming sporting authorities, including the early Olympic body, did not hamper physiological experiments or lead to anti-doping regulation.

The 'Home-Made' Phase—Doping in the Early Twentieth Century

In his discussion of drug use in cycling, Mignon (2003, 233) situates doping in two phases. It commenced with the "home-made stage," when doping practices resembled "kitchen recipes" passed from rider to rider and from *soigneur* to rider from the late nineteenth century through to the 1960s. While Mignon focuses his discussion on cycling, in the early decades of the twentieth century substance use in sport generally remained more closely aligned with earlier scientific exploration into the relationship between substance use and human physiology (see Hoberman 1992). Athletes were not generally labeled as deviant individuals engaged in illicit practices. Rather, they continued to be viewed as using whatever tools were at their disposal to cope with the extreme nature of sporting events. For example, at the 1924 Tour de France the Pélissier brothers, well-known cyclists of the time, detailed their doping practices:

> You have no idea what the Tour de France is like. . . . We suffer from start to finish. Do you want to see what we run on? . . . That's cocaine for the eyes, that's chloroform for the gums. . . . That is a cream to warm up my knees. And the pills, do you want to see the pills? . . . In short we run on "dynamite." (cited in Mignon 2003, 230)

There were concerns over doping, but these were underpinned by the belief that it was in conflict with the high ideals of amateur sport or the 'spirit of sport,' such as the unwritten rules of 'fair play,' especially in Olympic competition (Stokvis 2003). Doping was linked with professional sport, which was perceived as a degraded form of sport where the rewards associated with winning were the primary consideration (Cashman 1995; Dyreson 1998).

From the mid-twentieth century, and in contrast with earlier periods when sport provided a research forum for medical and scientific investigation, social and political events changed the relationship between science, medicine and sport. The political imperatives of World War II were a significant influence on the rapid development of medical and scientific technology and their incorporation into sport (Dimeo 2009; Williams 1975; Yesalis and Bahrke 2005). Military imperatives prompted governments' search for new drugs to benefit troops, resulting in organized and sanctioned drug use in the military, which "boosted the scientific efforts to synthesize drugs and . . . drew attention to the potential value of these drugs outside a therapeutic context" (Houlihan 2001, 125). As well as contributing to rapid pharmaceutical advances, this created moral ambiguity toward drug use that "continued into the Cold War period and entered the Olympic arena as sport emerged, along with space, as surrogates for military conflict" (Houlihan 2002, 57). The post-World War II period also saw the 'pharmacological revolution,' including the development of anti-bacterial drugs, the synthesis of new drugs and refinement of existing products (Houlihan 2002; Verroken 2005). Development of effective treatments for diseases previously considered fatal contributed to receptive public attitudes to substances such as antibiotics and more frequent use of prescription drugs (Dimeo 2009; Laure 2009). Attitudes toward the consumption of drugs changed as drug use became an increasingly accepted part of social life (Stewart 2007).

New drugs developed for legitimate medical purposes also provided a greater 'menu of choice' for post-war athletes. This enabled them to tailor drug use to meet particular training or sporting needs and removed some of the health risks associated with PED use (Houlihan 2002; Verroken 2005; Voy 1991). Also underpinning the sporting use of pharmacological discoveries was significant growth in institutional support for the scientific study of sport. For example, the British Association of Sports Medicine was established in 1953 and the American College of Sports Medicine in 1954 (Beamish and Ritchie 2005; Brissonneau 2010). From the mid-1960s, sports medicine took on a new disciplinary status, becoming "medicine for performance" (Brissonneau 2010, 2; Dimeo 2007). This period saw a new type of athlete, 'the trained athlete' (Williams 1962), supported by a medical regime including "specific treatments for specific injuries" and "medical staff as a necessary condition of sports preparation" (Mignon 2003, 233). Expanding revenue associated with sport facilitated this process, enabling the employment of medical and support staff specifically to improve performance (Waddington 2000). Drug use in sport can most effectively be examined in a broader social context that includes this increasing significance of pharmaceutical and medical technology, growth in the commercialization of sport as well as the political imperatives of the Cold War period (Verroken 2005).

The Second Doping Phase—A New Type of Amateur Athlete

The second phase of doping was given impetus by the political climate of the Cold War. The Union of Soviet Socialist Republics (USSR) reconceptualized the Olympic motto '*Citius, Altius, Fortius*' (faster, higher, stronger) into an "absolute performance principle" that became the "reigning doctrine of world sport" (Hoberman 1986, 10). In contrast with earlier periods when Olympic competition represented amateur ideals, the "Cold War athlete trained full-time . . . personifying the success and failures of capitalism and communism" (Wamsley and Young 2005, xix). In the 1960s, athletes from the German Democratic Republic (GDR), described as "sports diplomats in tracksuits" (Strenk 1980, 36), exemplified the politicization of Olympic sport. This included a rational, scientific approach to training and competition that incorporated systematic state-sanctioned PED use (see Franke and Berendonk 1997). The IOC was not aware of the extent of the GDR's state-sponsored doping program, with evidence only emerging after the fall of the Berlin Wall in 1989 (Teetzel 2004). Nevertheless, the Olympic inclusion of the GDR contributed to the promotion of science to sport. During the 1950s and 1960s, sport was driven by "strategic political objectives" and, as resources allocated to sport increased, this meant that "scientifically assisted, high-performance sport systems, and not individuals, became the main agents in world-class, high-performance sport in the post-war period" (Beamish and Ritchie 2005, 424).

The continued development of sporting technology and scientific knowledge, now applied to the body as a "sporting machine," changed the way that athletes trained (Cantelon 2005, 95). Broader social changes, such as the politically charged climate of the Cold War period, contributed to a new way of 'imagining' (Anderson 1991) elite sport. As Cantelon (2005, 95) states: "With the inclusion of the USSR in the Olympic 'family' . . . the new sibling confronted the older family members with a different type of amateur competition." This new way of imagining elite sport included a more rational approach to sports training, which Early (1998, x) described as ". . . the triumph of rationalism, the method, the quantification, the engineering mystique of science. Simply put, sports are about providing a context for the demonstration of the rationally engineered body." Potential financial rewards for athletes as 'skilled performers' meant that sport, including Olympic sport influenced by nationalistic imperatives, was increasingly approached in a work-like fashion (Cantelon 2005). However, despite the increasingly commercial nature of modern sport, at that time the IOC continued to formally maintain a commitment to amateur ideals. From that perspective, the main threat to Olympic sport was that presented by "perfidious professionals" (Tomlinson 2005; Torres and Dyreson 2005, 67). The IOC's failure to acknowledge the changing nature of modern sport hampered its ability to respond to drug use in sport.

The modern sporting environment rendered ideals of amateurism problematic because, rather than constituted by the principles of amateur competition, modern sport focused on winning. This was driven by increasing financial rewards and a record-breaking 'mania' in conjunction with appropriation of sport for political purposes. Emphasizing this point, Guttmann (1984, 119) asks: "When players become specialists . . . distinctions dissolve and categories are confounded. When the impulse to win . . . and to set records . . . are intensified by nationalism . . . where then is the amateur?" Nevertheless, under Brundage's presidency (1952 to 1972), the IOC maintained a strict amateur code (Espy 1979). Not only did Brundage resist any attempts to commercialize the Olympics, declaring up to his retirement that the IOC "should have nothing to do with money" (Barney et al. 2002, 100), he also viewed professional sportsmen as no better than "performing monkeys" (Allison 1993, 8). The IOC's strict adherence to amateur ideals—in contrast to professional sport, which was argued to debase and corrupt sport—made it difficult for the organization to recognize and take action to address doping in Olympic sport (Allison 1993; Cantelon 2005; Hill 1993; Hoberman 2005). Guttmann (1984, 123) notes that although taking the issue of doping seriously and condemning "athletes who popped pills" in order to gain a competitive advantage, "Brundage was never as concerned about doping as he was about professionalization . . . drugs never seemed quite the image of evil that Mammon did."

Underpinning these notions is the tendency to view amateurism as a "free-floating concept that every person, regardless of class, gender, race, age, wealth, national origin, in fact any social category can understand and, if [they] so desire, aspire to" (Cantelon 2005, 83). In other words, the imagined sporting community was based on a belief that members of that community, irrespective of their social position, adhered to an amateur ethos (Anderson 1991; Palmer 2001; Chapter 1, this volume). Such a view neglects the socially and historically contingent context in which sport takes place. For example, Pierre de Coubertin's Olympic Games idea reflected the class-based reality of the time that, for the most part, rendered those competitive spaces as inaccessible to the working classes (Brown 2005). Further, the concept of amateurism is itself open to contestation, as it is "contoured" differently by debates and broader social factors across time and space (Cantelon 2005, 84). Illustrating this point, Cantelon (2005, 84) explains that not all sporting participants experienced amateurism in the same manner and that "persons in positions of authority and influence were able to maintain notions of amateurism that contradicted the lived experiences of the majority of participants involved in high-performance sport."

As the driving force behind the Olympic Movement and with control over the Olympic Games, by the mid-twentieth century the IOC represented the "most powerful sporting organization in the world with global influence on the way that people understood, organized and played sport at a number of different levels" (Wamsley and Young 2005, xiii). This placed it in a position to take a significant leadership role in global sporting governance, including regulating or defining acceptable practices and behavior (Boyes 2001). However, the IOC's continuing insistence on the amateur nature of Olympic sport could not keep pace with the application of science and technology. This included PED use and the changing nature of how sport was 'played,' influenced by both political and commercial imperatives (Beamish and Ritchie 2005; Brohm 1978; Cantelon 2005; Hoberman 2005). Increasing commercialization of Olympic sport challenged the IOC's commitment to amateurism. This created a tension that transformed ways of imagining elite sport, with greater emphasis on bureaucratic rules and regulations, which began to challenge the IOC's claims to legitimacy and moral authority.

In this brief overview of the history of drug use in sport, we have seen that in the nineteenth and early twentieth century these practices were commonplace and did not negatively affect the legitimacy of the IOC or other early sporting bodies. As the twentieth century progressed, a more rational approach to drug use in sport was occurring, characterized by the increasing application of science and medicine to the sporting context. A combination of political imperatives, a more rational approach to sports training, pharmaceutical advances normalizing drug use and the medicalization of sport contributed to widespread non-medical uses of a range of drugs after World War II (Cantelon 2005; Dimeo 2009; Mignon 2003). There were, however, expressions of concern throughout the 1950s and 1960s over doping practices associated with negative health consequences for athletes as well as the threat doping presented to amateur ideals.

Rather than the IOC or other SGBs, mid-twentieth century concerns over doping emerged from public health reformers and members of the scientific community (Dimeo 2007; Woodland 1980). The optimistic spirit engendered by successful health reforms after World War II drew attention to attempts to address other public health concerns. Initiatives such as the establishment of the World Health Organization (WHO) in 1946 and the discovery of the link between smoking and lung cancer in 1950 reflected a global healthcare vision. This incorporated generic health and lifestyle interventions, including concerns over drugs in sport (Dimeo 2007, 2009; Mignon 2003). Some public health reformers were also concerned that the pressures associated with modern competitive sport influenced athletes' doping behavior (Dimeo 2009). Also influencing urgent calls for regulation of substance use in sport were the deaths of cyclists, soccer players and track athletes linked to amphetamines or other illicit substances (Dimeo 2007; Fife 1999; Hoberman 2005; Mignon 2003; Woodland 1980; Yesalis and Cowart 1998).

This prompted moves by (mostly European) governments, the (reluctant) IOC and SGBs to develop anti-doping rules. In 1963, for instance, the Council of Europe (CoE) held the first conference on doping, in which the IOC did not participate (Henne 2015), that included adoption of a resolution against doping, including a proposed list of banned substances and a definition of doping (Dimeo 2007; Houlihan 1999). The CoE definition of doping included concerns that doping undermined equality in competition (Houlihan 2002). Building on this view, during this period regulators and public health campaigners linked health concerns around doping to the value of sport, including ideals of fair play and a 'level' playing field and the claim that doping sports heroes were poor role models for youth (Dimeo 2007; Stokvis 2003). Several high profile sporting deaths heightened awareness of the dangers of doping and contributed to the introduction of anti-doping initiatives.

One of the first high profile sporting deaths linked to drugs commonly discussed was cyclist Knud Jensen (1960 Rome Olympics). Accounts of Jensen's death claim autopsy evidence of Ronicol, with two of his teammates also taken to hospital in a toxic condition (Donohoe and Johnson 1986; Houlihan 2002; Verroken 2005). Møller (2005) argues that Jensen died from a combination of heatstroke, concussion and lack of adequate medical attention. He further points out that as a list of prohibited substances was not even in the process of being compiled when Jensen died, attributing his death to doping is questionable at best (Møller 2005, 2010). Nevertheless, accounts discussing Jensen's death tend to focus on categorizations of drug use as deviant behavior. This type of approach, which conflates moral evaluations of doping with a concern for athletes' welfare, prevents a broader analysis of other factors in modern sport that present significant risks to athletes' health (see Henne et al. 2013; Henne and McDermott 2013). Irrespective of the debate surrounding Jensen's death, the incident contributed to the IOC's increased attention to anti-doping.[1] In 1964, the IOC formally adopted a (modified) 1963 CoE definition of doping, which stated that doping threatens sport ethics by providing an unfair advantage and jeopardizes athletes' health (Wrynn 2004).

Further heightening the regulation of drug use in sport was the death of Tommy Simpson in the 1967 Tour de France. Initial explanations cited heart failure from heat exhaustion, lack of oxygen and humidity. Examination later revealed amphetamines and cognac in Simpson's body, traces of amphetamine in his jersey pockets and drugs in his luggage (Cashmore 1990; Fife 2001; Fotheringham 2002; Voy 1991; Wheatcroft 2003). Simpson's death was the first *televised* doping death. Illustrating the power of the media to focus public attention, the highly public nature of Simpson's death meant that regulation of doping could no longer be neglected (Donohoe and Johnson 1986; Toohey and Veal 2000). Rather than simply discussing doping and passing resolutions against doping, Simpson's death led the IOC to implement anti-doping measures (Dimeo 2009; Stokvis 2003).[2] However, the IOC viewed its anti-doping role as primarily limited to supervision and, without the necessary resources, were not prepared to incur the expense or potential legal ramifications of testing (Hanstad et al. 2008; Hunt 2007). Prior to the 1968 Mexico Olympic Games, IOC President Avery Brundage clearly stated the organization's view and function, which was to alert National Olympic Committees (NOCs) and international federations and promote an educational campaign. The IOC was not prepared to take on the responsibility for testing control. Rather, the view was that the IOC's responsibility was defining doping and ensuring that adequate testing provisions were in place but that "the actual testing is left in the hands of others" (cited in Verroken and Mottram 2005, 310–311).

The point to note here is that the IOC's control of international Olympic amateur sport placed them in a position of sports leadership (Wamsley and Young 2005). From the perspective of the International Federations as well as NOCs, this meant that the IOC Medical Commission should be responsible for controls (Boyes 2001; Hunt 2007). NOCs pointed out that other groups, and particularly the media, looked to the IOC for a more active leadership role. For example, Dr. Daniel Hanley, chief medical officer of the US Olympic Committee (USOC), emphasized the importance of the IOC taking action regarding anti-doping because "dope control is becoming a very strong issue . . . I think we can ignore it, if you want to . . . but, more and more, many individuals and some important segments of our society, like the press, are looking to you for direction" (cited in Hunt 2007, 21). In this statement, Hanley was pointing to the potential for the IOC's failure to take a more active role in anti-doping regulation to adversely affect perceptions of their moral authority and legitimacy. Nevertheless, despite being constrained by a poor organizational structure and lack of resources, the IOC began to take a more active anti-doping policy leadership role (Dimeo 2007; Stokvis 2003). Although motivated by a concern for athletes' health, the IOC was also driven by other social actors' increasing concern over doping.

Other elite SGBs and governments introduced policies, regulations and testing initiatives prior to the IOC. The International Amateur Athletic Federation (IAAF) had banned the use of "stimulating substances" as early as 1928 (Douglas 2007; Healey 2003). The Amateur Squash Rackets Association had considered doping bans in 1938 (Woodland 1980). In 1962, the Austrian government passed a law against doping, followed in 1965 by France and Belgium. In 1966, the IAAF introduced random drug checks, FIFA introduced drug tests at the 1966 World Cup and the Union Cycliste International (UCI) took the same step at the 1966 Tour de France (Healey 2003; Houlihan 1999, 2002). In addition to anti-doping action taken by the CoE in 1963, Turkey and Italy introduced legislation on drugs in sport in 1971 (Beckett and Cowan 1978; Laure 2009; Todd and Todd 2001). From the mid-1960s, the British government began to implement a combination of sanctions and inducements to assist SGBs with the costs associated with testing (Houlihan 1999, 2002). This political involvement reminded the IOC and other SGBs that, as stakeholders in the modern political sporting context, governments had an interest in anti-doping. This was also influenced by growing evidence of drug use among North American footballers, suspicions of doping by unfeasibly muscular women from Eastern bloc nations and concerns over the effect of doping on youth behavior (Laure 2009; McArdle 2001; Mignon 2003; Yesalis and Cowart 1998).

Houlihan (2002) argues that this more active policy leadership role from the IOC was prompted mainly by a concern to maintain control of this high profile issue of PED use in international sport (see also Hanstad et al. 2008). Houlihan's claim is consistent with the argument I present in this book, which is that SGBs' effort to retain legitimacy is an important part of the debate over doping. This also brings interactions between stakeholder groups, such as the media, SGBs and government into the analysis. In other words, claims to legitimacy are multifaceted and contested, reflecting organizational power relationships.

Government anti-doping legislation also reflected changing attitudes toward the restorative value of drug use, driven by safety concerns such as the 1961 thalidomide scandal (Dimeo 2007). As Dimeo (2007, 88) notes, the view that "drugs offered opportunities in sport and society, gave way to a new paradigm in which drugs were something to be feared and regulated." Mehlman (2009, 131) links anti-doping initiatives to the larger "War on Drugs." Olympic drug testing in 1968 coincided with changing social attitudes and political initiatives to address public concern over drug use, such as Richard Nixon's 1968 presidential pledge to suppress the youth-oriented drug culture in the United States (Mehlman 2009). Five years later the North American Congressional hearings (Committee on the Judiciary 1973) continued to reflect anxiety over social drug use, including reports of athletes involved in "traffic and abuse" of drugs, investigation of claims of doping in athletic competition and efforts to curb athletes' improper drug use (Bowers 2002; Silver 2001).

From the 1950s onward, attitudes toward drug use in sport shifted from being a health-associated issue to "a moral panic that played on deeper social anxieties" (Dimeo 2007, 101), such as that sport was being over-run by "drug-crazed freaks" (Mehlman 2009, 131). Political, commercial, medical as well as scientific imperatives had generated a socially and historically new doping debate in the 1960s.

Anti-Doping—The IOC and Legitimacy

Through their control of the Olympic Games, the IOC was in a position to take a significant leadership role in anti-doping initiatives (Boyes 2001; Wamsley and Young 2005). However, into the 1970s inconsistencies between International Federations and the IOC in terms of banned substances and penalties created confusion and led to what some International Federations perceived as unfair treatment (Hunt 2007).[3] The IOC acknowledged that the reluctance of International Federations to cooperate with IOC-led anti-doping initiatives placed pressure on their legitimacy and moral authority. The need for direction from the IOC reflected the confusion resulting from the structure of the anti-doping framework at that time. The anti-doping regulatory system was a complex web of doping controls with the IOC, NOCs and International Federations all playing important roles, resulting in ambiguity of standards (Hunt 2007). Inconsistencies in regulations, as well as the substances banned, challenged perceptions of the IOC's moral authority and legitimacy, creating pressure for them to take a more proactive leadership stance.

Nevertheless, into the 1980s the IOC continued to see its role as essentially supervisory, such as emphasizing the need for NOCs to promote drug-free sport and implement appropriate drug testing arrangements. IOC involvement in anti-doping policy primarily took the form of publication and regular updating of lists of banned substances and practices to guarantee the integrity of the Olympics (Hanstad et al. 2008; Houlihan 1999). The IOC also advised the CoE on the anti-doping Charter, oversaw testing at IOC events, accredited testing laboratories and in 1983 created the Court of Arbitration for Sport (CAS) to deal with athletes' litigation (Hanstad et al. 2008; Houlihan 2002, 2008; Jacobs and Samuels 1995). Criticism of the IOC focused on claims of a lack of action against doping violations, a failure to detect PED use and suppression of positive tests (Teetzel 2004).

The ineffectiveness of the IOC was influenced, in part, by the lack of financial resources, a limited number of testing facilities and the medical view of the time that hormonal substances did not provide athletes with any competitive advantage (Christiansen 2009). The IOC also adhered to the widely held view that in-competition-testing would deter doping and hesitated to move to out-of-competition testing (Houlihan 1999). However, as limitations of in-competition testing became increasingly apparent, other institutional actors led the implementation of out-of-competition testing. The Norwegian Confederation was the first to introduce out-of-competition testing in 1977, followed by the United Kingdom in the early 1980s (Houlihan 2002; Verroken and Mottram 2005; Yesalis and Cowart 1998). Some of the constraints limiting IOC involvement in anti-doping, such as the cost associated with testing, would be addressed by the increasing commercialization of the Olympics, which gathered momentum in the 1980s (Stokvis 2003). Conversely, the commercialization of the Olympics also increased the stakes for the IOC as moral guardians of the Olympic Movement.

The Olympic Brand, Legitimacy and Doping

The Cold War consolidated the symbolic and political value of the Olympics as a forum for global politics. In the 1980s, a "more explicit economic logic emerged with the realization that Olympic events could be staged for . . . an international television audience" (Tomlinson 2005, 183). Under the Presidency of Juan Antonio Samaranch (1980 to 2001), the Olympics became a multi-billion dollar business driven by marketing of the Olympic brand and television broadcast rights. Income from television rights escalated from

US$25 million for the 1976 Montreal Olympics to US$309 million for the 1988 Calgary Winter Olympics (Stewart and Smith 2008; Tomlinson 2005; Wamsley and Young 2005; Whannel 2005). The 1984 Los Angeles Games, known as the 'Hamburger Olympics' because corporations such as McDonald's paid for Olympic venues, reflected an IOC leadership that specifically focused on strategies to increase commercial sponsorship (Tomlinson 2005).

The IOC's increasing involvement in commercial activity in the 1980s saw it develop into an international administrative authority reliant on routine regulation. This included anti-doping regulation under the authority of the *Olympic Charter* (Nafziger 1992) and, later, the IOC Medical Code (Boyes 2001). Weber's concept of legitimacy illustrates the significance of the *Olympic Charter* and the Medical Code, which the IOC used to extend their claims to legitimacy and moral authority over international amateur sport and as leaders against doping. For example, the 1980 *Olympic Charter* expressly stated that "every person or organization that plays any part whatsoever in the Olympic movement shall accept the supreme authority of the IOC and shall be bound by its Rules and submit to its jurisdiction" (IOC 1980, 6). For International Federations and NOCs, recognition by the IOC and thus inclusion in Olympic competition rested on their compliance with the criteria outlined in the *Olympic Charter* (IOC 1980).

However, despite claims to be leading the fight against doping, anti-doping requirements in the *Olympic Charter* receive limited attention compared to measures to protect the "philosophy" of Olympism and more commercial objectives. The *Olympic Charter* primarily protected the Olympics as the IOC's "exclusive property" and in particular their ownership of rights for the "organization ... exploitation ... transmission and reproduction by any means whatsoever" (IOC 1980, 8). The *Olympic Charter* also stipulated the appropriate use of the Olympic flag, motto, emblem and anthem with the IOC retaining all rights (IOC 1980, 7). These requirements remain in place (IOC 2014). Nevertheless, as the IOC's role is to promote "Olympism in accordance with the *Olympic Charter*" (IOC 1991, 8), the *Charter* constitutes a measure against which the IOC's claims to legitimacy can be evaluated, including for anti-doping regulation.

In conjunction with the *Olympic Charter*, the IOC sought to maintain authority and control of Olympic sport using the IOC Medical Code, which was underpinned by an intention to protect the spirit of fair play, to lead the fight against doping and safeguard athletes' health (Buti and Fridman 2001). The IOC's Medical Code clearly states International Federations' obligations:

> It is a condition for recognition of any international federation and any national Olympic committee that its statutes incorporate the IOC Medical Code by express reference and that its provisions apply, mutatis mutandis, to all persons and competitions under their jurisdiction. (cited in Siekmann et al. 1999, 8)

From this perspective, failure to incorporate the IOC's Medical Code renders International Federations ineligible for Olympic competition, carrying potentially disastrous financial consequences (Boyes 2001). More recent versions of the IOC Medical Code state that although it is "first adopted by the IOC. It is *not mandatory, but desirable*, that all members of the Olympic Movement adopt it" (IOC 2009, 14, emphasis added). This change may reflect the influence of the creation of WADA and the WADC, the adoption of which is mandatory for the whole Olympic Movement (Chapter 3, this volume). Nevertheless, while each International Federation is responsible for establishing its own eligibility criteria, these must be submitted to the IOC for approval (IOC 2013). This suggests that, at least for Olympic competition, the IOC remains concerned with maintaining the moral authority and legitimacy to regulate the Olympic community.

Inclusion in Olympic competition raises the profile and popularity of a sport, bringing with it a range of economic advantages. As Tomlinson (2005, 190) points out, while the various stakeholder groups engage in Olympic sponsorship in diverse ways, all "buy a universally recognizable badge, and the guarantee of inestimable media coverage and profile during the Olympic event itself." However, demonstrating that moral authority and legitimacy cannot be taken for granted; the IOC must maintain the support of NOCs and International Federations:

> Though the IOC has the power to withdraw recognition from NOCs and IFs, it is inconceivable that it would do so, except in cases of small and unimportant bodies which had few allies . . . the IOC would never expel from the Olympic programme the International Amateur Athletic Federation . . . the most powerful and richest of the federations. . . . The boot is on the other foot, for if the worst came to the worst the IAAF . . . could show their strength by withdrawing from the Olympic movement altogether. (Hill 1993, 88)

This illustrates that dominant groups, such as the IOC, must actively work to maintain stakeholder support. This supports the claim I make in this book, which is that power relationships between elite groups affect debates over social issues, such as drugs in sport. These contested relationships highlight the value of consensus-making as a moral panic criterion, because claims to legitimacy in an institutionalized moral panic cannot be taken for granted.

The importance of the *Olympic Charter* and the Medical Code to regulate behavior took on greater significance as the Olympics became an increasingly commercial enterprise. In 1974 the IOC replaced the term 'amateur' with 'nonprofessional' in the Olympic code and, in 1981, formally abandoned its commitment to amateurism (Donnelly 1996; Hill 1992). This process, which Donnelly (1996, 27, 30) describes as "Prolympism," saw Olympic and professional sport merge into "a single dominant sport ideology." Lucas (1992, 74) writes that "the dissolution of the unenforceable 'pure amateur code' was the first substantial and partially successful effort to blend the IOC, the NOCs, and all the international sport federations into a like-minded semi-democracy." This highlights the way that broader social factors influenced the way in which elite sport could be imagined (Anderson 1991) and emphasizes the multi-dimensional aspect of legitimacy (Suchman 1995; Chapter 1, this volume).

The more commercialized IOC could no longer rest their claim to legitimacy on assumptions that athletes, or SGBs, would adhere to amateur ideals to regulate their behavior and prevent drug use. This does not imply that the IOC no longer appealed to ethical ideas such as equality of competition or fair play. These continued to play an important ideological and normative role in anti-doping policy. The significance of a regulatory approach, including anti-doping policy, was that it provided a mechanism to impose specific ideals about behavior and ethics (Dimeo 2009). In other words, the legitimacy of modern sporting organizations, such as the IOC, became dependent upon a regulatory approach that, while founded on the values of amateurism, was measured against its ability to ensure 'clean' competition using a framework of codified rules and regulations.

During the 1980s, greater regulatory consistency between sporting federations and across international borders became increasingly important as the globalization of sport led to athletes training and competing outside their home country (Houlihan 2008). In such a context, the moral authority and legitimacy of the IOC was increasingly linked to its demonstrated ability to "catch some drug cheats" (Teetzel 2004, 217) using the *Olympic Charter* and the IOC Medical Code. The IOC used these regulatory mechanisms to maintain its status as a central actor in the anti-doping campaign and to deal with the changing nature of Olympic sport. As well as regulating sporting organizations and athletes, this placed a responsibility upon the IOC to perform that role to the highest ethical standards. The problem for the IOC was that pursuit of a strong commercial agenda potentially compromised their ability to adhere to those obligations. Critics of the IOC argue that commercializing the Olympics created "conditions conducive to cheating," including PED use, for which the IOC has failed to "assume any responsibility":

> . . . the historical evidence strongly suggests that the IOC has, indeed, profited from the long-celebrated exaggeration of the value of extreme human performance that provides the Games with much of its kudos in the first place. (Wamsley and Young 2005, xxii)

Throughout the 1980s, criticisms of the IOC's approach to anti-doping revolved around inconsistencies between their public statements and the efficacy of anti-doping controls, evidenced by a number of doping scandals

(Hoberman 2001). For example, Professor Arnold Beckett, a member of the IOC Doping Committee, speculated that the disappearance of nine positive drugs samples at the 1984 Los Angeles Olympics, after they had been sent to de Merode (head of the IOC Medical Commission), occurred to avert a public relations disaster:

> It would have done quite a lot of damage if . . . positives . . . had led to the medal winners, as undoubtedly it would have done . . . the federations and IOC are happy to show that they're doing something in getting some positives, but they don't want too many because that would damage the image of the Games. (cited in Hoberman 2001, 244)

In 1985, Wildor Hollmann (president of the German Association of Sports Physicians and Fédération Internationale Médicine-Sportive [FIMS]) criticized Samaranch for promoting "a totally commercialized professional sport circus" based on the view that professionalization of the Olympics significantly contributed to doping (cited in Hoberman 1992, 263). From the IOC's perspective, the shift to a more commercial approach was justified as a necessary step to ensure the survival of the Olympic Movement. Others argued that the "almost total commercializing of the Olympic Games" transformed the Olympic Movement into an "advertising vehicle for the multinational corporate sponsors and American television networks" (Hoberman 2001, 245; see also Tomlinson 2005; Whannel 2005). One consequence of this was that it created doubt over the integrity of the IOC's anti-doping program. Underpinning these concerns was the potential for the IOC's commercial relationships to create a conflict of interest for the organization that would jeopardize the legitimacy of the testing process. Despite ongoing evidence of doping, the IOC actively promoted itself as a vanguard in anti-doping. At the 1988 Calgary Winter Olympics, Samaranch stated:

> Above all such behavior makes a mockery of the very essence of sport, the soul of what we, like our predecessors, consider sacrosanct ideals. Doping is alien to our philosophy, to our rules of conduct. We shall never tolerate it. (cited in Hoberman 2001, 242)

Five days before the 1988 Seoul Olympics, Samaranch again positioned the IOC as firmly opposed to "this plague," stating that "doping equals death" (cited in Lucas 1992, 111). Casting doubt on the IOC's claims as leaders in anti-doping and questioning the efficacy of doping controls, Canadian sprinter Ben Johnson tested positive for anabolic steroid use at the 1988 Seoul Olympics (Buti and Fridman 2001). Illustrating the contested power relationships implicit in the doping debate, the IOC sought to deflect criticism and incorporate other International Federations into accountability for anti-doping controls. As Michelle Verdier, IOC press spokesperson, stated:

> Without the IOC the Ben Johnson affair . . . would never have come to light. It was the first body to tackle the problem of drugs in sport, and remember the IOC only runs the Games for a fortnight every four years. Who has the control of the competitors for the rest of the time? (cited in Stewart and Smith 2008, 123).

In this way, the IOC attempted to run onto moral high ground to deflect attention away from itself and onto International Federations. Into the 1990s, the IOC continued to claim that it was winning the war against doping, even though evidence suggested otherwise. Criticism of the IOC continued, including accusations of haphazard supervision of doping controls, inconsistent application of sanctions and suppression of positive tests (see Kidd, Edelman and Brownell 2001). Other concerns included a failure to detect 'designer' PEDs, particularly EPO (claimed to be responsible for the deaths of elite cyclists) and HGH (MacAloon 2001; Nafziger 1992; Parisotto 2006; Teetzel 2004). Nevertheless, the IOC continued to publicly and regularly promote a positive image of its own efforts as "winning the war on drugs" (Hoberman 2001, 242). Hoberman (2001) suggests that underpinning these public statements was the IOC's view of doping as a public relations issue and a concern to protect lucrative television and corporate contracts (Hanstad et al. 2008). As Jennings (1996, 234) more bluntly stated: "if the public ever catch on to how dirty elite sport has become, the sponsors and TV networks will pull the plug on the billions they pay the IOC for a clean, moral event."

The IOC's moral authority was also undermined by claims of the organization as a "plaything for corporate sponsors." The leadership was criticized as a "self-perpetuating oligarchy who travel the world like kings" (Cantelon and McDermott 2001, 33). Exacerbating doubts over the IOC's legitimacy was the 1998 Tour de France doping scandal, which led to Samaranch's comments in *El Mundo*, and accusations of bribery surrounding the Salt Lake City bid for the 2002 Winter Olympics. MacAloon (2001, 206) notes that "the two imbroglios were powerfully reinforcing each other, as the IOC plunged into a full-blown legitimacy crisis." Descriptions of these events as a "legitimacy crisis" for the IOC directly reflect one of the central claims made in this book, which is that doping events create a crisis of legitimacy for elite sporting organizations. A complementary area of analysis is the way in which a moral panic model helps to understand the significance of legitimacy in the debate over doping. In the Introduction, I pointed to the importance of the 1998 Tour de France doping scandal, Samaranch's *El Mundo* comments and the Salt Lake City bribery scandal because of their central role in the moral panic discourse over PEDs in sport. Next, I elaborate on those events and their relationship to a challenge to the IOC's legitimacy, which led to the creation of WADA and is discussed in more detail in the next chapter.

A CRISIS FOR THE IOC—LEGITIMACY AND THE WORLD ANTI-DOPING AGENCY

On July 11, 1998, just days before the start of the Tour de France, a Festina cycling team *soigneur* was caught by customs officers on the border between France and Belgium with large amounts of PEDs (Voet 2001). Police searched the hotels and vehicles of several teams. Banned substances were found in the hotels used by the Festina, TVM, ONCE and Casino teams, leading to the expulsion of one team and the withdrawal of another five. Police interrogated several of the world's leading cyclists, employing solitary confinement. After the Tour, three team doctors and one masseur were charged under the French *1989 Anti-Drugs Act* with supplying banned drugs at sporting events (Beamish 2009; Hanstad et al. 2008; Rasmussen 2005; Waddington 2000). The media reaction was scathing:

> In Britain, *The Times* described the race as the Tour de Farce while in France, the daily *Le Monde* demanded 'the Tour has to stop.' *Libération* carried a front page story saying that a 'Tour that runs from police station to the courtroom is too long,' while *L'Equipe* said the scandal highlighted how the doping issue had been swept under the carpet. *Le Figaro* wrote that the Tour was simply rotten. (Waddington 2000, 158)

Media coverage of the Tour focused on the doping scandals, conveying the impression that PED use was "completely out of control" (Møller 2009, 15) and that drug use in cycling was only the "tip of the iceberg" (Rasmussen 2005, 517) of a larger problem across elite sport. The quantity of drugs found, and the fact that the 'catch' was made by customs and police officers rather than anti-doping authorities, led to questions over whether doping controls and procedures were effective (Hanstad et al. 2008; Rasmussen 2005). This scandal suggested that doping was entrenched and systematic, raising doubts over the legitimacy of SGBs and their moral authority to maintain stability and order in modern sport. It is important to note that the IOC does not have responsibility for anti-doping initiatives outside the Olympics. However, professional cycling was an Olympic sport and the UCI, the governing body for cycling, was a signatory to the IOC's anti-doping agreements under the IOC Medical Code. As a result, and in conjunction with claims that the IOC Medical Commission knew, but ignored, doping in cycling, the Tour de France scandal raised concerns over the IOC's ability to enforce SGBs' anti-doping compliance (Hanstad et al. 2008; Teetzel 2004). Concerned by the potential for Tour de France riders to be subject to jail and police interrogation, and the possible spread of such actions to other (Olympic) sports, Samaranch attempted to diffuse the situation. However, his comments in the July 26, 1998 edition of the *El Mundo* newspaper exacerbated the issue:

> Doping is any product which, [sic] first damages the health of the sportsman and, second, artificially increases his performance. If it produces only this second condition, for me that's not doping. If it produces the first it is. . . . The current list of [banned] products must be drastically reduced. Anything that doesn't act against the athlete's health, for me that's not doping. (cited in Toohey and Veal 2000, 153)

This appeared to be a reversal of the IOC's public promotion of their strong anti-doping stance and drew harsh criticism from stakeholder groups (Hoberman 2005; MacAloon 2001). More significantly for this book, the IOC appeared to have failed to live up to its ideals. For many, the scandal suggested that the organization had forgotten its purpose as guardian of the Olympic Movement (MacAloon 2001; Schneider 2000).

To circumvent the growing tide of criticism, the IOC issued press statements on July 27 and 28 asserting its determination to address doping (MacAloon 2001). The IOC also announced a World Conference on Doping in Sport for 1999. Suggestions for the conference included the creation of an agency to coordinate the "worldwide fight against doping in sport, tentatively called the Olympic Movement Anti-Doping Agency (OMADA)" funded from the IOC's television profits (Teetzel 2004, 218). Before the conference could take place, criticisms of the IOC's leadership were exacerbated with allegations of bribery of IOC delegates by members of the Salt Lake City Winter Olympics organizing committee (Crowther 2002). In response to external pressure, the IOC established a Reform Commission, however, its recommendations primarily concerned internal IOC processes rather than public accountability and transparency (Houlihan 2005). The IOC's failure to respond appropriately to criticisms of its regulatory and policy frameworks created doubt over the legitimacy and moral authority of the organization. The 1998 Tour de France doping scandal, Samaranch's comments in *El Mundo* combined with the Salt Lake City accusations contributed to a public reaction that asked "the IOC to prove that *it* remains a part of the Olympic movement" (MacAloon 2001, 225, emphasis in original).

The Tour scandal was significant, as it acted as a catalyst for the institutional transformation of anti-doping regulation. According to Richard Pound, WADA Chairman from 1999 to 2008, the 1998 Tour "essentially led to the creation of WADA as the credibility of the IOC and the international federations had been greatly undermined" (*Reuters* 2007; see also Hanstad et al. 2008). In conjunction with doubts over the IOC's commitment to anti-doping, the Salt Lake City scandal exacerbated a growing loss of faith in the moral commitment of the IOC to international sport (MacAloon 2001; Stokvis 2003). The *Olympic Charter* and the IOC Medical Code played an important role as regulatory mechanisms used to bolster the IOC's moral authority and legitimacy. These provided the IOC with tools to govern and control elite international sport as the foundations of the IOC's legitimacy shifted from a focus on amateur ideals to a more bureaucratic approach in an increasingly commercial environment. However, the disjuncture between the IOC's public promotion of the organization as leaders in anti-doping in the face of ongoing doping events challenged their legitimacy and contributed to WADA's establishment. As well as highlighting the socio-historical nature of the doping debate, these events emphasize that claims to legitimacy are central elements of that debate.

CONCLUSION

In this chapter I have noted the socially and historically contingent nature of drug use in sport, influenced by political, commercial, medical as well as scientific imperatives. Broader social factors, such as the political climate of the Cold War and the medicalization of sport, as well as shifting concerns over drug use from a health issue to a "moral crisis" (Dimeo 2007, 93) influenced ideas and attitudes toward drugs in sport (Wrynn 2004). Although ideally situated to take an active leadership role, ongoing doping scandals, accusations of a failure to detect new PEDs, suppression of positive results and commercialization of the Olympics raised questions over the IOC's anti-doping commitment. The 1998 Tour de France doping scandal and Salt Lake City bribery scandal reinforced suspicions that the IOC failed to fulfill its role as guardian of Olympic sport. This led to the creation of WADA. The withdrawal of support for the IOC and the institutional transformation of anti-doping authority in the form of WADA demonstrate that claims to legitimacy cannot be taken for granted.

In the next chapter, I apply a Weberian framework to illuminate the role of WADA in the contemporary anti-doping debate, using a moral panic framework to highlight the significance of legitimacy in that debate. This is particularly relevant as the doping debate occurs in contested public and policy arenas where stakeholder groups hold diverse attitudes toward PEDs (Hanstad et al. 2010; Kidd et al. 2001). As well as providing an opportunity to consider the multifaceted nature of legitimacy, this illustrates that legitimacy requires consensus-making activities from, and between, elite groups to maintain support for WADA as the appropriate institutional response to doping. In other words, concerns to restore or maintain the legitimacy of SGBs contribute to the construction of doping as a moral panic.

NOTES

1   In 1960, the IOC commissioned Sir Arthur Porritt, a well-known British doctor, to report on doping solutions. In 1961, the IOC formed a Medical Committee and, in 1962, resolved to ban doping (Dimeo 2007; Stokvis 2003). At the 1964 Tokyo Olympics, under the auspices of the UCI, the IOC implemented

rudimentary tests for amphetamines in cycling. Also in 1964, Porritt presented recommendations from his report finding that doping was bad for athletes' health and constituted an unfair advantage and that doping sporting heroes were poor examples for youth (Wrynn 2004). Among other initiatives, the report recommended an educational program to warn against doping, rules in each sport to forbid its use and measures to control athletes' doping (Dimeo 2009; Stokvis 2003). Nevertheless, the IOC's 1964 recommendations and a later 1966 IOC Medical Committee declaration emphasizing education on the physical and moral aspects of doping aimed at monitoring rather than action (Dimeo 2007; Hoberman 2005; Houlihan 1999; Wrynn 2004).

2   In 1967, a formal Medical Commission was created and anti-doping rules drafted (Hoberman 2005; Yesalis and Cowart 1998). Acting on its earlier 1964 recommendations, the IOC introduced testing and regulations for the 1968 Mexico Olympics. These included establishing a medical center, developing a list of prohibited substances, adopting a Medical Code and requiring Olympic athletes to pledge that they would not use PEDs and to agree to gender verification examinations (Bowers 2002; Giulianotti 2005; McArdle 2001). This reflected the speculation of the time that Eastern bloc men were masquerading as women or hermaphrodites and gaining an unfair advantage (an idea that persisted into the 1970s) (Hunt 2007; McArdle 2001; Yesalis and Cowart 1998). According to Parisotto (2006, 15), these types of practices were evident from the 1930s, when German athlete Hermann Ratjen allegedly "concealed his genitals and called himself Dora" (see also Aitken 2002). Eva Klobukowska is said to be the first athlete to fail a sex test at the 1967 European Track and Field Championships because she had "one chromosome too many to qualify as a woman" (Wrynn 2004, 221–222). In contrast, McArdle (2001) argues that in approximately 30 years of sex testing at athletic events no case was ever documented. After her death in 1980, Stella Walsh, who won 41 AAU titles and two Olympic medals, was found to have the sex organs of a man and a woman (Donohoe and Johnson 1986; Wrynn 2004).

3   At the 1972 Munich Olympics, the positive test of a Puerto Rican basketball player did not result in team disqualification. In contrast, the entire Dutch cycling team had their bronze medal rescinded after one rider tested positive for a substance banned by the IOC, but not by the UCI (Hunt 2007). American swimmer Rich DeMont's use of asthma medication containing ephedrine was declared to team physicians but the American swim team failed to notify the Munich authorities. As a result, DeMont returned a positive drug test and was stripped of his medals and prohibited from participating in other events (Williams 1975). In contrast to the IOC's public accusations of misconduct addressed to the USOC, a doping scandal involving the Union Internationale de Moderne Pentathlon et Biathlon (UIPMB) did not attract sanctions (Hunt 2007).

REFERENCES

Aitken, C. 2002. "Lifting Your Game." *Meanjin* (Melbourne) 61 (2): 217–224.

Allison, L. 1993. "The Changing Context of Sporting Life." In *The Changing Politics of Sport*, edited by Allison, L., 1–14. Manchester: Manchester University Press.

Anderson, B. 1991. *Imagined Communities: Reflections on the Origin and Spread of Nationalism*. London: Verso.

Barney, R. K., Wenn, S. R., and Martyn, S. G. 2002. *Selling the Five Rings: The International Olympic Committee and the Tise of Olympic Commercialism*. Salt Lake City: University of Utah Press.

Battin, M. P., Luna, E., Lipman, A. G., Gahlinger, P.M., Rollins, D. E., Roberts, J. C., and Booher, T. L. 2008. *Drugs and Justice: Seeking a Consistent, Coherent, Comprehensive View.* Oxford: Oxford University Press.

Beamish, R. 2009. "Steroids, Symbolism and Morality: The Construction of a Social Problem and Its Unintended Consequences." In *Elite Sport, Doping and Public Health*, edited by Moller, V., McNamee, M. and Dimeo, P., 55–73. Odense: University of Southern Denmark.

Beamish, R., and Ritchie, I. 2005. "From Fixed Capacities to Performance-Enhancement: The Paradigm Shift in the Science of 'Training' and the Use of Performance-Enhancing Substances." *Sport in History* 25 (3): 412–413.

Beckett, A. H., and Cowan, D. A. 1978. "Misuse of Drugs in Sport." *British Journal of Sports Medicine* 12: 185–194.

Berg, C. 2008. "Politics, Not Sport, Is the Purpose of the Olympic Games." *Institute of Public Affairs* (July 2008): 14–18.

Birchard, K. 2000. "Past, Present, and Future of Drug Abuse at the Olympics." *The Lancet* 356: 1008.

Bowers, L. D. 2002. "Abuse of Performance-Enhancing Drugs in Sport." *Therapeutic Drug Monitoring* 24:178–181.

Boyes, S. 2001. "The International Olympic Committee, Transnational Doping Policy and Globalisation." In *Drugs and Doping in Sport: Socio-Legal Perspectives*, edited by O'Leary, J., 167–179. London: Cavendish Publishing.

Brissonneau, C. 2010. "An Interactionist Study of Phenomenon of Doping." In *Body Enhancement and (Il)legal Drugs in Sport—A Human and Social Science Perspective Conference.* University of Copenhagen.

Brohm, Jean-Marie. 1978. *Sport: A Prison of Measured Time.* London: Ink Links.

Brown, D. A. 2005. "The Olympic Games Experience: Origins and Early Challenges." In *Global Olympics: Historical and Sociological Studies of the Modern Games*, edited by Young, K. and Wamsley, K. B., 19–41. Amsterdam: Elsevier JAI.

Buti, A., and Fridman, S. 1994. "The Intersection of Law and Policy: Drug Testing in Sport." *Australian Journal of Public Administration* 53 (4): 489–507.

———. 2001. *Drugs, Sport and the Law.* Mudgeeraba, Queensland: Scribblers Publishing.

Cantelon, H. 2005. "Amateurism, High-Performance Sport, and the Olympics." In *Global Olympics: Historical and Sociological Studies of the Modern Games*, edited by Young, K. and Wamsley, K. B., 83–101. Amsterdam: Elsevier JAI.

Cantelon, H., and McDermott, L. 2001. "Charisma and the Rational-Legal Organisation: A Case Study of the Avery Brundage-Reginald Honey Correspondence Leading Up to the South African Expulsion from the International Olympic Movement." *OlyMPIKA: The International Journal of Olympic Studies* X: 33–58.

Cashman, R. 1995. *Paradise of Sport: The Rise of Organised Sport in Australia.* Melbourne: Oxford University Press.

Cashmore, E. 1990. *Making Sense of Sport.* London: Routledge.

Christiansen, A. V. 2009. "Doping in Fitness and Strength Training Environments—Politics, Motives and Masculinity." In *Elite Sport, Doping and Public Health*, edited by Moller, V., McNamee, M. and Dimeo, P., 99–118. Odense: University Press of Southern Denmark.

Committee on the Judiciary, United States Senate. 1973. "Proper and Improper Use of Drugs by Athletes." U.S. Government Printing Office, Washington D.C.: Subcommittee to Investigate Juvenile Deliquency.

Crowther, N. 2002. "The Salt Lake City Scandals and the Ancient Olympic Games." *International Journal of the History of Sport* 19 (4): 169–178.

Dimeo, P. 2007. *A History of Drug Use in Sport 1876–1976: Beyond Good and Evil.* New York: Routledge.

————. 2009. "The Origins of Anti-Doping Policy Sports: From Public Health to Fair Play." In *Elite Sport, Doping and Public Health*, edited by Moller, V., McNamee, M. and Dimeo, P., 29–40. Odense: University Press of Southern Denmark.

Donnelly, P. 1996. "Prolympism: Sport Monoculture as Crisis and Opportunity." *Quest* 48 (1): 25–42.

Donohoe, T., and Johnson, N. 1986. *Foul Play: Drug Abuse in Sports*. Oxford: Blackwell.

Douglas, T. 2007. "Enhancement in Sport, and Enhancement outside Sport." *Studies in Ethics, Law, and Technology* 1 (1): 1–15.

Dyreson, M. 1998. *Making the American Team: Sport, Culture, and the Olympic Experience*. Urbana: University of Illinois Press.

Early, G. 1998. *Body Language: Writers on Sport*. Saint Paul: Graywolf Press.

Espy, R. 1979. *The Politics of the Olympic Games*. Berkeley: University of California Press.

Fife, G. 1999. *Tour de France: The History, the Legend, the Riders*. Edinburgh: Mainstream.

Fife, G. 2001. *Inside the Peloton: Riding, Winning and Losing the Tour de France*. Edinburgh: Mainstream.

Fotheringham, W. 2002. *Put Me Back on My Bike: In Search of Tom Simpson*. London: Yellow Jersey.

Franke, W. W., and Berendonk, B. 1997. "Hormonal Doping and Androgenization of Athletes: A Secret Program of the German Democratic Republic government." *Clinical Chemistry* 43 (7): 1262–1279.

Giulianotti, R. 2005. *Sport a Critical Sociology*. Cambridge: Polity Press.

Goode, E., and Ben-Yehuda, N. 2009. *Moral Panics: The Social Construction of Deviance*. Chichester, West Sussex: Wiley-Blackwell Publishing.

Guttmann, A. 1984. *The Games Must Go On: Avery Brundage and the Olympic Movement*. New York: Columbia University Press.

————. 1992. *The Olympics: A History of the Modern Games*. Urbana: University of Illinois Press.

————. 2004. *From Ritual to Record: The Nature of Modern Sports*. New York: Columbia University Press.

Hanstad, D. V., Smith, A., and Waddington, I. 2008. "The Establishment of the World Anti-Doping Agency: A Study of the Management of Organizational Change and Unplanned Outcomes." *International Review for the Sociology of Sport* 43 (3): 227–249.

Hanstad, D. V., Skille, E. Å., and Loland, S. 2010. "Harmonization of Anti-Doping Work: Myth or Reality?" *Sport in Society* 13 (2): 418–430.

Healey, D. J. 2003. "The History of Drug Use in Sport." In *Drug Use in Sport*, edited by Healey, J., 1–5. Balmain: Spinney Press.

Henne, K. 2015. *Testing for Athlete Citizenship: Regulating Doping and Sex in Sport*. New Brunswick, NJ: Rutgers University Press.

Henne, K. E., Koh, B., and McDermott, V. 2013. "Coherence of Drug Policy in Sports: Illicit Inclusions and Illegal Inconsistencies." *Performance Enhancement and Health* (2): 48–55.

Henne, K. E., and McDermott, V. 2013. "Cruel Reality of Sport Business." 15 February 2013. http://www.canberratimes.com.au/comment/cruel-reality-of-sport-business-20130214–2efr0.html. Accessed 11 March 2015.

Hill, C. R. 1992. *Olympic Politics* Manchester: Manchester University Press.

————. 1993. "The Politics of the Olympic Movement." In *The Changing Politics of Sport*, edited by Allison, L., 84–104. Manchester: Manchester University Press.

Hoberman, J. 1986. *The Olympic Crisis: Sport, Politics and the Moral Order*. New Rochelle, NY: Aristide D. Caratzas.

————. 1992. *Mortal Engines: The Science of Performance and the Dehumanisation of Sport*. New Jersey: The Blackburn Press.

———. 2001. "How Drug Testing Fails: The Politics of Doping Control." In *Doping in Elite Sport the Politics of Drugs in the Olympic Movement*, edited by Wilson, W. and Derse, E., 241–274. Champaign, IL: Human Kinetics.

———. 2005. "Olympic Drug Testing: An Interpretive History." In *Global Olympics: Historical and Sociological Studies of the Modern Games*, edited by Young, K. and Wamsley, K.B., 249–268. Amsterdam: Elsevier.

Houlihan, B. 1994. *Sport and International Politics*. Hemel Hempstead: Harvester Wheatsheaf.

———. 1999. "Anti-Doping Policy in Sport: The Politics of International Policy Co-ordination." *Public Administration* 77 (2): 311–334.

———. 2001. "The World Anti-Doping Agency: Prospects for Success." In *Drugs and Doping in Sport: Socio-Legal Perspectives*, edited by O'Leary, J., 125–145. London: Cavendish.

———. 2002. *Dying to Win*. Strasbourg Cedex: Council of Europe.

———. 2005. "International Politics and Olympic Governance." In *Global Olympics: Historical and Sociological Studies of the Modern Games*, edited by Young, K. and Wamsley, K.B., 127–142. Amsterdam: Elsevier JAI.

———. 2008. "Detection and Eduction in Anti-Doping Policy: A Review of Current Issues and an Assessment of Future Prospects." *Hitotsubashi Journal of Arts and Sciences* 49: 55–71.

Hunt, T.M. 2007. "Sport, Drugs, and the Cold War The Conundrum of Olympic Doping Policy, 1970–1979." *Olympika XVI*: 19–42.

IOC (International Olympic Committee). 1980. "Olympic Charter." International Olympic Committee. http://www.olympic.org/Documents/OlympicCharter/Olympic_Charter_through_time/1980-Olympic_Charter.pdf. Accessed 24 June 2014.

———. 1991. "Olympic Charter." http://www.olympic.org/Documents/Olympic Charter/Olympic_Charter_through_time/1991-Olympic_Charter_June91.pdf.

———. 2009. "Olympic Movement Medical Code." International Olympic Committee. http://www.olympic.org/Documents/Fight_against_doping/Rules_and_regulations/OlympicMovementMedicalCode-EN_FR.pdf. Accessed 20 December 2010.

———. 2013. "Olympic Charter." International Olympic Committee. http://www.olympic.org/Documents/olympic_charter_en.pdf. Accessed 9 January 2015.

———. 2014. "Olympic Charter." http://www.olympic.org/Documents/olympic_charter_en.pdf. Accessed 24 June 2015.

Jacobs, J.B., and Samuels, B. 1995. "The Drug Testing Project in International Sports: Dilemmas in an Expanding Regulatory Regime." *Hastings International and Comparative Law Review* 18 (3): 557–589.

Jennings, A. 1996. *The New Lords of the Rings: Olympic Corruption and How to Buy Gold Medals*. London: Pocket Books.

Kennedy, M.C. 2000. "Newer Drugs Used to Enhance Sporting Performance." *Medical Journal of Australia* 173 (Special Olympic issue): 314–317.

Kidd, B., Edelman, R., and Brownell, S. 2001. "Comparative Analysis of Doping Scandals: Canada, Russia, and China." In *Doping in Elite Sport: The Politics of Drugs in the Olympic Movement*, edited by Wilson, W. and Derse, E., 153–188. Champgaign, IL: Human Kinetics.

Laure, P. 2009. "In Praise of the Non-Dominant Sense of Doping Behaviour." In *Elite Sport, Doping and Public Health*, edited by Moller, V., McNamee, M. and Dimeo, P., 119–133. Odensa: University Press of Southern Denmark.

Lucas, J.A. 1992. *Future of the Olympic Games*. Champaign, IL: Human Kinetics Books.

MacAloon, J. 1981. *This Great Symbol: Pierre de Coubertin and the Origins of the Modern Olympic Games*. Chicago: University of Chicago Press.

———. 1984. *Rite, Drama, Festival, Spectacle: Rehearsals Toward a Theory of Cultural Performance*. Philadelphila: Institute for the Study of Human Issues.

————. 2001. "Doping and Moral Authority: Sport Organisations Today." In *Doping in Elite Sport: The Politics of Drugs in the Olympic Movement*, edited by Wilson, W. and Derse, E., 205–224. Champaign, IL: Human Kinetics.

————. 2006. "The Mighty Working of a Symbol: From Idea to Organization." *The International Journal of the History of Sport* 23 (3–4): 528–570.

McArdle, D. 2001. " 'Say It Ain't So, Mo.' International Performers' Perceptions of Drug Use and the Diane Modahl Affair." In *Drugs and Doping in Sport: Socio-Legal Perspectives*, edited by O'Leary, J., 91–108. London: Cavendish.

Mehlman, M.J. 2009. *The Price of Perfection: Individualism and Society in the Era of Biomedical Enhancement*. Maryland: John Hopkins University Press.

Mignon, P. 2003. "The Tour de France and the Doping Issue." *The International Journal of the History of Sport* 20 (2): 227–245.

Møller, V. 2005. "Knud Enemark Jensen's Death During the 1960 Rome Olympics: A Search for Truth?" *Sport in History* 25 (3): 452–471.

————. 2009. "Conceptual Confusion and the Anti-Doping Campaign in Denmark." In *Elite Sport, Doping and Public Health*, edited by Moller, V., McNamee, M. and Dimeo, P., 13–28. Odense: University Press of Southern Denmark.

————. 2010. *The Ethics of Doping and Anti-Doping Redeming the Soul of Sport?* London: Routledge.

Nafziger, J.A.R. 1992. "International Sports Law: A Reply of Characteristics and Trends." *American Journal of International Law* 86 (3): 489–518.

Ordway, C., and Rofe, S. 1998. "Drugs in Sport." *The Law Society of South Australia Bulletin* (Nov 1998): 16–19.

Palmer, C. 2001. "Outside the Imagined Community: Basque Terrorism, Political Activism, and the Tour de France." *Sociology of Sport Journal* 18: 143–161.

Parisotto, R. 2006. *Blood Sports: The Inside Dope on Drugs in Sport*. Prahran: Hardie Grant Books.

Rasmussen, K. 2005. "The Quest for the Imaginary Evil: A Critique of Anti-Doping." *Sport in History* 25 (3): 515–535.

Reuters. 2007. "Ex-IOC Chief 'Not Interested in Doping.' " *The Sydney Morning Herald*, 25 October 2007. http://www.smh.com.au/news/Sport/ExIOC-chief-not-interested-in-doping/2007/10/25/1192941189806.html. Accessed 25 October 2007.

Riordan, J. 1993. "The Rise and Fall of Soviet Olympic Champions." *Olympika* 2: 25–44.

Schneider, A. 2000. *Olympic Reform, Are We There Yet?* Paper presented at the Bridging Three Centuries, Fifth International Symposium for Olympic Research, University of Western Ontario, London, Ontario, Canada.

Sheil, P. 1998. *Olympic Babylon: Sex, Scandal and Sportsmanship: The True Story of the Olympic Games*. Sydney: Pan Macmillan Australia.

Siekmann, R.R.C., Soek, J., and Bellani, A. 1999. *Doping Rules of International Sports Organisations*. Hague: T.M.C. Asser Press.

Silver, M.D. 2001. "Use of Ergogenic Aids by Athletes." *Journal of the American Academy of Orthopaedic Surgeons* 9: 61–70.

Stewart, B. 2007. "Drugs in Australian Sport: A Brief History." *Sporting Traditions* 23 (2): 65–78.

Stewart, B., and Smith, A.C.T. 2008. "Drug Use in Sport Implications for Public Policy." *Journal of Sport and Social Issues* 32 (3): 278–298.

Stokvis, R. 2003. "Moral Entrepreneurship and Doping Cultures in Sport." In *ASSR Working Paper Series*, 1–25. Amsterdam School for Social Science Research.

Strenk, A. 1980. "Diplomats in Tracksuits: The Role of Sport in the German Democratic Republic." *The Journal of Sport and Social Issues* 4 (1): 34–45.

Suchman, M.C. 1995. "Managing Legitimacy: Strategic and Institutional Approaches." *The Academy of Management Review* 20 (3): 571–610.

Teetzel, S. 2004. "The Road to Wada." In *Seventh International Symposium for Olympic Research*, 213–224. Windermere Manor, London, Ontario.

Todd, J., and Todd, T. 2001. "Significant Events in the History of Drug Testing and the Olympic Movement." In *Doping in Elite Sport: The Politics of Drugs in the Olympic Movement*, edited by Wilson, W. and Derse, E., 65–128. Champaign, IL: Human Kinetics.

Tomlinson, A. 2005. "The Commercialisation of the Olympics: Cities, Corporations, and the Olympic Commodity." In *Global Olympics: Historical and Sociological Studies of the Modern Games*, edited by Young, K. and Wamsley, K.B., 179–200. Amsterdam: Elsevier JAI.

Toohey, K., and Veal, A.J. 2000. *The Olympic Games: A Social Science Perspective*. Wallingford: CABI Publishing.

Torres, C.R., and Dyreson, M. 2005. "The Cold War Games." In *Global Olympics: Historical and Sociological Studies of the Modern Games*, edited by Young, K. and Wamsley, K.B., 59–82. Amsterdam: Elsevier JAI.

Verroken, M. 2000. "Drug Use and Abuse in Sport." *Bailliere's Clinical Endocrinology and Metabolism* 14 (1): 1023.

———. 2005. "Drug Use and Abuse in Sport." In *Drugs in Sport*, edited by Mottram, D.R., 29–63. New York, NY: Routledge.

Verroken, M., and Mottram, D.R. 2005. "Doping Control in Sport." In *Drugs in Sport*, edited by Mottram, D.R., 309–356. London: Routledge.

Voet, W. 2001. *Breaking the Chain: Drugs and Cycling: The True Story*. London: Yellow Jersey Press.

Voy, R. 1991. *Drugs, Sport and Politics*. Champaign, IL: Leisure Press.

WADA (World Anti-Doping Agency). 2006. "A Brief History of Anti-Doping." World Anti-Doping Agency. http://www.wada-ama.org/en/dynamic.ch2?pageCategory.id=31/ Accessed 11 March 2006.

Waddington, I. 2000. *Sport, Health and Drugs: A Critical Sociological Perspective*. London: E and FN Spon.

Wamsley, K.B., and Young, K. 2005. "Coubertin's Olympic Games: The Greatest Show on Earth." In *Global Olympics: Historical and Sociological Studies of the Modern Games*, edited by Young, K. and Wamsley, K.B., xiii–xxv. Amsterdam: Elsevier JAI.

Weber, M. 1969. *Economy and Society*. 2 vols. Berkeley: University of California Press.

Whannel, G. 2005. "The Five Rings and the Small Screen: Television, Sponsorship, and New Media in the Olympic Movement." In *Global Olympics: Historical and Sociological Studies of the Modern Games*, edited by Young, K. and Wamsley, K.B., 161–177. Amsterdam: Elsevier JAI.

Wheatcroft, G. 2003. *Le Tour: A History of the Tour de France*. London: Pocket Press.

Williams, J.G.P. 1962. *Sports Medicine*. London: Edward Arnold.

———. 1975. "Drugs and Sport." *Medicine, Science and the Law* 15 (1): 9–15.

Woodland, L. 1980. *Dope: The Use of Drugs in Sport*. Sydney: Reid.

Wrynn, A. 2004. "The Human Factor: Science, Medicine and the International Olympic committee, 1900–70." *Sport in Society* 7 (2): 211–231.

Yesalis, C., and Bahrke, M.S. 2005. "Anabolic Steroid and Stimulant Use in North American Sport between 1850 and 1980." *Sport in History* 25 (3): 434–451.

Yesalis, C., and Cowart, V.S. 1998. *The Steroids Game*. Champaign, IL: Human Kinetics.

3 The World Anti-Doping Agency
Legitimacy and a Moral Panic

Over the course of the twentieth century, broader socio-historical events led to new ways of imagining elite sporting communities. The influence of Cold War politics created new ideas of 'amateur' athletes and commercialization placed greater emphasis on global rules and regulations, which came to include anti-doping regulations. These changes had implications for the legitimacy of the IOC and, as guardian of Olympic sport, placed the organization under pressure to demonstrate leadership in the sporting community. Despite public statements emphasizing their commitment to anti-doping, ongoing doping scandals challenged the IOC's legitimacy. The 1998 Tour de France doping scandal and Salt Lake City bribery scandal exacerbated concerns that the IOC failed to fulfill its role and contributed to the creation of WADA. However, WADA also faces the challenge of maintaining legitimacy, as media reports reveal that doping continues to occur.

The focus of this chapter remains on the significance of legitimacy within a moral panic framework, applied to the role of WADA in the contemporary anti-doping debate. First, I overview the governance framework underpinning WADA and then discuss the World Anti-Doping Code (WADC). With the current WADC including more than 2,000 changes (WADA 2014d), I focus on several key aspects. Some of these are existing measures carried forward from earlier versions, while others elaborate on those measures or are new controls.

THE WORLD ANTI-DOPING AGENCY

Prior to WADA's formation, the anti-doping policies of governments and sporting authorities were fragmented rather than cohesive or coordinated. This reflected the fact that relationships between the IOC, International Federations and governments were characterized by low levels of trust, which hindered efforts to create and implement consistent anti-doping regulations. This also meant that anti-doping frameworks struggled to maintain legitimacy, and thus support and compliance from the sporting community, including athletes (Houlihan 2004). The primary task facing WADA was the global harmonization of anti-doping policies, which also necessitated attempts to improve relationships between sporting organizations, National Anti-Doping Organizations (NADOs)[1] and governments (Houlihan 2004). In other words, contested power relationships between organizational actors hampered a consistent global approach to anti-doping regulation. This required WADA to actively generate consensus amongst a range of diverse stakeholders. The long-term success of this task relies heavily on WADA's ability to establish and maintain positive perceptions of their legitimacy as the institution responsible for anti-doping policy coordination.

An important part of WADA's work is developing a framework of universally applicable sanctions, a list of prohibited substances and administrative coordination in the management of doping control (Soek 2003; WADA 2009). The central mechanism in this process is the WADC, first introduced in 2003–04, with revisions reached through a process of international stakeholder consultation that includes athletes (WADA 2006e, 2015b). Like the IOC, which supported education on the moral and physical dangers of doping, WADA also focuses on values-based education to change behavior and build a strong anti-doping culture (WADA 2010). As legitimacy rests on shared norms and values, WADA's emphasis on values-based anti-doping education provides a measure to gauge perceptions of organizational legitimacy (Chapter 6, this volume).

Unlike the IOC, which claimed a distinction between sport and politics (albeit in name only), WADA actively seeks political engagement with anti-doping initiatives. For example, an early body that was formed to facilitate a common governmental response to doping, including the public funding of WADA, was the International Intergovernmental Consultative Group on Anti-Doping in Sport (IICGADS) (CoE 2003; Houlihan 2002, 2004). WADA is a Swiss private law foundation and required a political document to enable governments to align domestic policy with the WADC (WADA 2009). The Copenhagen Declaration (March 2003) and, later, the UNESCO International Convention against Doping in Sport (October 2005) accomplished this task (WADA 2005, 2015d). More than 660 sport organizations have accepted the WADC and 170 governments have become signatories to the UNESCO Convention (UNESCO 2014; WADA 2014f, 2015c). WADA's two governing boards, the Foundation and Executive Boards, consist of representatives from the international sports movement and public authorities. The IOC continues to play a key role, with IOC members occupying central positions on both of WADA's Boards (WADA 2006a, 2014a, 2014b). Smith and Stewart (2008, 123–124) summarize WADA's characteristics:

> . . . WADA is funded jointly by the IOC and a group of national governments. This has provided the agency with both capital and influence. . . . WADA has secured a series of international declarations that have commended and ratified the policy code it has developed. . . . These achievements have consolidated WADA's position as the central international

agency for regulating drug use in sport. Currently, many sporting bodies seeking funding or competitive sanctioning from their international governing body, or national governments, must enact WADA policy.

WADA's ability to secure widespread support indicates a strong rational-legal basis for their legitimacy. However, in contrast with the IOC, which focused on doping in Olympic sport, WADA broadens anti-doping regulation to explicitly include professional sport. This has led to contentious issues of governance and control, as not all SGBs agree or consistently implement requirements under the WADC (Hanstad et al. 2010; Kidd et al. 2001). This creates tension around WADA's claims to legitimacy as the organization responsible for anti-doping harmonization. Failure to persuade audiences, in this case other organizational actors, carries the potential to damage claims to legitimacy (Throgmorton 1991). Looking at this issue from a moral panic perspective points to a further challenge linked to positive perceptions of organizational legitimacy. Here the challenge is to maintain the initial momentum in a moral panic. This requires dominant claim-makers (WADA) to demonstrate that although the policy framework is successfully catching 'folk devils' (PED-using athletes), the issue (doping) nevertheless remains significant and requires strong regulatory action. In other words, in the context of anti-doping regulation, WADA must actively engage in consensus-making work with a diverse range of stakeholders in order to successfully maintain support for their legitimacy and meet their objective of anti-doping harmonization.

The World Anti-Doping Code

From an administrative perspective, WADA and the WADC are important steps in reducing the complexity and inconsistency of former anti-doping frameworks. From a Weberian perspective, the WADC can be conceptualized as the "proper procedures" with which to negotiate "policies oriented towards the common good" (Wuthnow et al. 1984, 222) and restore order and stability to sport. The changing nature of modern sport, with increased application of medicine, science and the growth of commercialization, required a reformulation of values with which to tackle doping. Rather than a sporting community based on a shared amateur ethos, the WADC includes codified rules and regulations based on the ambiguous (Henne et al. 2013) 'spirit of sport.' WADA describes the spirit of sport as the "essence of Olympism" and the "celebration of the human spirit, body and mind" (WADA 2015g, 14). This includes a moral values-based component consisting of, amongst other elements, "Ethics, fair play and honesty, health . . . character and education . . . respect for rules and laws, respect for self and other Participants . . ." (WADA 2015g, 14).

Appeals to the "essence of Olympism" and placing the 'spirit of sport' values as principles of the WADC reminds stakeholders of the moral foundation of the Olympic Movement. This highlights that the values associated with Olympic competition provide the moral basis on which the WADC founds its legitimacy and authority. This is important because, although WADA is specifically concerned with implementing a new moral order in sport through the WADC, this remains integrally linked to Olympic competition. Not only is the IOC a WADC signatory, but WADC-compliant anti-doping polices are mandatory for International Federations seeking Olympic recognition and funding (IOC 2013; WADA 2015g). Further, WADA argues that the spirit of sport is "universal" and "practiced naturally, within the rules, and free from artificial enhancements" (WADA 2006d). Anti-doping regulation is necessary because doping is not fair, it is a danger to (athlete) health and athletes found to have used PEDs are poor role models for young people (WADA 2007a). Not only is doping considered problematic because it contravenes these values, but also because it threatens athletes' fundamental rights "to participate in doping-free sport and thus promote health, fairness and equality for Athletes worldwide" (WADA 2015g, 11). These ideas and values are integral parts of the "moral identity of sport" (Robinson 2007, 365).

The significance of WADA's claims is that they create a particular PED-free normative order based on values intrinsic to the spirit of sport. The stability of the new sporting order is regulated through the WADC. Such an approach is consistent with the Weberian ideal-type of rational-legal authority based on the implementation of bureaucratic, impersonal, all-inclusive and enforceable rules and regulations, or codes of conduct. These define the boundaries of a community while also providing a criterion against which claim-makers' legitimacy and moral authority is measured. The legitimacy of WADA, as the new institutional guardians of sport, rests on the ability of the WADC as a formal, codified regulatory framework to keep the spirit and bodies of sport PED-free.

Described as the "cornerstone in the fight against doping" (WADA 2006c), the WADC incorporates a number of rational-legal requirements together with the spirit of sport values. These include international standards[2] that are mandatory for all WADC signatories[3] and that concern administrative details related to the operationalization and harmonization of anti-doping policies (WADA 2015e). Also included are models of best practice and guidelines that, while not mandatory, are based on the WADC and the international standards and that signatories are "encouraged" to adopt (WADA 2015g, 122). In addition to the model rules, which allow SGBs (limited) flexibility, the WADC includes specific Articles that must be incorporated without substantive change (see Article 23.2.2 in WADA 2015g).[4] Part One of the WADC establishes the framework for its implementation:

> *All provisions of the Code are mandatory in substance* . . . followed as applicable by each Anti-Doping Organization and Athlete or other Person . . . *some provisions* . . . *must be incorporated without substantive*

change . . . other provisions . . . establish mandatory guiding principles that allow flexibility in the formulation of rules by each Anti-Doping Organization or establish requirements that must be followed. . . . (WADA 2015g, 16 emphasis added)

It is difficult to conceptualize the way in which '*guiding principles*' are simultaneously *mandatory* and how that might allow SGBs flexibility to construct anti-doping frameworks relevant to their particular sporting communities. Nevertheless, while some WADC provisions may not be mandatory, adoption of the international standards that support those provisions *is* mandatory for all WADC signatories. As well as monitoring athlete behavior, this approach brings other organizational actors, such as SGBs, anti-doping organizations and governments, under WADA's authority. This illustrates WADA's focus on maintaining the institutional authority to establish and police anti-doping regulation and brings issues of governance and control into the debate.

Revisions to the WADC include efforts to remove inconsistencies and better support anti-doping regulation, which is an important, and complex, task. However, anti-doping developments can also be considered through a Weberian-inspired moral panic lens. This highlights the dynamic nature of legitimacy as well as the evolutionary nature of institutional responses to behavior identified as threatening social order. From this perspective, a problem-specific institution (WADA) indicates that the issue (doping) requires a strong regulatory approach, thus justifying stronger measures of social control or the strengthening of existing measures (Cohen 2002; Goode and Ben-Yehuda 2009). Using a legitimacy-inspired moral panic lens, I next discuss six elements of the WADC 2015, commencing with the WADC's definition of doping (Article 1). Other elements discussed are the strict liability principle (Article 2.1); athletes' whereabouts failure (Article 2.4); rules concerning the manufacture, supply and trafficking of PEDs (Article 2.7); complicity (Article 2.9), prohibited association (Article 2.10) in conjunction with updated Article 21.2 that extends the roles and responsibilities of athlete support personnel; and, finally, the expansion of testing to include investigation (Article 5) supported by procedural requirements articulated in the international standard for testing.

Article 1: Definition of Doping

Transformation of anti-doping regulation from the IOC to WADA can be seen in the WADC's definition of doping (Article 1), which is mandatory for WADC signatories to adopt. It contrasts with the IOC's 2000 Olympic Movement Anti-Doping Code (OMADC) definition of doping as:

- The use of an expedient (substance or method) which is potentially harmful to the athlete's health and/or capable of enhancing their performance;

- The presence in the athlete's body of a prohibited substance or evidence of the use thereof or evidence of the use of a prohibited method. (IOC 2000, 6)

The OMADC applied to athletes and their support personnel involved in Olympic competition as well as competitions organized under the authority of an International Federation or NOC (IOC 2000, 4). In contrast, WADA's anti-doping approach brings a wider range of behaviors under observation. The WADC defines doping as "the occurrence of one or more of the anti-doping rule violations [ADRV] set forth in Article 2.1 through Article 2.10 of the Code" (WADA 2015g, 18).[5] Although representing important administrative aspects of effective anti-doping regulation, redefining doping as ADRVs also increases levels of surveillance of athletes and support personnel. From a Weberian perspective, redefining doping to ADRVs illustrates the tightening bureaucratic measures of social control (Chapter 1, this volume). An institutionalized moral panic lens is also useful, as stronger measures of social control increase the range of behavior subject to regulation, enabling progressively tougher sanctions. This also means that the legitimacy of WADA, and other anti-doping organizations, can be evaluated against their consistent and equitable application and enforcement of the anti-doping framework.

Article 2.1: Strict Liability Principle

Another measure transformed under WADA's regulatory framework is the strict liability principle. This refers to Article 2.1 of the WADC, which concerns the "Presence of a Prohibited Substance or its Metabolites or Markers in an Athlete's Sample" (WADA 2015g, 18). Strict liability means that athletes found with illegal substances in their bodies are responsible for the presence of those substances (see WADA 2015g, 141). The idea that athletes are responsible for ensuring that they avoid banned substances is not new. The OMADC stated that it is the "personal responsibility of any athlete . . . to ensure that he/she does not use or allow the use of any Prohibited Substance or any Prohibited Method" (IOC 2000, 5). The WADC uses ADRVs to "formalize" (WADA 2006b, 7) the idea of personal responsibility to the principle of strict liability, which removes the necessity to prove "intent, *Fault*, negligence or knowing *Use* . . . to establish an anti-doping violation under Article 2.1" (WADA 2015g, 18, emphasis in original). Strict liability implies all athletes are potentially 'cheats' or 'folk devils,' and this automatic presumption of guilt has been controversial.

Some athletes have argued that positive tests have resulted from contaminated or poorly labeled nutritional supplements or contaminated food. For example, in 2004 Australian triathlete Rebekah Keat received a two-year suspension for a positive drug test, which later retesting showed resulted from a contaminated nutritional supplement provided by her sponsor (Gardini 2010). In 2008, United States swimmer Jessica Hardy tested positive for clenbuterol, which was later ruled to have resulted from a contaminated supplement. Despite being 'cleared,' Hardy received a one-year suspension (Crouse 2010; Linden 2010; *Swimming World* 2009). In 2013, Australian cyclist Michael Rogers was provisionally suspended after returning a positive test for clenbuterol following the Japan Cup Cycle Road Race. Although cycling's international governing body, the UCI, later accepted Rogers' claim that the positive test was from eating contaminated meat in China where he had previously been competing, his Japan Cup results were automatically disqualified (Guinness 2014; Press Association 2014).

There is some scope for modification of sanctions based on "exceptional circumstances," such as evidence of sabotage by a competitor and where "No Fault or Negligence" can be established (WADA 2015g, 63).[6] Nevertheless, the primary responsibility to avoid an ADRV remains with the athlete. According to former WADA President, Richard Pound: "if you didn't know what was in there it's your own damn fault" (cited in Hiltzik 2006). Such an inflexible approach places athletes in a difficult position. For example, although initially reluctant to retest the supplements in the case of Rebekah Keat, later WADA retesting found contamination by norandrostenedione. Efforts to clear her name took over two years and cost Keat more than AUD$60,000 in legal fees (Gardini 2010; Krabel 2008). WADA unsuccessfully challenged the decision to clear Hardy, who later wrote about her battle with depression and post-traumatic stress disorder after the positive drug test and suspension (Dillman 2012; Futterman 2012). The severe sanctions attached to ADRVs and the personal costs for athletes, including to their health and well-being, heighten the importance of anti-doping information and education. Application of the strict liability principle has implications for SGBs' legitimacy based on their efforts in this area (Chapter 6, this volume).

Article 2.4: Athletes' Whereabouts Filing

The WADC, supported by the International Standard for Testing and Investigations (ISTI), requires sports federations to have a Registered Testing Pool (RTP) of elite athletes from which random individuals are chosen for testing, both in and out of competition (WADA 2014c; see Article 5.6 in WADA 2015g, 41, 140). Elite athletes are required to provide an up-to-date "quarterly Whereabouts Filing" (WADA 2012b, 42) that includes information such as their "home address, place and time of training, training camps and other plans to travel" (Hanstad and Loland 2009, 167–168). This means that athletes must advise sporting authorities where they will be for at least one hour per day, as well as any unforeseen changes to their schedule (WADA 2014c). Three missed tests "and/or filing failures" (WADA 2015g, 21) within a 12-month period (previously 18 months under the WADC 2009), based on a failure to be where athletes have stated they would be, incurs the risk of having committed an ADRV with or without a positive test (Kayser 2009; WADA 2014c). The whereabouts rule has been criticized on the basis that the system is unfair because the rule is not applied consistently by all countries or sporting bodies. It has also drawn concerns over athletes' privacy, autonomy and right to self-determination (Hanstad and Loland 2009). For example, elite tennis players Andy Murray and Rafael Nadal described the whereabouts regime as "draconian," showing a lack of respect for players' privacy, "completely pointless" and as an "intolerable hunt" (Gilmour 2009; Hodgkinson 2009; The Guardian 2009).

Concerns over the whereabouts rule and the strict liability principle illustrate that to maintain positive perceptions of legitimacy anti-doping regulations need to be seen as fair, and must acknowledge athletes' rights in terms of testing procedures as well as equitable application of sanctions (Donovan et al. 2002). As Houlihan (2004, 421) notes:

> The work of WADA in general, and the drafting of the World Anti-Doping Code in particular, provide important opportunities to regain athletes' confidence through the development of a policy framework which is consistent in its application, effective in its management, and which both respects and promotes the rights of athletes.

In other words, codes such as the WADC, which are designed to shore up the legitimacy of elite SGBs, can also severely test that very same legitimacy.

Article 2.7: Manufacture, Supply and Trafficking of PEDs

Under the authority of WADA and the WADC, anti-doping regulation targets not only PED-using athletes, but also those who facilitate and encourage doping (Article 2.7) and includes the manufacture, supply and trafficking of PEDs (Houlihan 2009). Again, this is not new, as the OMADC previously included provision for dealing with the trafficking and manufacture of PEDs (IOC 2000, 4, 8). WADA builds on this foundation to coordinate investigatory work with SGBs and multiple government agencies such as customs, drug and law enforcement (ISM 2007). For instance, in November 2008, WADA and Interpol reached a Memorandum of Understanding to formalize cooperation between the two organizations (WADA 2008). Other sporting stakeholders have taken a similar approach. In Australia, the Australian Sports Anti-Doping Authority (ASADA) has developed information-sharing networks with police, customs and immigration officers, Australia Post and the Australian Crime Commission (ACC) (Jeffery 2008; Lundy and Clare 2012; Magnay 2008; Lundy 2013).

Initiatives that incorporate other agencies of social control shift doping from a sporting infringement, with associated sporting sanctions, to criminal behavior and penalties ranging from court imposed fines to imprisonment (Møller 2009). Other changes under the WADC 2015 not only increase surveillance and monitoring of athletes, but also include a more explicit focus on athlete support personnel.

Article 2.9 and Article 2.10: Complicity and Prohibited Association

The WADC 2015 introduces two new ADRVs, which are Complicity (Article 2.9) and Prohibited Association (Article 2.10). Like Article 2.7, these changes are designed to counter the influence of members of the athletes' entourage or wider networks that might facilitate or encourage doping. WADA Director-General David Howman claims that 'cheats' can also be "coaches and trainers and lawyers and doctors and physiotherapists" (cited in Clarke 2015). It is now a potential ADRV for athletes to associate in a "professional or sport related capacity" with athlete support personnel that have been involved in doping activities but that are outside the jurisdiction of anti-doping authorities (WADA 2015f, 2015g, 23). These represent important procedural mechanisms intended to protect athletes from exploitation by outside influences. However, as well as stricter control of athletes' behavior, they also tighten control of athlete support personnel. There is further evidence of this in updates to Article 21.2, which concerns the Roles and Responsibilities of Athlete Support Personnel.

Article 21.2: The Roles and Responsibilities of Athlete Support Personnel
Previously under the WADC, athlete support personnel would be committing an ADRV by administering or trafficking prohibited substances to athletes. However, the *use* of PEDs by athlete support personnel was not addressed. A new sub-clause under WADC 2015 (Article 21.2.6) forbids athlete support personnel from using or possessing any prohibited substance "without valid justification" (WADA 2015g, 114). Similarly to the rationale applied to athletes as role models for young people, athlete support personnel are described as role models for athletes. According to WADA, this obligates them to ensure their conduct does not "conflict with their responsibility to encourage their Athletes not to dope" (WADA 2015g, 114). While not an ADRV, breaches by athlete support personnel are potentially subject to the disciplinary rules of the relevant sport (WADA 2015f, 4; 2015g, 114). New ADRVs as well as updated provisions in Article 21 are important measures aimed at countering any potential exploitation by or influence of broader doping networks. At the same time, however, these provisions tighten control over athletes and athlete support personnel, which potentially brings new groups of 'folk devils' into the regulatory framework. They also present WADA and sporting organizations with the challenge of ensuring the equitable and consistent application of such measures in order to maintain support for their authority and legitimacy to regulate the sporting community.

Article 5: Testing and Investigations

Article 5 concerns testing of athletes' samples, which is undertaken to determine compliance (or not) with the WADA List of Prohibited Substances or Methods. As well as addressing administrative details, Article 5 operates in conjunction with the International Standard for Testing, which was renamed the International Standard for Testing and Investigations (ISTI) to take effect from January 2015 (WADA 2014c). The ISTI defines procedures to facilitate effective testing and maintain the integrity of samples collected (WADA 2014c, 1; see Article 5.5 of WADA 2015g, 41). Article 5 is one of a range of WADC Articles[7] listed as "directly relevant" to the ISTI, which is an international standard forming part of the World Anti-Doping Program and is mandatory for WADC signatories (WADA 2014c, 1–2).

Testing for prohibited substances has long been a contentious issue, including concerns that some procedures constitute an infringement of athletes' civil rights (Black 2001; Houlihan 2004; Malloy and Zakus 2002; Rushall and Jones 2007; Schneider 2004). Testing technology has also faced the difficult task of 'keeping up' as drugs developed for legitimate medical purposes are used illegally in sport. Further challenges associated with drug testing technology concern the accuracy of doping controls and analytical ambiguities in doping results (Kayser, Mauron and Miah 2007). While there are claims that these limitations result in a "significant under-reporting bias" (Waddington 2005, 475), of more relevance is whether members of the sporting community perceive SGBs' legitimacy as "hamstrung by significant limitations in technology" (Waddington 2005, 475; Chapter 6, this volume). This point is highly relevant because, according to Donovan et al. (2002), a significant factor linked to SGBs' legitimacy is perceptions that drug testing procedures and technology are accurate.

To address issues associated with a reliance on testing, and in conjunction with the ISTI, the WADC 2015 expands testing controls to include "testing and investigations" (WADA 2014c, 2015g). There are two aspects informing investigations in WADC Article 5. The first of these concerns resolving analytical ambiguities in order to determine whether or not an ADRV has occurred (see Article 5.1.2 of WADA 2015g). This includes intelligence gathering, which here refers to determining whether correct procedures have been followed, such as those for therapeutic use exemptions, compliance with the ISTI or the International Standard for Laboratories (see Article 7.4 of WADA 2015g, 52). These are important procedural aspects of the anti-doping framework. However, the second aspect of investigations increases surveillance and monitoring of athletes and other individuals, as well as SGBs. Investigations now incorporate indications of *potential* ADRVs based on *non-analytical* intelligence or evidence (WADA 2015g, 37 emphasis added). This shift toward incorporating non-analytical intelligence gathering and evidence is also stressed in the ISTI, which as well as procedural elements noted above, establishes:

... mandatory standards for ... efficient and effective gathering, assessment and use of anti-doping intelligence and ... efficient and effective conduct of investigations into *possible* ... violations. (WADA 2014c, 1 emphasis added)

The expansion of testing controls to include investigations into *possible* non-analytical ADRVs brings a wider range of individuals and groups under the WADC and creates new obligations for SGBs.

Part 3 of the ISTI tasks WADC signatories and other anti-doping organizational stakeholders with doing "everything in their power" to gather anti-doping intelligence "from all available sources" (WADA 2014c, 57). This includes implementing policies and procedures to gather intelligence (including for the protection of athletes' rights, which is important for organizational claims to legitimacy) and ways to analyze and, if necessary, act on that information (see Article 11.2, 11.3 and 11.4 in WADA 2014c, 57–58; WADA 2015g, 116). As well as athletes and their support personnel, Part 3 of the ISTI defines 'all available sources' as including members of the public, individuals involved in sample collection as well as ". . . laboratories, pharmaceutical companies, National Federations, law enforcement, other regulatory and disciplinary bodies, and the media" (see Article 11.2.1 in WADA 2014c, 57). While not all these groups or individuals are bound by the WADC, such as pharmaceutical companies, the public or the media, they are nevertheless brought into the anti-doping regulatory framework as potential sources of information concerning possible ADRVs.

From a moral panic perspective, these changes constitute part of a 'widening the net process' as existing relationships between social actors are strengthened or new measures introduced. These measures also raise concerns around athletes' rights and, consequently, emphasize the importance of ensuring they are applied consistently and equitably. As such, this also means that these measures, and their application, provide opportunities to evaluate the legitimacy of WADA and other sporting authorities that implement these types of anti-doping controls. Modifications of ADRVs and the introduction of new anti-doping controls illustrate the dynamic and evolutionary nature of institutional responses to problematic issues, in this case drugs in sport. While this creates opportunities to enhance WADA's institutional legitimacy, it also means that such claims cannot be taken for granted. From a legitimacy-inspired moral panic perspective, maintaining positive perceptions of legitimacy means that WADA must engage in ongoing consensus-making work to persuade SGBs and other anti-doping stakeholders to adopt and implement these new measures.

THE WORLD ANTI-DOPING AGENCY, LEGITIMACY AND A MORAL PANIC

Weber's (1969) consideration of legitimacy highlights its subjective, evaluative nature and that claims to legitimacy cannot be taken for granted.

Dominant groups must actively work to maintain support for claims to legitimacy as well as compliance from other institutional actors and stakeholders. Like legitimacy, successful moral panics require that claim-makers engage in consensus-making activities, among both the public and other stakeholder groups, to secure support for institutional solutions for the deviant behavior. In a moral panic, in order to legitimate the ongoing provision of funding as well as public support, claim-makers must manage the 'delicate balance' (Zatz 1987) between showing that their efforts are effective, or legitimate, evidenced by detection and sanctioning of deviant individuals. As Hawdon (2001, 430) notes in his discussion of the role of rhetoric in the 'war on drugs' as a moral panic, claim-makers present stakeholders with "mixed results," because "if action is too successful, there is nothing left to fight. If not successful enough, public support for the crusade will likely erode."

In the case of WADA and drugs in sport, stakeholders include SGBs, governments, athletes and the public. Support for WADA provides opportunities for institutional actors, such as SGBs or governments, to enhance or restore perceptions of their legitimacy as making a genuine effort to maintain 'clean' sport. As Miah (2002, 359) writes:

> . . . WADA is supposed to be active at ensuring transparency about anti-doping practices and its existence as an independent body could give credibility and legal strength to any individual governing body that ascribes to its conditions.

Using an elites-engineered moral panic lens, this demonstrates that legitimacy based on the transparency of their regulatory approach is important to WADA and also speaks directly to issues of governance and control. While supporting WADA presents opportunities for SGBs to enhance their legitimacy, it also challenges their authority to control their particular sporting communities. For example, the WADC strengthens control over SGBs by linking access to funding and Olympic participation to implementation of WADC-aligned policies (AP 2007b; WADA 2015g). WADA's effort to maintain legitimacy and control over other organizational stakeholders is not limited to their interactions with SGBs, but also includes governments. This includes an expectation articulated in the WADC that governments will enact legislative frameworks that facilitate information sharing with anti-doping organizations and to "vigorously" pursue individuals involved in doping (see Article 22 in WADA 2015g, 116–117 and Article 20.6.6, 111). This expectation is in addition to obligations for governments to ratify the UNESCO Convention, the mechanism that aligns government policy with the WADC. Failure to do so means governments could potentially be ineligible to place bids to host Olympic Games, to hold World Championships or suffer other "symbolic" consequences (Aricle 20.6.6 and Article 22.8 in WADA 2015g, 111, 117). These measures bring power relationships between organizational actors, and contested claims to legitimacy, into the frame and emphasize WADA's concern to maintain the institutional legitimacy and authority to regulate the global anti-doping community.

A "key test" (Miah 2002, 359) for WADA is securing, and maintaining, support and commitment from a diverse group of sporting stakeholders, which includes SGBs as well as governments. The problematic nature of building consensus over anti-doping approaches reflects the fact that while "high performance sport may have become what some have called a global monoculture . . . attitudes toward the use of performance-enhancing drugs remain highly particular" (Kidd et al. 2001, 182). The challenge for WADA is to maintain support, resources and enthusiasm without "fracturing the fragile global consensus on anti-doping" (Houlihan 2009, 45). WADA's ability to generate stakeholder support, or build consensus, speaks directly to Weber's concept of legitimacy based on a rational-legal framework and fits neatly within an elites-engineered institutionalized moral panic framework.

On the one hand, WADA must work to build stakeholder agreement and support, and thus bolster claims to legitimacy, based on the demonstrated ability of their regulatory framework (the WADC and WADC-aligned policies) to 'catch' PED-using cheats. At the same time however, they must defend their legitimacy and justify their continued operation based on ideas that the problem (doping) remains and requires ongoing regulatory attention. This is an important point, as anti-doping policy has been largely reactive, driven by scandals such as the PED-related death of Simpson in 1967 and the 1998 Tour de France doping scandal, which substantially changed anti-doping approaches. However, reliance on scandal to generate support is not an effective strategy over the long-term. The dynamic nature of the broader social context presents claim-makers with the difficult task of maintaining commitment and momentum based on the tendency for problems or issues to "mutate" (Houlihan 2009, 45). For instance, debates over new PEDs or new technology, such as hyperbaric chambers or swimming bodysuits (Christie 2006; *Reuters* 2008), occur in policy and public arenas with competing claims for attention.

To address this, WADA emphasizes the importance of scientific research programs. However, these initiatives require public funding and WADA must compete with a range of other research priorities and groups also demanding attention and research funding. Professor Arne Ljungqvist[8] acknowledges that anti-doping research must compete for funding with more "prestigious" research areas, such as "cancer, AIDS, or malaria." Nevertheless, he argues anti-doping research is a "noble cause" with "significant benefits to public health" and thus obligates the "Olympic Movement and . . . public authorities to understand the importance of proper funding . . . I now think it is time to increase the WADA budget substantially" because this is an "inevitable evolution" in the "fight against doping" (WADA 2007b, 8). For WADA, securing funding to continue the development of detection technology is an essential part of the anti-doping framework, which also underpins the organizations' claims to legitimacy. Nevertheless,

WADA faces the ongoing task of maintaining or, ideally, increasing levels of funding, including from public authorities, to avoid any reduction in their anti-doping activities or negative affect on their overall objectives (see also WADA 2013a). From a moral panic perspective, this emphasizes the importance of a consensus-making process that not only identifies PED-using athletes as 'folk devils' but that also posits WADA and the WADC as the necessary institutional solutions in the anti-doping "fight."

Like the IOC, the legitimacy of WADA rests on the ability of a regulatory framework, in this case the WADC and WADC-aligned policies to keep sport PED-free. The WADC, supported by the international standards, underpins WADA's work toward the goal of anti-doping policy harmonization. These codified rules and regulations also enable WADA to retain claims to the institutional authority to police doping, including introducing more stringent measures of social control. These measures concern important administrative and procedural 'gaps' in the anti-doping framework, thus enhancing claims to organizational legitimacy. However, they also illustrate the dynamic nature of legitimacy where, from a Weberian perspective, measures of control tend to tighten around the individual (Weber 1969). An institutionalized moral panic theoretical lens is also useful here as it highlights the evolutionary nature of institutional responses to behavior identified as threatening social order. In this context, a problem-specific institution implies that the issue requires a strong regulatory approach. This enables implementation of greater control measures or the strengthening of existing measures, which the moral panic literature describes as processes of 'diffusion' and 'escalation,' a 'spiral of signification' or 'widening the net' (Cohen 2002; Goode and Ben-Yehuda 1994, 156; Goode and Ben-Yehuda 2009; Hall et al. 1978).These processes are clearly evident in the actions of WADA, using the WADC, as a problem-specific institutional response to doping.

Building on processes already in place under the IOC, the redefinition of doping as a range of ADRVs enabled incorporation of wider innovative methods of control, such as athletes' whereabouts rules and the strict liability principle. However, there are inconsistencies in the application of these protocols. For example, elite tennis player Andy Murray criticized the whereabouts system and its associated testing regime as unfairly targeting elite players, with "one system for the top players and another for the journey men" (Gilmour 2009). There are also issues around inconsistent application of the strict liability principle. Illustrating this point, in 2011 Mexico's governing body of football banned five soccer players after they tested positive for clenbuterol prior to the Gold Cup (Bhandari and Arce 2011). Similarly to China, Mexico also experiences significant issues with steroid contaminated meat. In contrast to cyclist Michael Rogers (described earlier in this chapter), WADA dropped an appeal against the players in the Court of Arbitration for Sport after accepting "compelling evidence" from FIFA supporting the players' claims that the tests were caused by contaminated meat. Mexico went on to defeat the United States in the Gold Cup final (AP 2011). As Donovan et al. (2002) have pointed out, consistent and equitable application of anti-doping protocols and sanctions are important for positive perceptions of organizational legitimacy (e.g., see Chapter 6, this volume).

WADA's incorporation of other agents of control, such as Interpol, 'diffused' anti-doping regulation and, by including government and law enforcement agencies, carries the potential to escalate doping to a criminal issue (Møller 2009). There is evidence that some SGBs and governments are supportive of criminal penalties for doping infringements. For example, referring to the 2012 London Olympic Games, Professor Arne Ljungqvist argued for the British government to criminalize doping, a stance taken by some European countries such as Italy, France and Spain (AP 2007a; Herman 2007). In 2014, the German government drafted a law aimed at top level professional athletes that included three year prison terms for doping athletes, with dealers and doctors who assist potentially facing prison sentences of up to 10 years (Clarke 2014a). These calls did not go uncontested, emphasizing that modern sport consists of a range of stakeholder groups, which includes athletes.

The German Athletes Commission indicated their significant concerns around the legitimacy of international anti-doping efforts, including doping controls at the 2014 Sochi Winter Olympics and consequences for athletes under the proposed German law. In an open letter to "NADO Germany, NOC Germany, Ministry of Internal Affairs/Sports, IOC Athletes Commission, EOC Athletes Commission, German Athletes and Public," the German Athletes Commission stated that German athletes lacked trust in anti-doping authorities' ability to address doping. Further, "as one national group of the main stakeholders in sport," German athletes demanded more "transparent result management . . . governance . . . and effectiveness" from WADA and other anti-doping organizations (Schreiber and Kassner 2014). While WADA has rejected jail sentences for PED use (Clarke 2014b), this emphasizes the point that, to enjoy positive perceptions of legitimacy, organizations must ensure that anti-doping frameworks are perceived as fair and as acknowledging athletes' rights (Donovan et al. 2002). This also demonstrates the significance of consensus-making underpinning positive perceptions of legitimacy, and thus support and compliance, with anti-doping regulatory initiatives.

New ADRVs of Complicity and Prohibited Association together with updated provisions in Article 21 are underpinned by efforts to counter the influence of broader doping networks on athletes' behavior and to close loopholes in anti-doping regulation. High profile examples of individuals alleged to have encouraged doping practices emphasize the challenge of this task. For example, in 2012 and as part of an investigation into the US Postal Service cycling team and Lance Armstrong, physician Michele Ferrari received a lifetime ban from the United States Anti-Doping Authority

(USADA) based on evidence of alleged doping practices (AP 2014; USADA 2012). The Italian Cycling Federation had previously banned Ferrari for life. Nevertheless, media reports suggest that Ferrari continues to have an influence with recent claims that, since his ban, he has been photographed meeting with other professional cycling teams (AP 2014; Pells 2015). These types of cases suggest that WADA's appeals to values associated with the 'spirit of sport,' codified in the WADC, are not shared by all in the sporting community.

The ADRVs of Complicity and Prohibited Association and the updated Article 21 are important procedural issues that also concern athlete well-being, including the prevention of potential exploitation by individuals or groups that might encourage doping for criminal purposes. However, this also means that anti-doping organizations, such as WADA, SGBs and governments must ensure that these measures are implemented in a manner that supports, rather than detracts from the goal of anti-doping regulations to maintain 'clean' sport and protect player welfare. There is also support for an elites-engineered moral panic framework here, as to successfully accomplish their objective of global harmonization, WADA must persuade SGBs and other anti-doping stakeholders to adopt and implement the new measures. Referring to Article 2.10 under the WADC 2015, Travis Tygart, CEO of USADA, stated: "These important changes advance the policy to most effectively protect clean athletes' rights, health and fair competition . . . the challenge is to ensure all countries and sports are fully implementing this gold-standard policy to ensure the real winners win" (cited in White 2015).

The WADC 2015 also 'widens the net' and escalates anti-doping regulation by expanding testing to include investigations based on non-analytical information. This shift could be seen, in part, as driven by high-profile doping scandals that were not revealed as a result of failed doping tests such as, for instance, seven-time Tour de France winner Lance Armstrong. In 2012, following an investigation by USADA, Armstrong was banned for life and stripped of all Tour de France titles by the UCI (*BBC* 2012; *CBS News* 2012; Macur 2012). Armstrong, who consistently denied PED use and was tested more than 200 times throughout his career with numerous allegations that failed tests had been concealed, was described as instrumental in "the most sophisticated, professionalized and successful doping program that sport has ever seen" (Benammar 2013). The significance of this for the legitimacy of WADA is that revelations of Armstrong's doping did not result from the actions of WADA, SGBs or event organizers that were signatories to, and bound by, the WADC. Rather, evidence from a long-term investigation by journalist David Walsh (see Macur 2014; Walsh 2007, 2012) combined with accusations in the media by Armstrong's former teammates ultimately led to the USADA investigation. Rather than analytical evidence from testing of athletes' samples, that investigation focused on affidavits and sworn evidence, including from other professional cyclists (*ABC* and *AFP* 2013; *CBS News* 2012). The Armstrong case raises further questions surrounding the legitimacy of elite SGBs, with claims that the UCI was complicit in concealing Armstrong's long-standing doping practices (AP 2013; Fotheringham 2015).

Questions must also be asked concerning whether the potential consequences of expanding testing controls can include investigations into *possible* non-analytical ADRVs. Not only can this be seen from a moral panic perspective, where a wider range of individuals and groups are brought under surveillance using the WADC, it also brings the issue of legitimacy into the analysis, as new compliance obligations around information gathering and reporting are created for SGBs. This brings power relationships as well as issues of governance and control into the frame, highlighting the dynamic and contested nature of claims to legitimacy and, from an elites-engineered moral panic perspective, the importance of consensus-making activities. According to WADA, their role as "custodian" (WADA 2015a) of the WADC includes a "duty to monitor stakeholder activities in relation to the Code and act to ensure the integrity of the Code" (WADA 2015a; see also WADA 2015g, 112). Notwithstanding this self-imposed obligation to monitor SGB compliance, WADA recognizes the need to ensure that policy frameworks meet and respond to "stakeholder needs and expectations" (WADA 2015g, 13). In other words, claims to legitimacy and moral authority require subjective acceptance by social actors based either on voluntary agreement or decisions by an authority held to be legitimate (Battin et al. 2008; Buti and Fridman 1994; Pakulski 1986; Suchman 1995). This applies equally to claims to legitimacy amongst organizational actors as it does to securing athlete support for, and compliance with, the anti-doping regulatory framework.

Investigation and anti-doping intelligence gathering requirements under the WADC also escalate and 'widen the net' of the moral panic by bringing organizations and individuals, such as pharmaceutical companies, the media and the public, into the anti-doping framework either as agents of social control or as sources of anti-doping intelligence. In either case, this approach emphasizes the Weberian point that bureaucratic measures of social control tend to tighten around the individual, which can include organizational actors. WADA also continually 'widens the net' by linking PED use to broader social issues easily conceptualized by the public. For example, in response to reports by Australian Customs that PEDs coming into Australia are appearing in gyms and sporting clubs, WADA President John Fahey used the media to argue for a public health campaign to "take the fight . . . directly into the community" (Silkstone 2008, *The Age*). This reflects long-standing claims by WADA that the necessary response to those types of situations is the WADC, as an "unprecedented triumph of Sport and Government joining forces to address a critical problem threatening public health and the integrity of sport" (ISM 2007, see also WADA President John Fahey in AFP 2008). Doping is presented not only as a "critical problem" (WADA 2006e, 5) for elite sport but one that "continues to threaten public health" (WADA 2012a) with the potential to permeate other parts of society (Howman 2012). This is illustrated by WADA's claims that the health of amateur athletes, particularly children, is threatened because more and more athletes are turning to doping:

> As a society we would be shocked at the amount of stuff . . . children are taking . . . this is a public health issue and we are supported by the World Health Organization and by many others who now see it's not just a sport issue. (WADA Director-General, David Howman cited in Clarke 2015)

This construction of doping fits within a moral panic framework, which notes the tendency for ideas about behavior described as deviant to shift from an issue isolated to a particular community, in this case elite sport, to one that "could happen any place" (Cohen 2002, xii). It also highlights the importance of legitimacy for WADA, supported by other dominant claim-makers such as the WHO, as the appropriate institutional solution to doping practices.

WADA's establishment entailed creating new, shared systems of meaning in which doping was cast as unacceptable behavior, a stance internalized and acted upon at every level of the sporting community (Girginov 2006). WADA is specifically concerned with implementing a new moral order in sport through the implementation of a global standard for anti-doping rules and regulations articulated in the WADC. Such an approach is consistent with the Weberian ideal-type of rational-legal authority based on the implementation of bureaucratic, impersonal, all-inclusive and enforceable rules and regulations, or codes of conduct. These define the normative boundaries of a community while providing a criterion against which claim-makers' legitimacy and moral authority is measured.

CONCLUSION

The transformation of anti-doping regulation in the form of WADA in response to claims that the IOC lacked legitimacy can be seen through a Weberian lens. From this perspective, the legitimacy of WADA is based on a combination of an appeal to shared values claimed to be inherent to sport (encapsulated in the 'spirit of sport') as well as a rational-legal foundation in the WADC. As Weber (1969, 944) noted, measures of the exercise of legitimacy can be given expression in regulations and include the creation of special agencies as well as more stringent measures of social control. There is evidence of this in the context of WADA and the WADC. The reclassification of already existing measures under the OMADC, such as redefining doping as a range of ADRVs, brings a greater range of behaviors under surveillance. This is evident in the strict liability principle and athletes' whereabouts ruling as well as the incorporation of other agencies of social control, such as customs and law enforcement, into the anti-doping framework.

A moral panic lens highlights that support for the moral authority and legitimacy to regulate the sporting community cannot be taken for granted. Rather, it is dependent upon ongoing concern that the particular issue, in this case doping, is problematic and requires a specific institutional response. Such a response includes a regulatory framework with the ability to detect and sanction deviants, which in turn enables application of increasingly strict measures of social control. An elites-engineered moral panic theoretical framework also helps to shed light on the role of legitimacy and highlights that contested power relationships between dominant groups are part of contemporary debates. In the context of anti-doping regulation, WADA's role as a global monitor of anti-doping polices simultaneously challenges the authority of SGBs and other institutional actors. While support for WADA provides an opportunity for SGBs to enhance claims to legitimacy, issues of governance arise, as these organizations are also subject to greater measures of control using the international standards, models of best practice and mandatory doping controls. Added to these existing measures, the WADC 2015 brings in new expectations and obligations around information gathering, including reporting possible non-analytical doping infringements to WADA. While information sharing between organizations is an important procedural element in effective anti-doping regulation, the incorporation of non-sporting groups and organizations 'widens the net.' Not only does this bring in new agents of control, it also creates potential new groups of 'folk devils' into the regulatory gaze.

The socio-historical case studies in this book, including in the next chapter, highlight the importance of expanding analysis of drugs in sport beyond a focus on the athlete-user. The transformation of anti-doping approaches in the form of WADA as well as the ability to maintain support, or build consensus, for their moral authority and legitimacy has implications for other elite SGBs. With WADA situated as the central anti-doping authority, support for its initiatives provides opportunities for SGBs to enhance perceptions of their legitimacy. At the same time, this demonstrates the multi-dimensional nature of legitimacy and moral authority, as WADA's role as a global monitor of anti-doping polices also challenges the authority of SGBs. This raises issues for SGBs in terms of maintaining governance and control of their particular sporting communities, with the possibility of resistance to the call to align with WADA's framework. I discuss these issues in the next chapter using an Australian sporting body, namely the Australian Football League (AFL), as a case study.

NOTES

1   The WADC defines a National Anti-Doping Organization (NADO) as: "the entity(ies) designated by each country as possessing the primary authority and responsibility to adopt and implement anti-doping rules, direct the collection of *Samples*, the management of test results, and the conduct of hearings at the

national level. If this designation has not been made by the competent public authority(ies), the entity shall be the country's *National Olympic Committee* or its designee" (WADA 2015g).

NADOs are not the same as anti-doping organizations (ADOs), which the WADC defines as: "a *Signatory* that is responsible for adopting rules for initiating, implementing or enforcing any part of the *Doping Control* process. This includes, for example, the International Olympic Committee, the International Paralympic Committee, other *Major Event Organizations* that conduct *Testing* at their *Events*, WADA, International Federations, and *National Anti-Doping Organizations*" (WADA 2015g, 130). Based on this definition, this book considers SGBs such as the Australian Football League (AFL) to be anti-doping organizations.

2   The international standards are: 1) The Prohibited List, 2) Testing and Investigations, 3) Laboratories, 4) Therapeutic Use Exemptions and 5) Protection of Privacy and Personal Information (WADA 2014e).

3   WADC signatories are defined as: "WADA, the International Olympic Committee, International Federations, the International Paralympic Committee, National Olympic Committees, National Paralympic Committees, Major Event Organizations, and National Anti-Doping Organizations. These entities shall accept the Code by signing a declaration of acceptance upon approval by each of their respective governing bodies" (WADA 2015g, 120). The Code also states that professional leagues that are not under the jurisdiction of a government or international federation will be "encouraged" to adopt the WADC (WADA 2015g, 120).

4   Articles to be implemented without substantive change are: Article 1 (Definition of Doping); Article 2 (Anti-Doping Rule Violations); Article 3 (Proof of Doping); Article 4.2.2 (Specified Substances); Article 4.3.3 (WADA's Determination of the Prohibited List); Article 7.11 (Retirement from Sport); Article 9 (Automatic Disqualification of Individual Results); Article 10 (Sanctions on Individuals); Article 11 (Consequences to Teams); Article 13 (Appeals); Article 15.1 (Recognition of Decisions); Article 17 (Statute of Limitations); Article 24 (Interpretation of the Code) (WADA 2015g, 121).

5   Anti-Doping Rule Violations: Presence of a Prohibited Substance or its Metabolites or Markers in an Athlete's Sample (Article 2.1); Use or Attempted Use by an Athlete of a Prohibited Substance or a Prohibited Method (Article 2.2); Evading, Refusing or Failing to Submit to Sample Collection (Article 2.3); Whereabouts Failures (Article 2.4); Tampering or Attempted Tampering with any part of Doping Control (Article 2.5); Possession of a Prohibited Substance or a Prohibited Method (Article 2.6); Trafficking or Attempted Trafficking in any Prohibited Substance or Prohibited Method (Article 2.7), Administration or Attempted Administration to any Athlete In-Competition of any Prohibited Substance or Prohibited Method, or Administration or Attempted Administration to any Athlete Out-of-Competition of any Prohibited Substance or any Prohibited Method that is prohibited Out-of-Competition (Article 2.8); Complicity (Article 2.9); Prohibited Association (Article 2.10) (WADA 2015g, 18–24).

6   No fault does not apply in cases such as contaminated or mislabeled vitamins or supplements, administration of a banned substance without the athlete's knowledge by another person, including trainers or medical personal, or sabotage of the athletes' food or drink by coaches, family members or friends. Athlete responsibility extends to their choice in medical personnel as well as the conduct of individuals with access to the athletes' food and drink (WADA 2015g).

7   Article 6 (Analysis of Samples), Article 7 (Results Management), Article 10 (Sanctions on Individuals), Article 13 (Appeals), Article 14 (Confidentiality

and Reporting), Article 20 (Additional Roles and Responsibilities of Signatories), Article 21 (Additional Roles and Responsibilities of Athletes and other Persons), Article 23 (Acceptance, Compliance and Modification) (WADA 2014c).
8   IOC Member (1987–2003), Chairman IOC Medical Commission (2003–2014) (IOC 2014), WADA Vice President and Vice Chairman of WADA Foundation Board (WADA 2013b, 2014b).

REFERENCES

ABC and AFP (Agence France-Presse). 2013. "Lance Armstrong: Career Timeline." ABC News, 18 January 2013. http://www.abc.net.au/news/2012–10–22/lance-armstrong-chronology/432796. Accessed 28 March 2015.
AFP (Agence France-Presse). 2008. "WADA Chief Warns Sports to Beat Drugs or Face Irrelevance." Agence France-Presse, 7 August 2008. http://afp.google.com/article/ALeqM5hispSXtLzWuSeW6IVKIYQLUgzzfA. Accessed 19 August 2009.
AP (Associated Press). 2007a. "Britain to Consider Criminalizing Doping in Sports." *International Herald Tribune*, 24 July 2007. http://www.iht.com/articles/ap/2007/07/24/sports/EU-SPT-OLY-Britain-Doping-Laws.php.   Accessed   25 July 2007.
———. 2007b. "WADA Chief Warns Lax Doping Rules Could Cost Slot in Olympics." *International Herald Tribune*, 6 July 2007. http://www.iht.com/articles/ap/2007/07/06/sports/LA-SPT-OLY-IOC-Doping.php. Accessed 16 July 2007.
———. 2011. "WADA Drops Case vs. Mexico Players." ESPN, 12 October 2011. http://espn.go.com/sports/soccer/news/_/id/7091999/world-anti-doping-agency-drops-case-mexico-soccer-players. Accessed 13 April 2015.
———. 2013. "Lance Armstrong Says Former UCI President Helped Cover Up Doing." *USA Today*, 18 November 2013. http://www.usatoday.com/story/sports/cycling/2013/11/18/lance-armstrong-coverup-doping-uci-tour-de-france/3628059/. Accessed 14 June 2015.
———. 2014. "Italian Cycling President: Police Must Act to Stop Michele Ferrari Influence." *The Guardian*, 19 December 2014. http://www.theguardian.com/sport/2014/dec/18/michele-ferrari-italy-police-must-act. Accessed 11 April 2015.
Battin, M.P., Luna, E., Lipman, A.G., Gahlinger, P.M., Rollins, D.E., Roberts, J.C., and Booher, T.L. 2008. *Drugs and Justice: Seeking a Consistent, Coherent, Comprehensive View*. Oxford: Oxford University Press.
BBC. 2012. "Lance Armstrong Stripped of All Seven Tour de France Wins by UCI." BBC, 22 October 2012. http://www.bbc.com/sport/0/cycling/2000852. Accessed 27 March 2015.
Benammar, E. 2013. "Stuart O'Grady, Lance Armstrong, Marco Pantani, Floyd Landis and Alberto Contador: Cycling's Doping Scandals." ABC News, 25 July 2013. http://www.abc.net.au/news/2013–07–25/cycling27s-infamous-doping-scandals/484206. Accessed 3 September 2014.
Bhandari, A., and Arce, L. 2011. "Five Mexico Stars Banned After Failing Drugs Test." CNN, 10 June 2011. http://edition.cnn.com/2011/SPORT/06/10/mexico.doping/. Accessed 24 April 2015.
Black, D.L. 2001. "Doping Control Testing Policies and Procedures." In *Doping in Elite Sport: The Politics of Drugs in the Olympic Movement*, edited by Wilson, W. and Derse, E., 29–42. Champaign, IL: Human Kinetics.
Buti, A., and Fridman, S. 1994. "The Intersection of Law and Policy: Drug Testing in Sport." *Australian Journal of Public Administration* 53 (4): 489–507.

CBS News. 2012. "Lance Armstrong Now Faces Justice Department in Lawsuit." CBS News, http://www.cbsnews.com/news/lance-armstrong-now-faces-justice-department-in-lawsuit/. Accessed 27 March 2015.

Christie, J. 2006. "WADA May Move to Ban Oxygen Tents." Canadian Sport Centre, Accessed 6 September 2006. http://www.canadiansportcentre.com/Communications/SportPerformanceWeekly/SPW2006/05_15_06.html. Accessed 6 September 2006.

Clarke, S. 2014a. "Germany Set to Introduce Jail Sentences for Doping Offences." *Cycling Weekly*, 12 November 2014. http://www.cyclingweekly.co.uk/news/latest-news/germany-set-introduce-jail-sentences-doping-offences-14404. Accessed 13 April 2015.

———. 2014b. "WADA President Denounces Jail Sentences for Doping Offenders." *Cycling Weekly*, 18 November 2014. http://www.cyclingweekly.co.uk/news/latest-news/wada-president-denounces-jail-sentences-doping-offenders-145219 — If4qPgZ72btyGwvM.9. Accessed 13 April 2015.

———. 2015. "Doping Is Becoming a Public Health Issue, Says WADA Chief." *Cycling Weekly*, 28 January 2015. http://www.cyclingweekly.co.uk/news/latest-news/doping-becoming-public-health-issue-says-wada-chief-15466. Accessed 10 February 2015.

CoE (Council of Europe). 2003. "Information Document Conclusions Regarding WADA Part IV International Consultative Group on Anti-Doping in Sport (IICGADS)." Council of Europe. https://wcd.coe.int/ViewDoc.jsp?id=34911&Site=COE—P589_4228. Accessed 31 March 2015.

Cohen, S. 2002. Folk devils and moral panics: the creation of the Mods and Rockers 3rd ed. Abingdon, Oxon, New York: Routledge.

Crouse, K. 2010. "For Swimmer, Ban Ends, but Burden Could Last." *The New York Times*, 7 August 2010. http://www.nytimes.com/2010/08/08/sports/08hardy.html. Accessed 24 April 2015.

Dillman, L. 2012. "Swimmer Jessica Hardy Gets Another Shot at the Olympics." *Los Angeles Times*, 25 April 2012. http://articles.latimes.com/2012/apr/25/sports/la-sp-oly-jessica-hardy-2012042. Accessed 24 April 2015.

Donovan, R. J., Egger, G., Kapernick, V., and Mendoza, J. 2002. "A Conceptual Framework for Achieving Performance Enhancing Drug Compliance in Sport." *Sports Medicine* 32 (4): 269–284.

Fotheringham, W. 2015. "Lance Armstrong and UCI 'Colluded to Bypass Doping Accusations.'" *The Guardian*, 9 March 2015. http://www.theguardian.com/sport/2015/mar/09/lance-armstrong-uci-colluded-circ-report-cycling. Accessed 14 June 2015.

Futterman, M. 2012. "Trials and Tribulations of the Angry Swimmer." *The Wall Street Journal*, 14 May 2012. http://www.wsj.com/articles/SB100014240527023042036045773965611903 1937. Accessed 25 April 2015.

Gardini, A. 2010. "Keat No Drug Cheat." *Gold Coast Bulletin*, 13 February 2008. http://www.goldcoast.com.au/article/2008/02/13/7716_gold-coast-sport.html. Accessed 17 September 2010.

Gilmour, R. 2009. "Andy Murray Awoken in New York Hotel Room by Early-Rising Drug-Testers." *The Telegraph*, 26 August 2009. http://www.telegraph.co.uk/sport/tennis/andymurray/6092431/Andy-Murray-awoken-in-New-York-hotel-room-by-early-rising-drug-testers.html. Accessed 27 March 2015.

Girginov, V. 2006. "Creating a Corporate Anti-Doping Culture: The Role of Bulgarian Sports Governing Bodies." *Sport in Society* 9 (2): 252–268.

Goode, E., and Ben-Yehuda, N. 1994. "Moral Panics: Culture, Politics and Social Construction." *Annual Review of Sociology* 20 (3): 149–171.

————. 2009. *Moral Panics: The Social Construction of Deviance*. Chichester, West Sussex: Wiley-Blackwell Publishing.

The Guardian. 2009. "Murray Attacks 'Draconian' Anti-Doping Rules." *The Guardian*, 6 February 2009. http://www.theguardian.com/sport/2009/feb/06/tennis-andy-murray-anti-doping. Accessed 8 January 2015.

Guinness, R. 2014. "Banned Australian Cyclist Michael Rogers Cleared to Ride Again." *The Sydney Morning Herald*, 23 April 2014. http://www.smh.com.au/sport/cycling/banned-australian-cyclist-michael-rogers-cleared-to-ride-again-20140423-zqybj.html. Accessed 1 April 2015.

Hall, S., Critcher, C., Jefferson, J., Clarke, J., and Roberts, B. 1978. *Policing the Crisis: Mugging, the State, and Law and Order*. London: MacMillan Press.

Hanstad, D. V., and Loland, S. 2009. "Where on Earth Is Michael Rasmussen?—Is an Elite Level Athlete's Duty to Provide Information on Whereabouts Justifiable Anti-Doping Work or an Indefensible Surveillance Regime?" In *Elite Sport, Doping and Public Health*, edited by Moller, V., McNamee, M. and Dimeo, P., 167–177. Odensa: University Press of Southern Denmark.

Hanstad, D. V., Skille, E. Å., and Loland, S. 2010. "Harmonization of Anti-Doping Work: Myth or Reality?" *Sport in Society* 13 (2): 418–430.

Hawdon, J. E. 2001. "The Role of Presidential Rhetoric in the Creation of a Moral Panic: Reagan, Bush and the War on Drugs." *Deviant Behaviour* 22 (5): 419–445.

Henne, K. E., Koh, B., and McDermott, V. 2013. "Coherence of Drug Policy in Sports: Illicit Inclusions and Illegal Inconsistencies." *Performance Enhancement and Health* 2 (2): 48–55.

Herman, M. 2007. "IOC Calls on Britain to Criminalise Doping." *The Guardian*, 24 July 2007. http://sport.guardian.co.uk/breakingnews/feedstory/0,,-6801161,00.html. Accessed 26 July 2007.

Hiltzik, M. A. 2006. "Athletes' Unbeatable Foe." *Los Angeles Times*, 10 December 2006. http://articles.latimes.com/2006/dec/10/sports/sp-doping10/. Accessed 7 January 2015.

Hodgkinson, M. 2009. "US Open: Britain's Andy Murray Frustrated by 'Intrusive' Tennis Drug-Testing Protocol." *The Telegraph*, 28 August 2009. http://www.telegraph.co.uk/sport/tennis/andymurray/6106682/US-Open-Britains-Andy-Murray-frustrated-by-intrusive-tennis-drug-testing-protocol.html. Accessed 27 March 2015.

Houlihan, B. 2002. *Dying to Win*. Strasbourg Cedex: Council of Europe Publishing.

Houlihan, B. 2004. "Civil Rights, Doping Control and the World Anti-Doping Code." *Sport in Society* 7 (3): 420–437.

————. 2009. "Doping, Public Health and the Generalisation of Interests." In *Elite Sport, Doping and Public Health*, edited by Moller, V., McNamee, M. and Dimeo, P., 41–54. Odense: University Press of Southern Denmark.

Howman, D. 2012. "Developing New Alliances to Tackle the Increasing Problem of Doping in Sport." In *Doping as a Public Health Issue Symposium*. Stockholm, Sweden: World Anti-Doping Agency.

IOC (International Olympic Committee). 2000. *Olympic Movement Anti-Doping Code*, 49. Lausanne: International Olympic Committee.

————. 2013. "Olympic Charter." International Olympic Committee. http://www.olympic.org/Documents/olympic_charter_en.pdf. Accessed 9 January 2015.

————. 2014. "Professor Arne Ljungqvist." International Olympic Committee. http://www.olympic.org/professor-arne-ljungqvist. Accessed 31 January 2015.

ISM (International Sports Movement). 2007. "World Anti-Doping Agency WADA Executive Committee and Foundation Board Advance Closer to Final Revision of the World Anti-Doping Code." Sports Features Communications, 14 May 2007. http://www.sportsfeatures.com/index.php?section=pp&action=show&id=3908. Accessed 24 May 2007.

Jeffery, N. 2008. "Performance Drug Fight Stepped Up." *The Australian*, 3 May 2008. http://www.theaustralian.news.com.au/story/0,25197,23636365-5013449,00. html. Accessed 13 February 2009.

Kayser, B. 2009. "Current Anti-Doping Policy: Harm Reduction or Harm Induction?" In *Elite Sport, Doping and Public Health*, edited by Moller, V., McNamee, M. and Dimeo, P., 155–166. Odense: University Press of Southern Denmark.

Kayser, B., Mauron, A., and Miah, A. 2007. "Current Anti-Doping Policy: A Critical Appraisal." *BMC Medical Ethics* 8 (2). doi:10.1186/1472-6939-8-2.

Kidd, B., Edelman, R., and Brownell, S. 2001. "Comparative Analysis of Doping Scandals: Canada, Russia, and China." In *Doping in Elite Sport: The Politics of Drugs in the Olympic Movement*, edited by Wilson, W. and Derse, E., 153–188. Champgaign, IL: Human Kinetics.

Krabel, H. 2008. "Meet Rebekah Keat." Slowtwitch.com. http://www.slowtwitch. com/Interview/Meet_Rebekah_Keat_415.html. Accessed 17 September 2010.

Linden, J. 2010. "WADA Loses Bid to Hike Suspension of Swimmer Hardy." Reuters, 21 May 2010. http://www.reuters.com/article/2010/05/21/us-swimming-hardy-doping-idUSTRE64K49Y2010052. Accessed 25 April 2015.

Lundy, Senator the Hon Kate, and The Hon Jason Clare MP. 2012. Media release: New partnership to tackle doping in sport. Australian Government http://www.asada.gov.au/publications/media/ministerial_media_releases/ministerial_release_121016_new_partnership_to_tackle_doping.pdf. Accessed 15 April 2015.

Macur, J. 2012. "Lance Armstrong Is Stripped of His 7 Tour de France Titles." *The New York Times*, 22 October 2012. http://www.nytimes.com/2012/10/23/sports/cycling/armstrong-stripped-of-his-7-tour-de-france-titles.html?_r=. Accessed 27 March 2015.

———. 2014. *Cycle of Lies: The Fall of Lance Armstrong*. London: William Collins.

Magnay, J. 2008. "Baggaley Faces Drugs Charges in Two States." *The Sydney Morning Herald*, 2 May 2008. http://www.smh.com.au/news/sport/baggaley-faces-drugs-charges-in-two-states/2008/05/01/1209235055647.html. Accessed 13 February 2009.

Malloy, D.C., and Zakus, D.H. 2002. "Ethics of Drug Testing in Sport—An Invasion of Privacy Justified?" *Sport, Education and Society* 7 (2): 203–281.

Miah, A. 2002. "Governance, Harmonisation, and Genetics: The World Anti-Doping Agency and Its European Connections." *European Sport Management Quarterly* 2 (4): 350–369.

Møller, V. 2009. "Conceptual Confusion and the Anti-Doping Campaign in Denmark." In *Elite Sport, Doping and Public Health*, edited by Moller, V., McNamee, M. and Dimeo, P., 13–28. Odense: University Press of Southern Denmark.

Pakulski, J. 1986. "Legitimacy and Mass Compliance: Reflections on Max Weber and Soviet-Type Societies." *British Journal of Political Science* 16 (1): 35–56.

Pells, E. 2015. "Associating with Drug Cheats Forbidden in'15 Olympics code." *The China Post*, 4 January 2015. http://www.chinapost.com.tw/sports/other/2015/01/04/425592/Associating-with.htm. Accessed 7 April 2015.

Press Association. 2014. "Michael Rogers Cleared to Race as UCI Accepts Contaminated Meat Claim." *The Guardian*, 23 April 2014. http://www.theguardian.com/sport/2014/apr/23/michael-rogers-uci-contaminated-meat. Accessed 1 April 2015.

Reuters. 2008. "FINA to Tackle Super Swim Suit Issue." *The Sydney Morning Herald*, 25 March 2008. http://news.smh.com.au/fina-to-tackle-super-swim-suit-issue/20080325-21bd.html. Accessed 25 March 2008.

Robinson, S. 2007. "Drugs in Sport: A Cure Worse than the Disease?" *International Journal of Sports Science and Coaching* 2 (4): 363–368.

Rushall, B.S., and Jones, M. 2007. "Drugs in Sport: A Cure Worse Than the Disease?" *International Journal of Sports Science and Coaching* 2 (4): 335–358.

Schneider, A. 2004. "Privacy, Confidentiality and Human Rights in Sport." *Sport in Society* 7 (3): 438–456.

Schreiber, C., and Kassner, S. 2014. "Open Letter and Statement." German Athletes Commission. http://www.dosb.de/fileadmin/fm-dosb/arbeitsfelder/leistungssport/Antidoping/WADA_final_17122014__3_.pdf. Accessed 13 April 2015.

Senator the Hon Kate Lundy. 2013. Media Release: Important New Anti-Doping Powers for ASADA Pass Through Parliament. Australian Government http://www.asada.gov.au/media/ministerial.html. Accessed 15 April 2015.

Silkstone, D. 2008. "Steroids Scourge Leaps from the Sports Field into the Community." *The Age*, 20 September 2008. http://www.theage.com.au/national/steroids-scourge-leaps-from-the-sports-field-into-the-community-20080919-4k8r.html?page=. Accessed 14 November 2008.

Smith, A. C. T., and Stewart, B. 2008. "Drug Policy in Sport: Hidden Assumptions and Inherent Contradictions." *Drug and Alcohol Review* 27: 123–129.

Soek, J. 2003. "The WADA World Anti-Doping Code: The Road to Harmonisation." *The International Sports Law Journal* 2: 2–11.

Suchman, M. C. 1995. "Managing Legitimacy: Strategic and Institutional Approaches." *The Academy of Management Review* 20 (3): 571–610.

Swimming World. 2009. "Jessica Hardy Suspension Reduced to One Year, Supplement Ruled as Contaminated: USA Swimming Releases Statement: USADA Press Release; AdvoCare Disputes Findings—Updated." Swimming World. http://www.swimmingworldmagazine.com/news/jessica-hardy-suspension-reduced-to-one-year-supplement-ruled-as-contaminated-usa-swimming-releases-statement-usada-press-release-advocare-disputes-findings-updated/. Accessed 24 April 2015.

Throgmorton, J. A. 1991. "The Rhetorics of Policy Analysis." *Policy Sciences* 24 (2):153–179.

UNESCO (United Nations Educational Scientific and Cultural Organization). 2014. "Background to the Convention." United Nations Educational Scientific and Cultural Organization. http://www.unesco.org/new/en/social-and-human-sciences/themes/anti-doping/international-convention-against-doping-in-sport/background/. Accessed 3 September 2014.

USADA (United States Anti-Doping Agency). 2012. "Members of the United States Postal Service Pro-Cycling Team Doping Conspiracy, Dr. Garcia Del Moral, Dr. Ferrari and Trainer Mart Receive Lifetime Bans for Doping Violations." USADA (United States Anti-Doping Agency).

WADA (World Anti-Doping Agency). 2005. "UNESCO International Convention against Doping in Sport—Overview." World Anti-Doping Agency. http://www.wada-ama.org/en/dynamic.ch2?pageCategory.id=39. Accessed 5 February 2007.

———. 2006a. "Chairman's Message." World Anti-Doping Agency, http://www.wada-ama.org/en/dynamic.ch2?pageCategory.id=25. Accessed 5 October 2006.

———. 2006b. "The Code and Sanctions." *Play True* 3: 7–8.

———. 2006c. "Letter of Ratification—UNESCO International Convention Against Doping in Sport." World Anti-Doping Agency. http://www.wada-ama.org/rtecontent/document/WADA_Letter_Ratification_Convention_En.pdf. Accessed 5 February 2007.

———. 2006d. "Logo Story." World Anti-Doping Agency. http://www.wada-ama.org/en/dynamic.ch2?pageCategory.id=26. Accessed 9 January 2008.

———. 2006e. "The World Anti-Doping Code: A Guide." *Play True* 4 (3): 3–6.

———. 2007a. "Q&A: The World Anti-Doping Agency." World Anti-Doping Agency. http://www.wada-ama.org/rtecontent/document/QA_The_World_Anti-Doping_Agency.pdf. Accessed 9 January 2008.

———. 2007b. "Essential Partnerships." *Play True* 5 (2): 5–8.

———. 2008. "WADA Advances Cooperation with Interpol, Athlete Passport Development." World Anti-Doping Agency. http://www.wada-ama.org/en/news article.ch2?articleId=311574. Accessed 24 November 2008.

———. 2009. "World Anti-Doping Program—Governments." World Anti-Doping Agency. http://www.wada-ama.org/en/World-Anti-Doping-Program/Governments/. Accessed 11 December 2009.

———. 2009 (Jan). "WADA History." World Anti-Doping Agency. http://www. wada-ama.org/en/dynamic.ch2?pageCategory.id=31. Accessed 30 January 2009.

———. 2010. "Education and Awareness." World Anti-Doping Agency. http:// www.wada-ama.org/en/Education-Awareness/. Accessed 2 January 2011.

———. 2012a. "Code and International Standards (IS) Review." World Anti-Doping Agency. http://www.wada-ama.org/en/world-anti-doping-program/ sports-and-anti-doping-organizations/the-code/code-review/. Accessed 7 December 2012.

———. 2012b. "The World Anti-Doping Code International Standard for Testing." World Anti-Doping Agency. https://wada-main-prod.s3.amazonaws.com/ resources/files/WADA_IST_2012_EN.pdf. Accessed 3 September 2014.

———. 2013a. "2013 Anti-Doping Testing Figures—Sport Report." World Anti-Doping Agency. https://wada-main-prod.s3.amazonaws.com/resources/files/WADA-2013-Anti-Doping-Testing-Figures-SPORT-REPORT.pdf. Accessed 7 April 2015.

———. 2013b. "WADA Appoints Sir Craig Reedie as Its New President." World Anti-Doping Agency. https://www.wada-ama.org/en/media/ news/2013–11/wada-appoints-sir-craig-reedie-as-its-new-president. Accessed 31 January 2015.

———. 2014a. "Governance—Executive Committee." World Anti-Doping Agency. https://elb.wada-ama.org/en/who-we-are/governance/executive-committee. Accessed 3 September 2014.

———. 2014b. "Governance—Foundation Board." World Anti-Doping Agency. https://elb.wada-ama.org/en/who-we-are/governance/foundation-board. Accessed 3 September 2014.

———. 2014c. "International Standard for Testing and Investigations." https:// wada-main-prod.s3.amazonaws.com/resources/files/WADA-2015-ISTI-Final-EN.pdf. Accessed 8 January 2015.

———. 2014d. "A Strong, Fair Set of Rules." *Play True* (2): 12–13.

———. 2014e. "What we Do—International Standards." World Anti-Doping Agency. https://elb.wada-ama.org/en/what-we-do/international-standards. Accessed 3 September 2014.

———. 2014f. "What we Do—The Code." World Anti-Doping Agency. https:// www.wada-ama.org/en/what-we-do/the-code. Accessed 3 September 2014.

———. 2015a. "Anti-Doping Community." World Anti-Doping Agency. http:// www.wada-ama.org/en/Anti-Doping-Community/. Accessed 19 March 2015.

———. 2015b. "Code Review Process." World Anti-Doping Agency. https:// www.wada-ama.org/en/what-we-do/the-code/code-review-process. Accessed 18 March 2015.

———. 2015c. "Copenhagen Declaration—List of Signatories." World Anti-Doping Agency. https://www.wada-ama.org/en/who-we-are/anti-doping-community/gov ernments/copenhagen-declaration-list-of-signatories. Accessed 18 March 2015.

———. 2015d. "Governments." World Anti-Doping Agency. https://www.wada-ama. org/en/who-we-are/anti-doping-community/governments. Accessed 19 March 2015.

———. 2015e. "International Standards." World Anti-Doping Agency. https://elb. wada-ama.org/en/what-we-do/international-standards. Accessed 31 March 2015.

———. 2015f. "Significant Changes Between the 2009 Code and the 2015 Code." World Anti-Doping Agency. https://www.wada-ama.org/en/resources/the-code/

significant-changes-between-the-2009-code-and-the-2015-code. Accessed 24 April 2015.

———. 2015g. "World Anti-Doping Code 2015." https://wada-main-prod. s3.amazonaws.com/resources/files/wada-2015-world-anti-doping-code.pdf. Accessed 3 September 2014.

Waddington, I. 2005. "Changing Patterns of Drug Use in British Sport from the 1960s." *Sport in History* 25 (3): 472–496.

Walsh, D. 2007. *From Lance to Landis Inside the American Doping Controversy at the Tour de France*. New York: Ballantine Books.

———. 2012. *Seven Deadly Sins My Pursuit of Lance Armstrong*. London: Simon and Schuster.

Weber, M. 1969. *Economy and Society*. 2 vols. Berkeley: University of California Press.

White, R.J. 2015. "New Code Prohibits Olympic Athletes from Working with Drug Cheats." CBS Sports.com, 2 January 2015. http://www.cbssports.com/general/eye-on-sports/24931946/new-code-prohibits-olympic-athletes-from-working-with-drug-cheats. Accessed 22 March 2015.

Wuthnow, R., Hunter, J., Bergesen, A., and Kurzweil, E. 1984. *Cultural Analysis*. London: Routledge.

Zatz, M.S. 1987. "Chicano Youth Gangs and Crime: The Creation of a Moral Panic." *Contemporary Crises* 11 (2): 129–158.

4   The Australian Football League
Legitimating the War on Drugs in Sport

In response to a crisis of legitimacy for the IOC exacerbated by the 1998 Tour de France doping scandal, the creation of WADA can be conceptualized as an institutionalized moral panic to regulate PED-using 'folk devils.' WADA's establishment as the institution responsible for the global harmonization of anti-doping policy, including in professional sport, brings structural issues and power relationships between organizations, including governments, into the analysis. This reflects the complex nature of modern sport, which is constituted by a range of stakeholders with diverse interests and objectives (see Kidd et al. 2001). In this chapter, I continue to focus on contested claims to legitimacy evident in the doping debate using the Australian Football League (AFL), described as a national sporting organization (NSO), and tensions over policy approaches to drugs in sport with the Australian federal government as a case study. I specifically examine policy responses in the period following the creation of WADA and the AFL's introduction of a policy explicitly concerned with addressing the issue of illicit drug use.

Rather than a limited focus on the behavior of athlete-users as deviant individuals, this socio-historical case study approach broadens analysis of the debate to consider the influence of structural factors, such as power relationships between organizations, in the doping debate. This enables us to broaden the types of questions asked in the doping debate to include those that consider the impact of doping on sporting organizations, such as whether media reports of doping challenge the legitimacy and authority of those groups. From that perspective, implementing strict anti-doping measures is an opportunity for sporting organizations to enhance their authority by positioning themselves as 'doing the right thing' or as leaders in protecting the health or integrity of the sporting community. However, this also presents them with the challenge of ensuring their anti-doping efforts meet and support community expectations, using a rational-legal framework such as anti-doping regulations or codes of conduct. In other words, sporting and anti-doping organizations cannot take legitimacy for granted but must actively work to maintain community support.

The development of anti-doping policy by the Australian federal government and sporting organizations in Australia, including the AFL, has been well canvassed in the literature (in particular, see Stewart et al. 2004). I draw on the existing literature to discuss some key developments in order to illustrate the multi-dimensional nature of legitimacy and, by including other stakeholders and media reports, examine how claims to legitimacy are made and challenged. I begin by briefly outlining the emergence of the Australian anti-doping policy up to 1998, including the AFL's introduction of an anti-doping policy, as PED use in Australian sport became an issue of government concern. The discussion does not attempt to detail every policy initiative or drug-related event in Australian sport, but rather demonstrates that the debate around doping must be considered in the context of the broader sociopolitical environment in which it is situated. I then examine the interactions between the AFL and the Australian government, specifically in the period following WADA's establishment.

ANTI-DOPING POLICY IN AUSTRALIAN SPORT

For much of the twentieth century, little attention was paid to doping in Australian sport, including in professional sporting codes such as the AFL. This lack of concern reflected the belief that, in contrast to other nations, Australian sport was drug-free (Stewart 2006). Prior to the 1970s, the Australian federal government tended to view sport as a "purely private affair," with management left mainly to national sporting organizations (NSOs) (Booth and Tatz 2000, 163; Green 2007). However, by the latter half of the twentieth century sport had become increasingly politicized, illustrated by socialist governments' sports development models (Chapter 2, this volume) and global reactions to apartheid (Nixon 1992; Stewart et al. 2004). Providing significant impetus for greater government involvement in sport was Australia's poor 1976 Montreal Olympic performance—one silver and four bronze medals—the lowest medal count since 1936 (AOC n/d; Buti and Fridman 2001; Opie 2004). Growing evidence of links between sedentary lifestyles and preventable disease also meant that governments were increasingly aware of the role sport could play in community well-being (Stewart et al. 2004). These factors, but primarily Australia's poor Olympic performance, prompted a more interventionist government approach to sport policy (Green and Houlihan 2006). This increased government involvement in sport came to include anti-doping policy.

Recognizing that Australian athletes were part of a global sporting community in which doping took place, the Australian government instituted drug testing programs in the 1980s. These early initiatives focused on national athletes and athletes associated with the Australian Institute of Sport (AIS), which was created in 1981 in response to Australia's poor Olympic performance (Buti and Fridman 2001; Opie 2004). Commencing in January 1982, and as part of a code of ethics, all AIS scholarship holders were required to agree to undertake random drugs tests. However, tests were not carried out until 1986, when random testing was introduced first with professional athletes and then, in 1988, with all potential Australian Olympians (Buti and Fridman 1994, 2001; Green 2007; Stewart et al. 2004). Complementing the AIS, the Australian Sports Commission (ASC) was established in 1985 to deliver increased funding to NSOs, consolidate sport development programs and coordinate the government's National Program of Drugs in Sport (Anti-Drugs Campaign) (Buti and Fridman 1994). The AIS and ASC transformed the structure and operation of Australian sport and, parallel with international sport, strengthened the application of science to sport. In contrast to their earlier 'arms-length' relationship, the federal government recognized the significance of funding NSOs in order to create a pool of elite athletes, which was essntial if Australia was to restore their international reputation for sporting excellence (Stewart et al. 2004).

By the end of the 1980s, sport was an integral part of the Australian federal government's social and economic policy framework (Green 2007; Green and Houlihan 2006). Sport became tied to a range of issues that included reducing national health costs, driving economic growth and, as I discuss shortly, Australia's national identity linked to their international sporting reputation and profile (Stewart et al. 2004). Linking sporting regulation and policy to broader social issues enabled the Australian government to criticize other organizations, such as the AFL, for taking what they saw as a lax approach to drugs in sport, which I discuss later in this chapter. The AIS and ASC were central elements of a more interventionist governmental approach to sport policy, including anti-doping initiatives. However, in 1987, allegations in the media of a 'PED culture' at the AIS challenged perceptions of Australian sport as drug-free. This became a major public issue, as the AIS was intended to improve Australia's declining Olympic performance, which was widely attributed to other nations' PED use (Opie 2004). Those allegations resulted in a Senate Committee Inquiry, which led to the creation of the Australian Sports Drug Agency (ASDA) in 1990 as Australia's official drug testing body (Senate Standing Committee on Environment 1989, 1990). The response of the Australian government to the AIS doping scandal had implications for the AFL's approach to drugs in sport. The AFL recognized the potential for that scandal to challenge their legitimacy and moral authority and, as I next discuss, this contributed to their introduction of anti-doping policies.

THE AUSTRALIAN FOOTBALL LEAGUE AND
ANTI-DOPING POLICY

In 1990, after the AIS scandal and creation of ASDA, the AFL implemented an Anti-Doping Code (ADC) (Stewart 2006, 2007). Although Australian football is not an Olympic sport, the ideology underpinning the ADC closely followed that of the IOC, namely, protecting athletes' health, respect for medical and sport ethics and equality for competing athletes (AFL 2006). Like the IOC, commercialization of Australian sport during the latter half of the twentieth century saw the AFL become an administrative authority with centralized decision-making. This included a framework of rules, regulations and codes of conduct addressing a range of issues, such as racial vilification, that were binding on the clubs (e.g., see Linnell 1995; Nadel 1998a, 1998b; Pascoe 1995; Stewart et al. 2005). As part of that framework, the ADC applied to players, clubs and officials and incorporated both in and out of season testing using ASDA, with a strong focus on player education. Not only did these initiatives position the AFL as a leader in sports governance (Stewart 2006, 2007), but the ADC also played a significant role in underpinning the AFL's legitimacy. In particular, the ADC demonstrated the AFL's concern to ensure players provided positive role models in sport and the community and to maintain the image of Australian football as drug-free.

These issues would play a significant role in interactions between the AFL, the Australian government and WADA. Drawing on a figurational analysis of violence in sport, Hemphill (2002, 22) has also suggested that protecting the image and appeal of sport has become increasingly important in the modern sporting environment:

> As the sporting marketplace becomes increasingly commercial and professional, competition for broader (especially television) audiences is forcing sport leagues to deal with the more 'illegitimate' rough edges of sport and make them palatable to larger, especially younger audience members.

Thus, claims to legitimacy have become linked to sport's commercial viability and the ability of sporting organizations, including the AFL, to attract and maintain audience support.

During the 1990s, the AFL pursued a commercial agenda, expanding into a 16-team national competition, raising match attendances and increasing broadcasting rights (Andrews 2000; Pascoe 1997). This success at the elite level had consequences for the grassroots development of the game, as national expansion and increased television coverage led to a "serious slide in the numbers playing amateur football and attending local games" (McKay 1996, *The Age*). Coupled with growth in the number of sporting 'choices,' this meant that maintaining the image and appeal of the AFL was increasingly important in terms of building participation rates and developing the sport. In this context, and as reports of PED use emerged in other Australian sports, the ADC became a central part of the regulatory processes supporting the AFL's legitimacy. In 1991, Australian cyclists Carey Hall, Stephen Pate and Martin Vinnicombe received two-year suspensions after testing positive for steroids. In 1995, Australia's leading track sprinter, Dean Capobianco, as well as a Western Reds rugby league player tested positive for Stanozolol. An internal Western Reds investigation revealed that between six to 15 of their players had been taking steroids (Stewart 2007). Despite ongoing reports that professional and Olympic athletes were testing positive for PEDs, the AFL at this time successfully kept the appearance of Australian football as PED-free. Nevertheless, incidents of drug use did eventually emerge in Australian football, challenging its status as a drug-free community and the legitimacy of its anti-doping policy.

Drug related incidents in this early period of the ADC that are most commonly discussed are Justin Charles (Richmond Football Club) and Alastair Lynch (Brisbane Lions Football Club), the only two AFL players to appear before the AFL Tribunal for PED use (Lane 2006a, *The Age*). Stewart et al. (2008) note the cases of Steven Koops (Freemantle Dockers Football Club) and Nick Stone (West Coast Eagles Football Club), which are also relevant to consider in terms of the AFL's claims to organizational legitimacy underpinned by the ADC. In 1997, Charles tested positive for Boldanone (a steroid). Although arguing its use was to assist in recovery from a muscle tear, he received a suspension for the first 16 premiership matches of the 1998 season (Stewart et al. 2008). What was significant in terms of the AFL's legitimacy was that inconsistencies under the ADC soon became apparent. Only days after announcing Charles's result, *The Age* newspaper revealed that Ilija Grgic (West Coast Eagles Football Club) had tested positive for an over-the-counter cold remedy, resulting in a club fine (Linnell 1997; Stewart et al. 2008). Grgic was not the first player to test positive for a stimulant with claims that a third player, whose identity 'remained a mystery,' also returned a positive test (Johnson 1997, *The Age*; Murphy 1997). In contrast to Charles's 16-match ban, a club fine and failure to reveal a player's identity suggested inconsistent applications of sanctions under the ADC.

These events enabled the AFL to introduce tougher controls against players as well as clubs, illustrating that the introduction of stricter measures of control underpins attempts by dominant groups to maintain the legitimacy to exercise their authority (Weber 1969). The amended rules were presented as part of a "streamlined process" intended to reduce complexity and provide "the league with greater flexibility." At the same time they also increased the AFL's power over clubs and players (Linnell 1998, *The Age*). Previously, players had been permitted to play in feeder competitions while waiting to appear before the AFL Tribunal. Under the new rules, a positive test meant an automatic playing ban until their Tribunal appearance. The new provisions also meant that clubs could be brought before the Tribunal with club doctors or other officials "automatically deemed to have breached the code" and "liable for hefty penalties" (Linnell 1998, *The Age*). The cases of Charles and Grgic were not the only drug-related events in the late 1990s that highlighted inconsistencies under the ADC leading the AFL to regulatory reform.

Further inconsistencies in the ADC became apparent in 1998 when Alastair Lynch appeared before the AFL Tribunal for Dehydroepiandrosterone

(DHEA) use. Lynch claimed that ASDA advised him DHEA was permissible to assist in recovery from chronic fatigue syndrome. At that time the ADC did not include therapeutic use exemptions and an exemption was denied. The fact that Lynch was held accountable for receiving treatment for a non-football related illness raised questions over players' rights to legitimate medical treatments available to the wider community (Lane 2006a, *The Age*; Stewart et al. 2008). As Lynch stated, "as there is no flexibility in the AFL drug code, all matters relating to this aspect of the game must be referred to the AFL Tribunal . . . my only intention . . . was to fight for my quality of life" (cited in Rielly 1998, *The Age*). In 1999, less than 24 hours after knee surgery, Steven Koops (Freemantle Dockers Football Club) tested positive for Pethidine. This again raised questions surrounding players' rights under the ADC to use legitimate medication available outside football. Pethidine was prohibited due to its potential to place athletes' health at risk and its restricted access in the community (Blair 2005, *The Bulletin*; Stewart et al. 2008). The AFL Tribunal did not sanction Koops. However, like Lynch, his case suggested inequities in the ADC over players' rights to make use of medication that, while restricted, was available to the wider community (Stewart et al. 2008).

The AFL responded to these cases by modifying the ADC. Pethidine became a restricted 'in-competition' substance and rules were introduced to prevent players in circumstances similar to Koops from being tested (Duffield 2002, *The Age*; Hagdorn 2001, *Sunday Herald-Sun*; Timms 2002, *Herald Sun*). Modifications linked to the Lynch case included adding therapeutic use exemptions to the ADC and changing sanctions to a two-year suspension for a first offense for steroids, stimulants and diuretics used as masking agents. A second offense would result in a life-time suspension (Stewart 2006). Amendments to the ADC suggest that the AFL recognized the implications for their legitimacy of an inconsistent anti-doping policy. The Lynch incident was particularly significant, as it not only prompted changes to the ADC but also exposed inconsistencies across anti-doping policies in Australian sport more broadly, contributing to a government review of anti-doping policy (Stewart 2007).

Consideration of the Charles, Grgic and Lynch events is also useful in terms of considering the doping debate as a moral panic. After the Charles incident and details of Grgic's positive test became public, media reports suggested that drug use in the AFL was a problem of increasing proportions. One report described the Grgic incident as the "latest AFL drug furor" (Linnell 1997, *The Age*). Another said that AFL had a "a serious problem with steroids" with "increasing numbers of players . . . turning to performance-enhancing substances" (Schwartz and Connolly 1997, *Sunday Age*). Reinforcing suggestions that drug use was widespread in the AFL, the report cited claims from the Victorian Director of the International Federation of Body Builders that AFL players regularly approached him for advice about beating the drugs tests and that Charles was "the tip of the iceberg" (Schwartz and Connolly 1997, *Sunday Age*). Reports surrounding the 1998 Tour de France doping scandal also implied drug use in cycling was symptomatic of a larger problem across elite sport (Chapter 2, this volume). Media coverage described the Lynch case as "the possibility of another drug scandal" and "the specter of a third scandal" (Rielly 1998, *The Age*). These types of reports created a "public relations disaster" for the AFL (Stewart 2007, 70). Exaggerated claims that drug use was widespread in the AFL fit within a moral panic framework and, by creating the impression that a drug culture permeated Australian football, implied that the AFL's anti-doping approach was flawed. This raised doubt over their legitimacy and moral authority to govern the game.

Illustrating the contested nature of claims to legitimacy and stakeholders' use of the media to respond to those challenges, the AFL used media reports to emphasize that their drug-testing program was effective. They pointed out that "tests in relation to recreational drugs . . . show that 2 per cent of footballers showed some sort of residue—which is very low in regard to community standards" (Schwartz and Connolly 1997, *Sunday Age*). Using statistics to respond to the panics, the AFL tried to emphasize that their anti-doping policy successfully met community expectations regarding illicit drug use. As I noted earlier in this chapter, maintaining the image of Australian football as a 'clean' and safe sporting environment was an important part of building participation rates and developing the sport.

Different stakeholders respond to PEDs in ways that reflect the diverse objectives relevant to their particular communities. The AFL responded to the government's reaction to the AIS doping scandal by introducing the ADC as one of a range of rules and regulations that underpinned the AFL's legitimacy. This helped maintain their position as a leader in sporting administration, including drug free sport. Drug-related incidents in Australian football in the late 1990s demonstrated that this legitimacy could not be taken for granted. These events also reveal that media reports constitute a site where stakeholders' claims to legitimacy can be challenged and defended. Moral panic criteria, such as exaggerated or disproportional claims of the extent of drug use, are also evident in media reports discussing drug use in Australian football. For the Australian federal government, the AIS scandal contributed to a strengthening of Australian sport policy, which, as I discuss in the next section, included linking sport explicitly to community welfare. This enabled them to question the legitimacy of the AFL's anti-doping policy based on the role of sport in community well-being. Also at issue for the Australian federal government were the implications for their global reputation as a leader in anti-doping, which was emphasized in their response to the 1998 Tour de France scandal and establishment of WADA. These issues are discussed in the next section, with a focus on AFL's interaction with the Australian federal government in the period after WADA's creation.

ANTI-DOPING POLICY IN AUSTRALIAN FOOTBALL:
POST-1998 TOUR DE FRANCE

In the wake of the 1998 Tour de France doping scandal, the Australian federal government strongly supported tougher anti-doping measures, co-chairing the International Intergovernmental Consultative Group on Anti-Doping in Sport (IICGADS 1999; Chapter 3, this volume). In 1999, the Australian federal government implemented the *Tough on Drugs in Sport* policy to deliver a national drug education and enforcement strategy (ASDA 1999; Commonwealth of Australia 2001a; ISR 1999c; Parham 2008; Stewart 2007). This also reflected the government's zero tolerance of illicit drug use in the community under the National Illicit Drug Strategy (also known as 'Tough on Drugs'), which was launched in 1997 and focused on catching drug traffickers, rehabilitation and community drug prevention education (AAP 2006; AIC 2009). Delivered through the ASC, *Tough on Drugs in Sport* strengthened sport policy to require that NSOs implement a government-defined anti-doping policy to access federal funding (ASC 1999; Stewart 2006). The Australian government understood the potential for negative perceptions of legitimacy should NSOs fail to meet community expectations around 'clean' sport. Thus, the *Tough on Drugs in Sport* policy "encouraged" professional sporting organizations, "such as Rugby League and Australian Rules," to continue testing in order to "protect the image of these high profile sports" (ISR 1999b). More specifically, this policy positioned the Australian federal government as world leaders in anti-doping, which enhanced their authority to question the legitimacy of other organizations' anti-doping approach, such as the AFL, as I discuss shortly.

The *Tough on Drugs in Sport* policy was an important tool used to promote Australia's international reputation by delivering a model of sporting administration and technology that developed elite athletes while also keeping sport PED-free. The timing of the *Tough on Drugs in Sport* launch in 1999 was directly concerned with ensuring that no drug scandals would tarnish Australia's anti-doping reputation at the 2000 Sydney Olympics (ISR 1999a). As the first Olympics after the creation of WADA, the 2000 Sydney Games took place during a time of heightened public and regulatory attention to PEDs. This also provided the Australian federal government a "unique" opportunity to "push a strong 'tough on drugs' agenda" (ISR 1999c). The government exploited this opportunity, promoting Australia's sports delivery systems to a worldwide audience (ISR 1999a; see also Hanstad and Loland 2009). Further, the "comprehensive" *Tough on Drugs in Sport* strategy bolstered Australia's international reputation as a "world leader in the fight against drugs in sport" by providing the "clearest example for the world to follow" (ISR 1999a). Then Minister for Sport and Tourism, Jackie Kelly, stressed the government's opposition to doping on the basis that it "violates the integrity of sport" and "strikes at the heart of fair play and the true spirit of competition" (ISR 1999a). However, positioning

Australia as a 'clean' sporting nation meant balancing marketing of their efforts as leaders in sports technology while downplaying any reliance on "technologies to enhance bodily performance" (Magdalinski 2000, 307). This required the Australian government to take a strong anti-doping stance.

Illustrating the political dimension of the doping debate, the Australian federal government linked 'clean' sport to Australia's national identity. Sport is often presented as integral to Australia's "collective identity" and "sense of self" associated with values such as "mateship" and an egalitarian tradition of a "fair go" (Booth 1995; McKay 1986, 347; McKay and Roderick 2010; Stewart et al. 2004, 9; Stoddart 1986, 71). A more critical analysis reveals that these values are not unique to the Australian context and that sport in Australia, as elsewhere, is far from egalitarian (Toohey and Taylor 2009). Sport can also be associated with social division and conflict as structural issues, such as socioeconomic status and gender inequality, continue to restrict participation (McKay 1986; Tonts and Atherley 2010). Nevertheless, popular presentations describe Australians as "the most sports-obsessed people on the planet" (Chandrasekaran 2000) and sport as the "opiate of the Australian masses . . . to be uninterested . . . is to be an outcast in the land of the unending quest for sporting glory" (Barker 2004, 62, cited in Tonts and Atherley 2010, 384). Stewart et al. (2004, 9) note that for Australia, as a "small country with only 20 million inhabitants . . . geographically isolated from the rest of the world, sporting success is a highly visible and potent way of achieving global media exposure and international awareness."

The government linked the *Tough on Drugs in Sport* policy to the centrality of 'clean' sport in the Australian national identity. Australia's sporting achievements were constructed as integral to Australia's way of life and national pride and, consequently, there was "no place . . . for cheats . . . especially those who try to gain some advantage by using banned drugs" (ISR 1999a). The ASC also drew on the notion that sport was integral to the Australian national identity and also linked sport to providing health, social and economic benefits for the Australian community (ASC 1999). By linking the *Tough on Drugs in Sport* policy to qualities at the core of Australian national identity, the government added weight to the importance of a strong stance against doping.

The Australian federal government claimed to be the legitimate representative of Australia's interests and community expectations to achieve sporting success, including drug-free sport, associated with a "progressive, egalitarian" Australian society (ASC 1999). To maintain Australia's status as a "world-leading nation in the fight against drugs in sport," the ASC was charged with the responsibility for a "national policy which requires all NSOs to have an anti-doping policy as a condition of funding" (ASC 1999). These claims demonstrate that particular objectives influenced the Australian federal government response to PED use in sport. From this perspective, drug scandals in Australian sport, such as the AIS scandal, not only carried the potential to damage Australia's international reputation, but also suggested that the Australian federal government had failed to meet community expectations of 'clean' international sporting success. Community expectations around drug-free sport formed part of the Australian government's challenge to the AFL's policy responses to drugs in sport, which I discuss later in this chapter.

Importantly, maintaining Australia's reputation as a world leader against doping also had an economic dimension. The ASC (1999, 37) noted that sport played a significant role in meeting the government's economic goals, such as "increased employment . . . and overall economic growth rate of 4 per cent per annum over the next decade." With sport seen as a significant contributor to the Australian economy, and the government committed to supporting the sport and leisure industry in reaching an AUD$1.3 billion per year export target by 2006, keeping sport drug-free was important (Commonwealth of Australia 2001b, iii, v). One policy initiative centrally linked to this process was the 2001 *Backing Australia's Sporting Ability: A More Active Australia* policy (Green 2007). As part of connecting Australia's sporting success to a "thriving sport and leisure industry," the policy included working with NSOs to "escalate the fight against drug cheats" (Commonwealth of Australia 2001a, 4, 10). The policy emphasized the Australian government's support for WADA, demonstrated by membership on the WADA Board, executive and sub-committees and funding of AUD$1,000,000 (Commonwealth of Australia 2001a, 10–11). As well as economic goals, the *Backing Australia's Sporting Ability* policy was underpinned by two other objectives.

On the one hand, the policy worked to improve community well-being by increasing community participation in organized sport. Sport was described as a "vital factor" in building strong communities by preventing socially unacceptable behavior, including drug use, and providing "an enduring message of . . . healthy, drug-free lifestyles to school children and local communities" (Commonwealth of Australia 2001a, 1, 6–7). This reflected the Australian government's conservative approach to issues of law and order, including a 'zero tolerance' approach to illicit drugs (Dept. of Health and Ageing 2001; Mendes 2001). The other, and primary, policy focus was to maintain Australia's status as a successful sporting nation by identifying a future pool of elite sporting talent (Commonwealth of Australia 2001a; Stewart et al. 2004; Toohey 2010). Also at work here was the notion that successful elite sport would create a 'trickle down' effect and increase participation in recreational sport, thus helping to address declining levels of physical fitness and rising obesity levels in the community (Green and Houlihan 2006; Toohey 2010, 2772). However, Toohey (2010) writes that although federal sport funding had reached record levels, elite sport was the primary beneficiary, receiving approximately 75 percent of available funding. As Green (2007) points out, this policy approach suggests a greater concern on the part of government with securing a better return on investment in the form of (medal-winning) Olympians rather than any 'trickle down' community benefit. Nevertheless, positioning sport as important for social well-being provided a foundation for presenting drugs in sport as threatening social order or, in other words, as a moral panic.

For the AFL, there were significant consequences flowing from the government's policy approach, as discussed above, and support for WADA. The AFL had implemented the ADC in 1990, well before the establishment of WADA, with reports from ASDA suggesting they were successful in this area. For example, the *2000–01 ASDA Annual Report* noted that of 534 tests, one player tested positive for amphetamines and one for methamphetamine (ASDA 2001). In 2001–02, ASDA carried out 523 tests on Australian footballers, with no positive tests for either PEDs or illicit drugs (ASDA 2002). However, as we have seen, the Australian government used policy mechanisms to associate PED-free sport with reducing illicit drug use and community cohesion.

In such a context, and problematically for the AFL, rather than PEDs, reports of illicit drug use in Australian football emerged as an issue. Although none of ASDA's 522 tests for PEDs in 2003–04 returned a positive result, the AFL's private testing agency reported 31 positive tests for illicit drugs (14 in 2003 and 17 in 2004) (Albergo 2007; ASDA 2003). In 2004, two Carlton Football Club players, Laurence Angwin and Karl Norman, attended training under the influence of recreational drugs (*ABC Premium News* 2004). Angwin was sacked from the club. While not delisted, Norman agreed to sign a 'legally-binding document' with stringent conditions including counseling and regular drug testing (Stevens 2004, *The Daily Telegraph*; Stevens and Barrett 2004, *Herald Sun*). The ADC did not include disciplinary measures for illicit drug use, with only out-of-competition "statistical testing" conducted for those substances (AFL 2007, 2). The AFL used the media to deny widespread drug use in Australian football, pointing out that no more than three percent of players had tested positive for recreational drugs (Stevens, Phillips and Cunningham 2004, *The Mercury*).

Nevertheless, incidents of illicit drug use in the AFL had implications for their legitimacy. In contrast to the Australian government's zero tolerance approach, the AFL saw illicit drug use as a social issue, and focused on player anonymity, education, rehabilitation and counseling. This approach created tension between the AFL and the Australian government, with WADA criticizing the AFL's approach to illicit drug use as 'soft.' The Australian government's approach was linked to their promotion of drug-free sport using the *Tough on Drugs in Sport* and *Backing Australia's Sporting Ability* policies, in which athletes were presented as positive role models who contributed to the elimination of illicit drug use and building healthy, cohesive communities (ASC 1999; Commonwealth of Australia 2001a). The federal government had also pointed out in the *Tough on Drugs in Sport* policy the potential negative impact on NSO's legitimacy for any failure to meet community expectations to keep sport drug-free (ISR 1999b). Consequently, in February 2005 and to complement the ADC (which remained in place), the AFL introduced a *separate* Illicit Drugs Policy (IDP), the first professional sporting body in the world to do so (Davies 2005, *The Bulletin*). The AFL's response to incidents of illicit drug use demonstrates that negative perceptions of legitimacy tend to generate regulatory mechanisms that are presented as in accordance with community expectations (Chapter 1, this volume).

The IDP dealt specifically with out-of-competition illicit drug use, including cannabis, cocaine and ecstasy (Davies 2005, *The Bulletin*). As well as rehabilitation and counseling, the IDP focused strongly on player anonymity and education and recognized their responsibility as positive role models for young athletes as well as others in the community (Gleeson 2006, *The Age*; Horvath 2006; Smith 2006a, *The Australian*). In line with the ADC, the IDP included in and out of competition testing as well as pre-and post-match testing and what came to be described as the 'three strike' ruling. Under the IDP, a first offense required private counseling, a second offense meant attendance at a rehabilitation program, with a third offense resulting in club notification, referral to a disciplinary tribunal and possible suspension (Stewart 2006). The AFL maintained a strong anti-PED approach, with a two-year suspension for a first offense and a lifetime suspension for a second offense. According to the AFL's medical officers, after the introduction of the IDP there had been a "significant fall in cannabis detection and . . . none in the match-day testing" (cited in Demetriou 2005a, 6). From the perspective of the AFL, these results suggested success in keeping Australian football drug free, bolstering perceptions of their legitimacy and moral authority.

The AFL took a strong regulatory approach to illicit and PED use in Australian football. This suggests recognition of the implications for their legitimacy if they failed to implement a framework that met community expectations. However, illustrating the contested nature of claims to legitimacy, critics of the AFL, such as the Australian federal government and WADA, argued that the relatively small number of positive tests demonstrated a flawed policy that failed to detect "doping cheats" (Stewart et al. 2008, 69). As I discuss shortly, the use of statistics in this debate also fits within a moral panic framework, where figures can be used to support, or challenge, claims to legitimacy. Along with the AFL's reluctance to recognize WADA's authority to regulate Australian football for PEDs, the primary area of disagreement between the AFL, WADA and the Australian government surrounded illicit drugs. The media played an important role by providing opportunities for different stakeholders to challenge claims to legitimacy and respond to those challenges.

MEDIATING THE AFL, WADA AND THE AUSTRALIAN FEDERAL GOVERNMENT

Taking a punitive public naming and shaming approach, WADA applied the same penalty to illicit and PED use, underpinned by the view that illicit drugs are equally contrary to values that are intrinsic to sport (Horvath 2006; Stewart 2006). The Australian federal government supported the WADC and agreed that both illicit drugs and PEDs were cheating, against the spirit of sport and damaging to athletes' health (Stewart 2007). Ensuring that all local sporting codes, including the AFL, adopted a WADA-aligned model had significant implications for the Australian government's reputation as world-leaders in anti-doping, both domestically and internationally. As Davies (2005, *The Bulletin*) reported: "With an eye to Australia's anti-drugs reputation . . . the three codes [the AFL, National Rugby League (NRL) and Cricket Australia] . . . will lose all Federal funding if they fail to sign [the WADC]." However, all three codes disputed WADA's authority to regulate their respective sporting communities and were reluctant to sign the WADC (Horvath 2006). A main point of contention for these professional sports was the use of legal drugs, such as probenecid and glucocorticoid-steroids, commonly used in football and cricket. The codes argued that these drugs were rehabilitative rather than performance enhancing even though they were prohibited under the WADC. Heightening the debate were the WADC's sanctions for cannabis use, which the codes argued was non-performance enhancing (*ABC Sport* 2005; Davies 2005, *The Bulletin*).

Professional sports organizations, such as cricket, AFL, NRL and rugby union, were also concerned over WADA's more punitive approach in the 'three strikes and out' policy. In contrast to the AFL's three strike rule, under the WADC a first offense could mean a three- to 12-month suspension, a second offense attracted a maximum two-year penalty and a third offense could mean a lifetime ban (Stewart 2006). Players could also receive a mandatory two-year ban if they failed to make themselves available for testing on three successive occasions (Masters 2004, *The Sydney Morning Herald*; Chapter 3, this volume). Although contesting WADA's approach to illicit drugs, the AFL publicly supported the principles underpinning WADA's framework that PEDs were unfair and unethical. The AFL also supported the government's zero tolerance of illicit drug use in sport (Demetriou 2005a; Horvath 2006). However, the AFL argued that, as WADA was created with a focus on countering drug-taking in Olympic sports, it was better suited for sports other than Australian football, which was not an Olympic sport.

From the perspective of the AFL, not only was the IDP more appropriate for Australian football but it also complied with the spirit and intention of the WADC and, in some areas, was more rigorous (Demetriou 2005a). For example, testing for illicit drugs under the AFL's IDP covered a 44-week period, a timeframe that exceeded other Australian sporting codes as well as WADA's testing regime (Demetriou 2005a; Horvath 2006). Under the WADC, out-of competition testing did not test for amphetamines, cocaine, ecstasy and cannabis and, despite claiming to incorporate a concern with athletes' health, did not contain any rehabilitation measures (Horvath 2006). In contrast, the AFL views illicit drug use as a social issue requiring counseling and education rather than heavy sanctions. The AFL continued to view PEDs as the more "insidious drug problem" (Stewart 2006, 111), but remained determined to enforce their authority to govern the Australian football community. AFL CEO, Andrew Demetriou (2005a, 7), clearly stated that the organization maintained the "right to create rules and regulations . . . for the good of our competition, while being keenly aware of our social responsibilities and our responsibilities to our players . . . at all levels." These comments reveal how this debate is concerned with issues of governance and control.

The AFL presented their right to authority in terms of a concern with player welfare, which is a central part of the AFL's claim to legitimacy under the IDP. The AFL stressed that they took an inclusive approach to drug use in sport that did not simply focus on elite competition but incorporated all levels of the Australian football community. In other words, the AFL argued that they were concerned with building healthy communities, an element that was central to the approach of the Australian federal government to sport policy. The interactions between the Australian federal government and the AFL demonstrate that different stakeholders bring particular objectives to the debate around drugs in sport, which is also influenced by contested power relationships between organizational actors.

The AFL's reluctance to become WADA-compliant had implications for the Australian government's focus on building healthy communities using sport, as indicated in *Backing Australia's Sporting Ability* policy. At the same time, the AFL's resistance to implementing a WADC-aligned anti-PED framework risked the loss of government funding for sport development initiatives, such as the Auskick grassroots sport program (Horvath 2006; Stewart et al. 2008). Under the ASC's Targeted Sports Participation Growth (TSPG) initiative, the AFL received AUD$1,000,000 for Auskick, which focused on primary-school aged children (Green 2007; Stewart et al. 2004). The AFL's position in the TSPG program was significant because they had a demonstrated ability to help the government achieve their policy goals of increased sporting participation (Stewart et al. 2004). The AFL also risked the loss of an estimated AUD$10 million in grants from a range of government departments for initiatives that focused on indigenous support and welfare as well as issues such as childhood obesity, anti-smoking and multicultural development (Johnson 2005, *The Age*; Lane 2005a, *The Sunday Age*). The federal government attempted to use this as leverage in order to secure the AFL's compliance, stating: "if they [the AFL] don't come on board we will find other ways. It's not as if we won't fund those programs any more, it just means we won't fund them through the AFL" (in Lane 2005a, *The Sunday Age*). This highlights that contested power relationships between organizational actors are part of the debate around drugs in sport.

The government continued to emphasize that their strong anti-drugs approach was fundamentally concerned with ensuring community welfare and building strong communities. WADA criticized the AFL for failing to sign the WADC and for the decision to adopt a separate illicit drugs policy:

If they've got such a big problem that they have to run a separate program to counsel all of those who are playing . . . to be off illicit drugs . . . I think they've got a big problem . . . they should be addressing that in a more aggressive and more positive approach. (WADA Director-General David Howman in *ABC Sport* 2005)

This is a tautological statement. Nevertheless, it shows how 'a big problem' can be amplified, and it challenged the legitimacy of the AFL's anti-doping framework. It was symptomatic of the production of doping as a moral panic with suggestions that drug use in Australian football was a growing problem that required a strong regulatory approach. The potential loss of federal government funding for sports development programs, which are important for the ongoing sustainability of the code, was a significant issue for the AFL. Consequently, and with both the NRL and Cricket Australia finally acquiescing to the WADC, in 2005 the AFL agreed to become WADC-compliant for PEDs for the 2006 season (*ABC Sport* 2005; Demetriou 2005b). Although the AFL is not an international or Olympic sport, the government linked the AFL's WADC-compliance to Australia's international reputation as a leader in anti-doping. As then Minister for Arts and Sport, Senator Kemp (2005) stated:

The AFL now joins all major sporting codes in Australia in becoming WADA code compliant. Australia has been acknowledged as world leaders in fighting drugs in sport and will continue to pursue a sporting environment in which athletes are able to compete fairly.

The Australian government continued to strengthen policy and legislation to regulate the Australian sporting community and maintain their international reputation as leaders in drug-free sport. For example, in 2006 ASDA was renamed the Australian Sports Anti-Doping Authority (ASADA) with its powers and responsibilities extended to incorporate investigation into drug trafficking and possession (DCITA 2005; Stewart 2007). Since its establishment, ASADA has developed extensive information-sharing networks with police, customs and immigration officers (Jeffery 2008, *The Australian*; Magnay 2008, *The Sydney Morning Herald*). As well as enhancing the government's anti-doping reputation, strengthening regulation against drug use challenged the claims of other stakeholders to legitimacy, such as the AFL. From a moral panic perspective, this also demonstrates the 'widening the net' principle when connections between and among enforcement agencies are activated or strengthened (Cohen 2002; Goode and Ben-Yehuda 2009).

The AFL again came under pressure in 2006, as claims emerged that three senior players had twice tested positive for illicit drugs in out-of-competition testing. Despite demands to reveal the players' identities, and although details had been leaked to the media, the AFL won a court injunction preventing publication of the players' names (Hedge 2006, *Sunday Times*;

Wilson 2006a, *Herald Sun*). The leaking of players' names to the media had significant implications for the legitimacy of the IDP, which enjoyed player support based on the AFL's assurances of strict confidentiality and focus on player health and welfare (Cooper 2006, *AAP Sports News Wire*; *The Australian* 2006). Senior players, such as Peter Bell (AFLPA President and Freemantle Dockers Football Club captain) indicated their concerns: "Now that the confidentiality has been undermined, the integrity of the system as a whole is seriously in question" (Cooper and Fiamengo 2006, *AAP Sports News Wire*). The AFL also came under pressure from high profile AFL coaches, who called for club notification of any positive drug tests (*ABC Premium News* 2006; Lane 2006b, *Sunday Age*).

Media reports drew on these concerns to claim that the IDP lacked public support. As one report stated: "the fans consider it absurdly over-protective, secretive and a sham" and described (unidentified) drug-using players as "lame-brains" (Roach 2006, *The Advertiser*). Other reports categorized the AFL's illicit drug policy as "devised purely for the protection of AFL players who have recreational drug habits . . . they really treat all drug users with a feather instead of a cane" (Wilson 2006e, *The Advertiser*). Some media reports criticized the AFL's policy as "tacit approval of recreational drug abuse . . . the biggest problem in . . . elite sport full of young men earning a lot of money" (Wilson 2006d, *The Advertiser*). Other reports used former players to support claims that the "use of recreational drugs is more widespread than ever" and that the leaked tests were the "tip of an iceberg" (Pierik 2006, *The Mercury*; see also Murphy 2006, *The Australian*). Several elements of a moral panic are evident in these reports. In a moral panic there are suggestions that the dangerous behavior is widespread, or as the report suggests, 'the tip of an iceberg.' Similar claims were made in the media following the 1998 Tour de France scandal, with implications for the IOC's legitimacy (Chapter 2, this volume). In the media reports discussing the AFL's IDP, a 'folk devil' responsible for the problematic behavior, in this case drug-using 'lame brains,' is clearly identified. These individuals challenge the stability of sport by failing in their responsibilities as positive role models for youth.

An elites-engineered moral panic framework is useful in this context, as it illustrates that to enhance or challenge claims to legitimacy, stakeholder groups use media reports to construct 'folk devils.' These socially constructed 'folk devils' took the form of individual performance-enhancing or illicit drug-using athletes as well as institutional actors. Claims that the AFL failed to implement anti-doping regulations that upheld community values and ideals associated with drug-free sport raised questions about their legitimacy and constructed the AFL as an institutional 'folk devil.' There was bipartisan political support for the view that the AFL's anti-doping approach failed to meet community expectations and, more specifically, was undermining the government's zero tolerance approach (Magnay 2006, *The Sydney Morning Herald*). This challenged the legitimacy of the AFL and put pressure on them to "show leadership" (Magnay 2006, *The Sydney Morning Herald*). According to the Federal Minister for Arts and Sport, the IDP was not:

> . . . rigorous enough . . . I have called on the AFL to have another look at their code . . . and look more closely at how the sanctions are applied and how the reporting arrangements are applied . . . and have some tougher sanctions and a more open and transparent reporting process. (in Magnay 2006, *The Sydney Morning Herald*)

In a moral panic, linking the deviant behavior to broader social issues reinforces the idea that the social order is threatened. The media reports on illicit drug use in Australian football created the idea that not only was the problem widespread and tolerated in that sporting community but explicitly linked this to drug addiction in the wider community. One report suggested that the AFL's CEO should consider the "thousands of kids" that "have stuffed their lives using these so-called recreational drugs" and that the AFL should "start again on its drugs policy and fall into line with other sports and codes. Defending the indefensible is starting to wear very thin indeed" (Wilson 2006d, *The Advertiser*). Another report argued that ". . . the three AFL players (so far unnamed) who took illegal drugs should be matters for the criminal justice system, not just for sports administrators. . . . Not only are the drug-takers afforded complete privacy, there is almost no chance that their suppliers will be caught" (*The Gold Coast Bulletin* 2006). There are implications here for the legitimacy of dominant groups, in this case the AFL. These types of constructions suggest that drug use in sport has the potential to spread to the wider community and is a particular problem that necessitates a specific response in the form of strong anti-drug regulations to meet community expectations. In other words, these reports illustrate doping as an institutionalized moral panic underpinned by elite claim-makers' concerns for maintaining positive perceptions of legitimacy.

The AFL was committed to retaining their authority to govern and control Australian football while also meeting community expectations around drug-free sport. They continued to apply the WADA compliant in-competition ADC as well as the separate out-of-competition IDP with a focus on education and rehabilitation: "We think the community expects a tough stance and that's why we've implemented out-of-competition for illicit drugs" (in Wilson 2006b, *Herald Sun*). Nevertheless, the IDP drew significant criticism from a range of stakeholders, such as the Australian Olympic Committee (AOC), government, media, clubs, players and others. The media and stakeholders, such as the AOC, criticized the IDP focus on player welfare as deflecting attention from 'the real issue.' They claimed that irrespective of whether it was illicit drugs or PEDs, these substances symbolized cheating and were against the fundamental values of sport. For example, although congratulating the AFL for a focus on player welfare, nevertheless, the code was criticized because despite an education program that included alcohol and drugs and that cost "1.5 million annually . . . at some stage they [players] must take responsibility . . . they are protected to such an extent the good health of the competition is at risk. The AFL's determination to be seen as the sport with the keenest social conscience has led to bad policy . . . " (Smith 2006b, *The Australian*).

Media reports cited stakeholders, such as AOC official Kevan Gospar, that were critical of the AFL because "any drug use is cheating . . . putting players' health at risk." Not only was the AFL "protecting the cheats" but this was also the "wrong message to send to children." Fundamentally, however, the issue was the "damage" to Australia's international "reputation . . . the AFL can't have it both ways and set their own rules. . . . Cocaine and cannabis are illicit drugs . . . there are significant health and social issues with these drugs . . . " (AOC official Kevan Gospar in Wilson 2006c, *The Australian*). These challenges to the AFL's legitimacy were based on claims that their policy framework failed to deal effectively with the problem of drug use in the Australian football community. More specifically, however, these claims suggest that the AFL's tolerant approach to drug use in sport threatened the social order and challenged Australia's international reputation as a world leader in anti-doping regulation. As we have seen in this chapter, Australia's reputation as a successful, and 'clean,' sporting nation plays a central role in constructions of the Australian national identity.

Demonstrating the contested and multi-dimensional nature of legitimacy, in addition to the Australian federal government and WADA, stakeholders from within the Australian football community also criticized the IDP. For example, the Hawthorne Football Club 'strongly requested' greater sharing of information by notifying at least one club official of a positive test. The Adelaide and Port Adelaide Football Clubs called for a reduction of the 'three strikes rule' to two strikes (Barrett and Williams 2007, *Fox Sports*). Some players, such as Geelong Football Club captain Tom Harley, also felt that the IDP contained 'loopholes.' This was perceived as a particular issue in a code comprised of young men, which Harley described as "risk takers" that would "look for loopholes and find them" (Anderson 2007, *Herald Sun*). Harley was here referring to West Coast Eagles Football Club star player Ben Cousins, who was sacked in 2007 following a range of alcohol and behavior related issues. The AFL banned Cousins for 12 months for bringing the game into disrepute (AAP 2009; Wilson 2007, *The Daily Telegraph*). Cousins later admitted being a 'drug addict,' although he never failed a drug test for either illicit drugs or PEDs under the IDP or ADC. The federal government drew on Cousins as a 'folk devil' to claim the AFL's policies were flawed and pressured the AFL to adopt the government's model of zero tolerance. For example, referring to Ben Cousins, Sports Minister George Brandis stated:

> . . . It's not tenable for any national sporting organization to be dragging the chain on drugs in sport. We expect all sporting organizations to

be aware of the problems. We look to the AFL to come on board with the government's protocol. (cited in AAP 2007c, *The Age*)

Media reports also described the IDP as a 'joke.' Cousins's ability to "get away with a drug habit . . . smacks of a football culture . . . happy to hide behind a seriously flawed policy that gives players too many reasons to become drug users" (Wilson 2007, *The Daily Telegraph*). Other incidents of drug use in Australian sport, such as the 2007 London arrest of Andrew Johns (former Newcastle Knights Australian rugby league player) for possessing an ecstasy tablet, led to media reports critical of NSO's anti-drugs policies. Johns claimed that he had taken drugs throughout his 14-year football career to help battle depression and had regularly "ran [sic] the gauntlet" with drugs testers, with his drug use known by officials and teammates (Walter 2007, *The Age*). Media reports argued that these incidents revealed that elite football in Australia was "awash with a drug problem that authorities are struggling to counteract" (Chesterton 2007, *The Daily Telegraph*). These types of reports created doubt over the legitimacy of the AFL, as well as other football codes, to address drugs in sport.

As we have already seen, government criticism of the IDP in the media included claims that the AFL's sanctions and reporting arrangements were out of touch with community expectations and that "athletes have a responsibility as role models" (Masters 2007, *The Sydney Morning Herald*). The federal government's 2007 *Illicit Drugs in Sport Policy*, with a 'Tough on Drugs in Sport' approach, was presented as a contrast. That policy stressed athletes' obligations as role models, arguing that athletes have a "revered role" with an "important influence on the community—and on our youth in particular—in representing courage, health, excellence, teamwork and integrity" (Australian Government 2007, 1). These are values aligned with the spirit of sport statement articulated in the WADC.

From the perspective of the Australian government and WADA, the IDP lacked transparency and, as a result, "a growing body of evidence" showed that "social drugs is rising [sic] in the major football codes" (Masters 2007, *The Sydney Morning Herald*). Of particular concern for the government and WADA was that "a three-strike policy is not a zero tolerance policy" (AAP 2007a, *The Age*) and the "three strikes and you-may-be-out policy doesn't send the right messages" of the dangers of illicit drug use to the community (AAP 2007b, *The Age*). These unsupported exaggerated claims of rising drug use in Australian football point to a moral panic. Critics claimed that the AFL disregarded sport's role in contributing to social well-being by not sufficiently emphasizing the dangers of drug use. WADA's Director General David Howman complained: "Three strikes before you're out? That's . . . a wet bus ticket for the first (offence) and two wet bus tickets for the second." The AFL, he argued, needed to be "more transparent and more aggressive in ensuring the players, who are well respected in this country, continue to be role models" (in AP 2007, *The Globe and Mail*). These types of claims had the potential to erode the AFL's legitimacy.

Other groups involved in anti-drugs campaigns, such as the National Drug and Alcohol Research Centre (NDARC), had also indicated the view that the AFL's policy failed to meet community expectations. According to NDARC director, Paul Dillon, the most talked about topic when he visits schools to deliver lectures regarding "the danger of drugs" is the "latest drug scandal." He further argued that the AFL's "three strikes policy" failed to address the influence on youth of the poor behavior of their sporting "idols" (in Kogay and Read 2006, *The Australian*). Dr. Joseph Santamaria from Drug Free Australia claimed that the three strikes rule created a "pool of infected players spreading their illness. . . . To simply name and shame players and abandon them would be intolerable. But merely helping an elite athlete decrease their illicit drug use . . . is nowhere near what the community expects" (in Edmund and Dunn 2007, *Herald Sun*). These types of reports identified drug-using 'folk devils' as 'infected players' failing to fulfill their obligations as positive role models and threatening social order. The AFL's anti-drug policy aimed to reduce rather than eliminate drug use, but was presented as contrary to community expectations that drug use threatens social well-being. The message was that drug use required a stronger punitive approach than the AFL mandated.

However, the AFL used the media to defend itself. Other health professionals and drug authorities publicly supported the education and rehabilitation focus of the IDP. According to Australian Drug Foundation (ADF) chief executive Bill Stronach, the AFL recognized that "players are young people" and that "like it or not, some will experiment with drugs." The aim of the AFL's policy, he stated, was to prevent drug use from becoming a long-term problem, particularly as "these drugs are unlikely to be performance-enhancing, the best response is one that places player health and welfare at the forefront" (Kogay and Read 2006, *The Australian*). These comments illustrate that the AFL faced the task of implementing a regulatory approach that balanced the conflicting demands of "clubs, officials, and the media on one hand, and players, their agents, and unions on the other" (Stewart et al. 2008, 59). This included ensuring that anti-drugs in sport policies were effective and acknowledged players' responsibilities as role models while at the same time recognizing, and respecting, the civil liberties of players (AFL 2007, 2; Horvath 2006; Lane 2005b, *The Age*). In other words, the AFL sought to balance conflicting demands on their legitimacy from external as well as internal stakeholders. A fundamental part of this process was the AFL's guarantee of player confidentiality for positive tests for illicit drugs.

Maintaining support for the legitimacy of a regulatory framework requires that dominant groups build stakeholder consensus with the underlying goals of that approach (Battin et al. 2008; Buti and Fridman 1994). As internal stakeholders in the game, the AFL required player support to legitimately exercise their authority over the Australian football community using the IDP as a legally enacted regulatory framework. The IDP is a voluntary code and, with a focus on education and rehabilitation rather than naming and shaming (AFLPA 2008), enjoys player agreement and strong support. This suggests that the AFL successfully established their internal legitimacy to regulate player behavior. Voluntary participation was significant because it indicates that players, as active social agents, recognized the potential for their conduct to influence others as well as a desire to keep the game 'clean' and uphold community expectations. For example, Luke Power (Brisbane Lions Football Club) described the IDP as "over and above any other sporting organization's policy" (AFLPA 2008). Other players also voiced their support for the IDP and indicated their awareness, as active social agents, of their responsibilities as role models in the community. For example, Freemantle Dockers Football Club captain, Matthew Pavlich, emphasized that players were committed to ensuring that the community, including the parents of young players and fans, understood that "players are steadfast in ensuring that it's a clean sport, it's a healthy sport and it's one that everyone should be involved in" (in AFLPA 2008).

Supporters of the IDP, within the Australian football community as well as other stakeholder groups, emphasized that responsibility for addressing drug use in sport should not be placed solely upon athletes' shoulders. Some stakeholders and media reports criticized the unrealistic expectations placed on athletes and sporting groups. For example, one media report cited the Brisbane Lions Football club coach as questioning why the responsibility for addressing the problem of illicit drug use should be placed on sports' shoulders, particularly as spending "billions of dollars in the wider society . . . achieved absolutely nothing." The report went on to argue that the government's "tough on drugs" approach threatened to undermine broader, voluntary, player support for anti-drugs policies: "players are happy with an illicit drugs code but if the Government wants to chase votes by enacting a thoughtless zero tolerance policy . . . then they might have a rethink" (Lalor 2007, *The Australian*). Other reports described the "rush to test sportspeople" as an "expedient exercise to devolve . . . responsibility for the drug scourge in society onto the shoulders of sporting heroes. It smacks of turning a hobgoblin into a witch and . . . hunting it. . . . Authorities rail against drugs because it is easy to rail against drugs" (Baum 2007, *Real Footy*).

These reports explicitly reveal how the debate over doping became a moral panic with PED-using 'folk devils.' They also provide evidence of an elites-engineered institutionalized moral panic, as they point out that 'authorities' have a vested interest in constructing drug-using athletes as 'witches' that are then the focus of regulatory action. The reports demonstrate that the moral panic over drugs in sport opens opportunities for elite groups, such as the Australian government, to enhance their claims to legitimacy or to challenge the claims to legitimacy made by other stakeholder groups, such as the AFL, to control the 'problem.' The AFL had clearly identified using illicit drugs and PEDs as unacceptable behavior for the Australian football community. From the introduction of the IDP until February 2007, there were 28 positive tests for illicit drugs (Demetriou 2007; Slattery 2007). In other words, they had taken measures to meet 'community expectations' to regulate and monitor Australian football. Nevertheless, critics continued to argue that the AFL conducted an insufficient number of tests and that a 'narrow' definition of in and out of competition contributed to their failure to prevent high profile cases of drug use (such as Ben Cousins) (McAsey 2007, *The Australian*). There is a parallel with the IOC here, where external stakeholders and media reports drove organizational change. Reforms to the AFL's IDP resulted from pressure from the media as well as stakeholders such as the Australian government.

The AFL recognized that addressing criticism of their anti-drugs regulations and engaging in ongoing actions to address the socially defined 'problem' were essential for perceptions of their legitimacy and, in 2008, reviewed and modified the IDP (Holroyd 2007, *Real Footy*).[1] From the perspective of the AFL, the revised IDP represented a stronger approach to both illicit drugs and PEDs using new drug-testing technologies, such as hair-testing players following the holiday (i.e., out of competition) period (Phelan 2008). The AFL continued to emphasize that their policy approach to drug use in sport focused on player welfare, as Demetriou stated: "Our illicit drugs policy is above and beyond the WADA policy . . . backed by Australia's leading drug and medical experts . . . and the evidence shows that our policy is working. We refuse to have a policy that is 'name and shame' and which benefits no one" (cited in Phelan 2008). As well as demonstrating that contested power relationships are part of the debate, this comment reveals how the AFL drew on 'socially accredited experts' (Becker 1963) linked to concern with player welfare to bolster their claims to legitimacy.

There were strong expressions of support for the revised IDP from many stakeholders, including players, clubs and ASADA. For example, speaking on behalf of players, AFLPA President and Richmond Football Club veteran Joel Bowden supported out-of-competition testing, including holiday hair-testing, because players "want to send a message to all young people that it's not ok" (in AFL and AFLPA 2008). Other internal stakeholders, such as Essendon Football Club CEO Peter Jackson, supported reforms that "improved" the IDP, which was "on the right path to start with" but was now a "good policy and it's transparent" (in Ralph 2008, *Herald Sun*). Jackson went on to state that, together with a continued focus on education and rehabilittion, the fact that positive tests lapsed after four years instead of players potentially carrying "the stigma of a positive result forever" meant that the policy would "allow players to be role models" (in Ralph 2008, *Herald Sun*). External stakeholders, such as ASADA Chairman Richard Ings, also supported reforms to the IDP, describing the AFL's approach as "world's best practice." He went on to highlight the AFL's leadership role and "significant financial and operational commitment to anti-doping," including a collaborative working relationship with ASADA (in AFL and AFLPA 2008). These supportive statements emphasized the key claims underpinning the AFL's regulatory approach to drugs in sport, which focused on player welfare, including education and rehabilitation, and that recognized the importance of players as positive role models in the community.

The results of the IDP suggested that the AFL had been successful in stopping the moral panic from escalating, with no players recording a third failed test in the four years of the IDP since 2005 (AFL 2009). Nevertheless, the IDP continued to experience criticism. Media reports claimed that the new policy simply highlighted that the code was "dirty" and did not enjoy public perceptions of legitimacy. Reports dismissed the AFL's appeal to medical advice and counseling as flawed because it "pertains to rehabilitating players, not protecting the integrity of the game" and that player support for the code was "self-serving," allowing the AFL space to "manage its image." The report continued, arguing that the AFL's claims to be a 'clean sport' were unfounded because their rules allowed "players to take myriad drugs that are potentially performance enhancing. . . . This is not a code, it is a catastrophe" (Smith 2008, *The Australian*). Media reports cited survey data to indicate that the AFL's policy failed to meet community expectations. For example, according to a *Herald Sun Issues* 2007 survey, a minority of respondents, "only 11 per cent," supported the AFL's policy, while "more than 64 per cent" were in favor of "zero tolerance or a one-strike-and-you're-out . . . 24 per cent back a two-strike policy . . . 72 per cent believe the league is out of touch . . . almost 80 per cent want drug cheats banned for life" and nearly "57 per cent" thought sports stars failed as role models (Kelly 2008, *Herald Sun*).The use of numbers and the exaggerated language place these responses within a moral panic framework.

As Goode and Ben-Yehuda (2009) note, statistics, or exaggerated facts and figures, are often used in the construction of a moral panic to emphasize the extent of the particular problem. In this case, the media reports drew on (questionable) statistics to question the legitimacy of the AFL's anti-doping policy and to indicate that it did not enjoy public support. In terms of interactions with the Australian federal government, although the incoming Labor government indicated some support for the AFL's approach, the view remained that "there's clearly an ongoing problem," which required "some strengthening of that [IDP] policy" (AAP 2007d, *The Age*). Irrespective of claims that the AFL's approach failed to meet community or government expectations, the AFL's results for illicit drug tests in 2009 showed that positive tests continued to fall, despite an increase in the number of tests conducted. In 2009, there were 14 failed tests and, although no players failed a third test, two players returned a second positive result (Whitham 2010). For the AFL, these results demonstrated not only an effective policy approach but also support for community expectations concerning the regulation of drug use in sport. This bolstered its claims to legitimacy.

The AFL continued to monitor their policies aimed at modifying player behavior around a range of issues, including drug and alcohol use. For example, in 2010 the AFL modified the IDP[2] to include mandatory referrals to a drug and alcohol specialist for any player with a failed test. Clubs also supported the AFL's framework by working to identify 'at risk' individuals that required extra support (Essendon Football Club 2011). While this suggests support for the AFL's legitimacy from internal stakeholders, claims to legitimacy remained contested. Media reports argued that the IDP did not meet its stated objective of player welfare, as it failed to adequately address drug use by players struggling with mental health issues. Underpinning these claims was the media attention devoted to the 2010 case of Travis Tuck (Hawthorne Football Club), who became the first player sanctioned under the IDP. When he was found by police unconscious in his car with drug paraphernalia, it was revealed that he suffered from clinical depression. Media reports argued that penalizing Tuck under the IDP illustrated that "as a welfare policy it has failed. . . . It must protect the sick and desperately ill" (Smith 2010, *The Australian*). Player welfare was a cornerstone of the AFL's anti-drugs in sport policy and claims that they failed to consider issues surrounding players' mental health potentially challenged their legitimacy.

The Tuck case is significant in terms of the legitimacy of the IDP. Suggesting that the policy was accomplishing its objective of player welfare, Tuck's need for treatment for depression (which he had been receiving) had come to light as a result of positive tests under the IDP (3AW Football 2010; Munckton 2010). Tuck was one of 14 positive test results for illicit drugs in 2010 and the only player to fall into the 'third strike' category of the policy framework. There were no positive test results for PEDs under the ADC (AAP 2011, *The Australian*; Warner 2011, *Herald Sun*). The AFL stressed that player support was essential for the success of the policy in terms of changing player behavior, demonstrated by the continuing fall in positive test results. Further emphasizing the significance of player welfare with a focus on education, including for social issues such as responsible use of alcohol as well as drug use, as part of the AFL's regulatory approach, Demetriou stated:

> You'll be educated from the day you walk in . . . about racial vilification, illicit drugs, responsible alcohol, respect and responsibility with women. . . . We promote that. . . . Come and play our code! . . . We can't offer internationals . . . we are . . . this code that develops you as people beside your sporting prowess. (cited in Macintyre 2011, *The Conversation*)

This bolstered the AFL's claims to legitimacy and demonstrated how contested power relationships need to be considered in the debate over doping. AFL Football Operations Manager Adrian Anderson stated that the policy attracted "considerable interest" from international sporting organizations based on its "cutting edge approach" that was "above and beyond the WADA code" and, "with a drop in the number of failed tests despite increases in the number of tests," the "focus on education, intervention, rehabilitation and welfare . . . has shown to be effective" (cited in McNicol 2011). Similarly to the Australian federal government, the AFL positioned their approach to illicit drugs in sport as 'cutting edge' and world leading. More than that, by 'going above and beyond the WADA code,' this statement enhances the AFL's claims to legitimacy to be effectively protecting the integrity of sport from illicit drug use.

Results continued to suggest that the IDP was successful. Test results for the 2011 season revealed a drop in positive results, with only six players failing out-of-competition tests for illicit drugs and no players failing a test twice. From the perspective of the AFL, these results demonstrate that the IDP is effective (AAP and *ABC News* 2012). However, in 2012 there were 26 out-of-competition detections for illicit drugs. These results led the AFL, again with the support of internal stakeholders, including the AFLPA and players, to modify the IDP.[3] The AFL claimed that amending the IDP demonstrated their commitment to player welfare as well as addressing illicit drug use across society (AFL 2013a). Ongoing support from players and the AFLPA indicates that the AFL's strong anti-drugs in sport framework has successfully generated support from internal stakeholders for the organization's legitimacy. However, positive perceptions of legitimacy from external stakeholders, such as the media and the public, are also important, as the AFL continues to work toward becoming the number one football code in Australia (AFL 2014a). This is a constant challenge as, according to the ABS, outdoor soccer enjoyed a stronger participation rate for boys in the year ending April 2012 (22 percent) compared to AFL (15 percent) (ABS 2012). Nevertheless, there were indications suggesting the AFL enjoys strong support for their legitimacy from external stakeholders.

In 2014, the AFL commenced negotiations for broadcasting rights with bids reportedly starting at anything from AUD$1.5 up to $1.8 billion (Davidson 2014, *The Australian*). This represented an increase on the 2011 television broadcasting arrangement, which at AUD$1.25 billion (Whitham 2011) had been the largest in Australian sporting history history (Nicholson 2006). Match day attendances for the 2014 season reached 6,954,585, an increase of 28,205 on 2013 (AFL 2014b). There was a 24 percent growth in the number of women playing Australian football and community level participation rates reached 938,069, with 129,775 people participating in the game in various countries around the world (AFL 2013b). Grassroots development through the Auskick program saw growth in junior sport, with "Auskickers transitioning to clubs at a younger age" (AFL 2013b, 85), which is an important element for the future development of the code. With significant financial returns at stake, the ongoing task facing the AFL involves maintaining public support for their moral authority and legitimacy. This rests on supporting its own regulatory framework of consciously made rational-legal rules that meet and support community expectations that drug use in sport is unacceptable while also safeguarding athlete welfare. These rules, however, are under constant challenge from other authorities, such as the Australian federal government and WADA, demanding their own rules are applied.

CONCLUSION

As this chapter has described, the debate over policy approaches to drug use in Australian football illustrates how issues of governance and control based on particular regulatory frameworks influence claims to legitimacy. However, claims to legitimacy are both contested and multi-dimensional. The debate between the Australian federal government and the AFL illustrates that different stakeholder groups pursue different agendas in terms of their anti-doping regulatory approaches. For the Australian government, it consisted of policies such as the *Tough on Drugs in Sport* policy, which reflected a conservative 'Tough on Drugs' law and order approach, and the *Backing Australia's Sporting Ability* policy, aimed primarily at building a pool of elite sporting talent, together with building grassroots community participation rates in organized sport.

For the AFL, participation and development of Australian football were important and they worked to maintain the image of the game as free of PEDs and illicit drugs by using the ADC and the IDP. The AFL recognized the potential implications for their legitimacy if the issue of PEDs was not addressed and, using codes of conduct including the ADC, sought to protect the image and appeal of Australian football. The AFL responded to challenges to their legitimacy and moral authority as instances of illicit drug use emerged in the code. To restore order to their sporting community and address community criticism, the AFL introduced, refined and strengthened an illicit drugs policy. This was important for perceptions of its legitimacy, which required regulatory mechanisms that meet and support community expectations over acceptable behavior, including identifying and sanctioning deviance (Ericson et al. 1991; Habermas 1976; Wuthnow et al. 1984).

The interactions between the AFL and the Australian government, particularly in relation to the issue of illicit drug use in sport that are debatably not performance-enhancing, also reveal the wider political dimensions of the anti-doping debate. The Australian government associated implementation of a WADA aligned anti-doping policy, for both illicit drugs and PEDs, with maintaining Australia's status as a world leader against doping. Clean sport was linked to national identity, strong national economic growth as well as community cohesion and healthy lifestyles. Along with other stakeholders, the Australian government argued that the AFL's approach to drugs in sport undermined this message and had the potential to damage Australia's international reputation as a leader in anti-doping. Of particular concern for both WADA and the Australian government was the focus of the AFL's IDP on rehabilitation, education and counseling rather than a punitive naming and shaming approach. The AFL's insistence on implementing a separate IDP, in conjunction with the WADC-aligned ADC, illustrated that interactions and power relationships between organizations are important elements of the debate. The AFL's position challenged WADA's authority and legitimacy, which was based on the WADC as formally constituted rules and regulations underpinned by values articulated in the 'spirit of sport' statement (Chapter 3, this volume).

The media provided a site where competing claims to legitimacy were made and challenged. The Australian federal government drew heavily on the media to present drug use in sport as damaging to community cohesion and a threat to social order and stability. In contrast, the AFL used the media to promote the ADC and IDP as the most appropriate regulatory response for the Australian football community. This also served to enhance their internal legitimacy and moral authority as guardian of a 'clean' code with a focus on player welfare. In other words, media reports carry the potential to create a crisis of legitimacy for organizations by constructing particular issues as problematic while also providing opportunities for those organizations to enhance legitimacy as providers of solutions to the particular problem. In this way, media reports of the debate between the Australian government and the AFL highlight the value of an elites-engineered moral panic framework to understand the role of legitimacy in the context of PEDs.

Media reports presented drug use in Australian football, both illicit drugs and PEDs, as widespread and increasing in severity. Like the reports over doping in the 1998 Tour de France, the media suggested that instances of drug use in Australian football were 'the tip of the iceberg.' The reports cited throughout this chapter used melodramatic language to create concern over doping and identify those responsible as 'folk devils' or 'lame brains.' This language normalizes expressions of hostility toward individuals who, by failing to provide positive role models, threaten to 'infect' the wider community. The perceived threat to the social order justifies stricter measures of social control and specific institutional responses, such as WADA and the WADC, to regulate the problem. Media reports provided opportunities for stakeholders, such as the Australian government, to pressure the AFL into compliance with WADA's global framework in order to protect sport as a social institution as well as the community more broadly. Implicitly, these contestations involved power relationships between organizational actors, as they each aimed to secure and maintain the legitimacy and moral authority to regulate and control sport, using the media to make and contest those claims.

The evidence presented in this chapter has demonstrated that the doping debate can be conceptualized as an elites-engineered moral panic, driven by challenges to SGBs' legitimacy due to continued reports of doping. The discussion has also highlighted the media's role in that process. While I have drawn on media reports in this chapter to explore and illustrate these points,

I extend that discussion in the next chapter by presenting a review of media reports of doping using a legitimacy-inspired elites-engineered moral panic framework.

NOTES

1   The number of tests increased to 1,500 with a hair-testing trial introduced to detect illicit drug use over the off-season (identified as a high-risk period for illicit drug use). The three-strike rule remained, with modifications addressing club requests for increased information sharing. For example, a first failed out-of-competition test meant consultation with the AFL medical commissioner to undertake education, counseling and treatment, with players subject to ongoing target testing and a suspended sanction of $5,000. A second offense meant immediate referral by AFL medical commissioners to a more intense program of education, counseling and treatment, ongoing target testing and a suspended sanction of six matches. A third offense meant appearing before the AFL Tribunal, a possible suspension of 18 matches (six for the second offense and an additional 12 for the third offense) and enforcement of the suspended sanction of $5,000 from the first test (AFL and AFLPA 2008).

2   Tuck was banned for 12 matches and fined $5000 (AAP and ABC News 2012).

3   Some of the amendments included permitting players to self-report illicit drug use only once during their career. Clubs could draw on their own observations to request AFL Medical Directors to target test players and, across the game, there would be more target testing at more targeted times and increased levels of hair-testing during the 'high-risk' off-season period. Players exhibiting attitudes contrary to the objectives and spirit of the IDP could be directed to undergo more intense education and counseling with the Club CEO notified of any failure to change their behavior. The amendments also allowed for AFL Medical Directors to provide greater de-identified feedback regarding IDP results and trends to the clubs. Changes also extended to club CEOs and player leadership groups to include mental health 'first aid,' and the regular drug education programs would continue to be revised and enhanced (see AFL 2013a).

REFERENCES

3AW Football. 2010. "AFL Statement on Travis Tuck." 3AW, 1 September 2010. http://www.3aw.com.au/blogs/3aw-football-blog/afl-statement-on-travis-tuck/20100901–14frl.html. Accessed 18 February 2011.

AAP. 2006. "Howard Defends 'Tough on Drugs' Policy." *The Sydney Morning Herald*, 4 May 2006. http://www.smh.com.au/news/National/Howard-defends-tough-on-drugs-policy/2006/05/04/1146335863149.html. Accessed 25 May 2011.

———. 2007a. "AFL Letter Defends Drug Policy." *The Age*, 28 March 2007. http://www.theage.com.au/realfooty/news/afl/afl-letter-defends-drug-policy/2007/03/27/1174761475630.html. Accessed 10 April 2007.

———. 2007b. "Banned for Life Under New Drugs Policy." *The Age*, 6 October 2007. http://www.theage.com.au/news/National/Banned-for-life-under-new-drugs-policy/2007/10/06/1191091408100.html. Accessed 21 November 2007.

————. 2007c. "Change AFL Drug Policy, Repeats Brandis." *The Age*, 17 October 2007. http://www.theage.com.au/articles/2007/10/17/1192300834795.html. Accessed 24 October 2007.

————. 2007d. "New Government to Keep Drugs Pressure on AFL." *The Age*, 26 November 2007. http://www.theage.com.au/news/Sport/Swans-looking-at-inhouse-drug-policy/2007/11/26/1196036782057.html. Accessed 27 November 2007.

————. 2009. "Cousins Facing Testing Future." WWOS.com.au, 6 January 2009. http://wwos.ninemsn.com.au/article.aspx?id=70694. Accessed 7 January 2009.

————. 2011. "AFL Says Number of Positive Tests for Recreational Drugs Down from 14 in 2009." *The Australian*, 22 June 2011. http://www.theaustralian.com.au/news/sport/afl-says-number-of-positive-tests-for-recreational-drugs-down-from-14-in-2009/story-e6frg7mf-122607988333. Accessed 28 July 2011.

AAP, and *ABC News*. 2012. "AFL Applauds Drug Testing Results." ABC News, 21 June 2012. http://www.abc.net.au/news/2012–06–21/afl-applaud-drug-testing-results/408404. Accessed 14 February 2015.

ABC Premium News. 2004. "Carlton Sacks Angwin, Keeps Norman." *ABC Premium News*, 7 April 2004.

————. 2006. "AFL's Drug Policy Flawed: Coaches." *ABC Premium News*, 30 March 2006.

ABC Sport. 2005. "WADA Attack AFL Over Failure to Sign Code." *ABC Sport*, 1 July 2005. http://www.abc.net.au/sport/content/200507/s1404945.htm. Accessed 29 May 2007.

ABS (Australian Bureau of Statistics). 2012. "Sport and Recreation: A Statistical Overview, Australia 4156.0." Australian Bureau of Statistics. http://www.ausstats.abs.gov.au/ausstats/subscriber.nsf/0/6E28777ED2896A2BCA257AD9000E2FC5/$File/41560_2012.pdf. Accessed 17 February 2015.

AFL (Australian Football League). 2006. "Australian Football Anti-Doping Code January 2006." AFL Official Web page. Australian Football League. http://www.aflpa.com.au/media/Anti-DopJan06.pdf. Accessed 7 March 2006.

————. 2007. "Illicit Drugs Policy." Australian Football League. http://afl.com.au/Portals/0/afl_docs/afl_hq/Policies/Illicit Drugs Policy Feb 2007.pdf. Accessed 13 June 2008.

————. 2009. "2008 Illicit Drugs Policy Results." Australian Football League. http://www.afl.com.au/news/newsarticle/tabid/208/newsid/77745/default.aspx. Accessed 29 May 2009.

————. 2013a. "AFL / AFLPA Amendments to AFL Illicit Drugs Policy (IDP) / Release of 2012 Testing Results." Australian Football League. http://www.afl.com.au/news/2013–05–16/afl-aflpa-amendments-to-afl-illicit-drugs-policy-idp-release-of-2012-testing-results-. Accessed 14 February 2015.

————. 2013b. "Annual Report 2013." Australian Football League. http://www.afl.com.au/staticfile/AFL%20Tenant/AFL/Files/Annual%20Report/2013%20AFL%20Annual%20Report.pdf. Accessed 14 February 2015.

————. 2014a. "2014 Toyota AFL Premiership Season Fixture Released." Australian Football League. http://www.afl.com.au/news/2014–10–30/max-4-words. Accessed 14 February 2015.

————. 2014b. "AFL CEO Gillon McLachlan Thanks AFL Supporters." Australian Football League. http://www.afl.com.au/news/2014–09–29/afl-ceo-gillon-mclachlan-thanks-afl-supporters. Accessed 14 February 2015.

AFL (Australian Football League), and AFLPA (Australian Football League Players' Association). 2008. "AFL Players Say 'No' to Drugs." Australian Football League and Australian Football League Players' Association. http://www.afl.com.au/Portals/0/afl_docs/AFLPlayersSayNoToDrugs.pdf. Accessed 12 January 2009.

AFLPA (Australian Football League Players' Association). 2008. "AFL Players and the AFL Have a Simple Message: Say NO to Drugs." Australian Football League Players' Association. http://www.afl.com.au/Default.aspx?tabid=1221. Accessed 29 August 2008.

AIC (Australian Institute of Criminology). 2009. "National Illicit Drug Strategy." Australian Institute of Criminology. http://www.aic.gov.au/crime_types/drugs_alcohol/illicit_drugs/strategy/illicit.html. Accessed 10 February 2015.

Albergo, L. 2007. "Demetriou Defends Drug Code." Australian Football Association of North America, 1 April 2007. http://www.afana.com/drupal/node/43. Accessed 15 November 2007.

Anderson, J. 2007. "Tom Harley Revved Up Over Drug Loopholes." *Herald Sun*, 22 November 2007. http://www.news.com.au/heraldsun/story/0,21985,22801005-11088,00.html. Accessed 28 December 2007.

Andrews, I. 2000. "From a Club to a Corporate Game: The Changing Face of Australian Football 1960–1999." *International Journal of the History of Sport* 17 (2/3): 225–254.

AOC (Australian Olympic Committee). N.d. "Montreal 1976." Australian Olympic Committee. http://corporate.olympics.com.au/games/montreal-197. Accessed 19 February 2015.

AP (Associated Press). 2007. "WADA Official: Gap Closing Between New Drugs and Testing." *The Globe and Mail*, 1 June 2007.

ASC (Australian Sports Commission). 1999. "The Australian Sports Commission—Beyond 2000." Australian Sports Commission. http://www.ausport.gov.au/publications/ascbeyond_2000s.pdf. Accessed 15 November 2006.

ASDA (Australian Sports Drug Agency). 1999. *1998–99 Annual Report*. Canberra: Commonwealth of Australia. https://secure.ausport.gov.au/_data/assets/pdf_file/0007/247858/ASDA_AR_1998-1999.pdf. Accessed 11 February 2015.

———. 2001. *Annual Report Australian Sports Drug Agency 00:01*. Canberra: Australian Sports Drug Agency. http://www.asada.gov.au/resources/reports/previous/ar01/asda_ar01.pdf. Accessed 20 November 2007.

———. 2002. *Australian Sports Drug Agency Annual Report 2001–02*. Canberra: Australian Sports Drug Agency. http://www.asada.gov.au/resources/reports/previous/ar02/index.htm. Accessed 20 November 2007.

———. 2003. *Australian Sports Drug Agency Annual Report 03:04*. Canberra: Australian Sports Drug Agency. http://www.asada.gov.au/resources/reports/previous/ar04/_docs/asda_ar04.pdf. Accessed 20 November 2007.

The Australian. 2006. "Drugged AFL Men to Remain Unnamed." *The Australian*, 23 March 2006.

Australian Government. 2007. "Illicit Drugs in Sport Policy—Tough on Drugs in Sport." Australian Government. http://www.sport.gov.au/_data/assets/pdf_file/0003/74982/Illicit-Drugs-in-Sport-policy-Oct-07.pdf. Accessed 10 April 2008.

Barker, G. 2004. "Sporting a Lesser Culture." *Australian Financial Review*, February 16, 2004, 62 cited in Tonts, M., and Atherley, K. 2010. "Competitive Sport and the Construction of Place Identity in Rural Australia." *Sport in Society* 13 (3):381–398.

Barrett, D., and Williams, R. 2007. "AFL Delay on Drugs Policy." *Fox Sports*, 17 December 2007. http://www.foxsports.com.au/story/0,8659,22935225–23211,00.html. Accessed 21 December 2007.

Battin, M. P., Luna, E., Lipman, A. G., Gahlinger, P. M., Rollins, D. E., Roberts, J. C., and Booher, T. L. 2008. *Drugs and Justice: Seeking a Consistent, Coherent, Comprehensive View*. Oxford: Oxford University Press.

Baum, G. 2007. "Sporting Heroes Carry Extra Burden in Drug Witch-Hunt." *Real Footy*, 7 September 2007. http://www.realfooty.com.au/news/news/sporting-heroes-carry-extra-burden-in-drug-witchhunt/2007/09/06/1188783414288.html?page=fullpage—contentSwap. Accessed 7 September 2007.

Becker, H. S. 1963. *Outsiders*. New York: Free Press.

Blair, T. 2005. "Shame and Disgrace." *The Bulletin*, 18 May 2005. http://bulletin.ninemsn.com.au/bulletin/site/articleIDs/EE4EODCFFFF092D0CA25700300 11865B5. Accessed 7 March 2006.

Booth, D. 1995. "Sports Policy in Australia: Right, Just and Rational?" *The Australian Quarterly* 67 (1): 1–10.

Booth, D., and Tatz, C. 2000. *One Eyed: A View of Australian Sport*. St. Leonards, Australia: Allen and Unwin.

Buti, A., and Fridman, S. 1994. "The Intersection of Law and Policy: Drug Testing in Sport." *Australian Journal of Public Administration* 53 (4): 489–507.

———. 2001. *Drugs Sport and the Law*. Mudgeeraba, Queensland: Scribblers Publishing.

Chandrasekaran, R. 2000. "Sports Crazy: On the Fields, in the Stands and in the Betting Parlors, Australians May Be the Most Sports-Obsessed Nation on Earth." *Washington Post*, 3 September 2000.

Chesterton, R. 2007. "Drugs Use in Sport Is Out of Control." *The Daily Telegraph*, 3 October 2007. http://www.news.com.au/story/0,23599,22520718-2,00.html. Accessed 4 October 2007.

Cohen, S. 2002. Folk devils and moral panics: the creation of the Mods and Rockers 3rd ed. Abingdon, Oxon, New York: Routledge.

Commonwealth of Australia. 2001a. "Backing Australia's Sporting Ability a *More* Active Australia." Sport and Tourism. Commonwealth of Australia. http://www.dbcde.gov.au/_data/assets/pdf_file/0009/7677/BASA.pdf. Accessed 16 November 2006.

———. 2001b. "Game Plan 2006 Sport and Leisure Industry Strategic National Plan." Department of Industry Science and Resources. Canberra: Commonwealth of Australia. http://fulltext.ausport.gov.au/fulltext/2001/feddep/gp2006.pdf. Accessed 15 November 2006.

Cooper, A. 2006. "AFL Demanding Answers from Government Over Drug Test Details." *AAP Sports News Wire*, 14 March 2006.

Cooper, A., and Fiamengo, M. 2006. "AFL: Identities Remain Secret, But Anger at System Continues." *AAP Sports News Wire*, 16 March 2001.

Davidson, D. 2014. "AFL Eyes as much as $1.6bn for Television Rights Deal." *The Australian*, 27 October 2014. http://www.theaustralian.com.au/business/media/afl-eyes-as-much-as-16bn-for-television-rights-deal/story-fna045gd-122710286382. Accessed 14 February 2015.

Davies, J. 2005. "White Line Fever." *The Bulletin*, 18 May 2005. http://bulletin.ninemsn.com.au/bulletin/site/articleIDs/7E2DAF12F1A64903CA25700200 72D07. Accessed 7 March 2006.

DCITA (Dept. Communications Information Technology and the Arts). 2005. "New Anti-Doping Body Legislation Introduced (media release)." Department of Communications Information Technology and the Arts. http://www.minister.dcita.gov.au/kemp/media/media_releases/new_anti-doping_body_legislation_introduced. Accessed 6 March 2006.

Demetriou, A. 2005a. "The AFL and WADA: Room for Compromise." *AFL Record* (Melbourne, Aust) (8–10 July): 6–8.

———. 2005b. "How the Final Decision Was Made." *AFL Record* (Melbourne, Aust) (22–24 July 2005): 6.

———. 2007. "AFL Response to Behaviour." *AFL Record* (Melbourne, Aust) (May 4–6): 20–21.

Dept. of Health and Ageing. 2001. "Federal Health Minister Announces New Funding Commitments for *Tough on Drugs*." Commonwealth of Australia. http://www.ocs.gov.au/internet/main/publishing.nsf/Content/health-mediarel-yr2001-kp-kp01002.htm. Accessed 25 May 2011.

Duffield, M. 2002. "Koops Is Absolved by Tribunal Football." *The Age*, 30 April 2002.

Edmund, S., and Dunn, M. 2007. "Groups Split on AFL Drug Policy." *Herald Sun*, 18 October 2007. http://www.news.com.au/heraldsun/story/0,21985, 22604881–662,00.html. Accessed 10 December 2007.

Ericson, R. V, Baranek, P. M., and Chan, J. B. L. 1991. *Representing Order*. Toronto: University of Toronto Press.

Essendon Football Club. 2011. "AFL Releases Illicit Drugs Policy Results." Essendon Football Club. http://www.essendonfc.com.au/news/2011–06–22/afl-releases-illicit-drugs-policy-results. Accessed 14 February 2015.

Gleeson, M. 2006. "Footy Drugs Testing Finds 15 Under the Influence." *The Age*, 10 March 2006. http://www.theage.com.au/realfooty/articles/2006/03/09/1141701634085.html. Accessed 10 March 2006.

The Gold Coast Bulletin. 2006. "AFL and the Court Just Don't Get Tt." *The Gold Coast Bulletin*, 1 September 2006.

Goode, E., and Ben-Yehuda, N. 2009. *Moral Panics: The Social Construction of Deviance*. Chichester, West Sussex: Wiley-Blackwell Publishing.

Green, M. 2007. "Olympic Glory or Grassroots Development?: Sport Policy Priorities in Australia, Canada and the United Kingdom, 1960–2006." *The International Journal of the History of Sport* 24 (7): 921–953.

Green, M., and Houlihan, B. 2006. "Governmentality, Modernization, and the "Disciplining" of National Sporting Organizations: Athletics in Australia and the United Kingdom." *Sociology of Sport Journal* 23: 47–71.

Habermas, J. 1976. *Legitimation Crisis*. London: Heinemann Educational.

Hagdorn, K. 2001. "Hope on Koops." *Sunday Herald-Sun*, 6 May 2001.

Hanstad, D. V., and Loland, S. 2009. "Where on Earth Is Michael Rasmussen?—Is an Elite Level Athlete's Duty to Provide Information on Whereabouts Justifiable Anti-Doping Work or an Indefensible Surveillance Regime?" In *Elite Sport, Doping and Public Health*, edited by Moller, V., McNamee, M. and Dimeo, P., 167–177. Odensa: University Press of Southern Denmark.

Hedge, M. 2006. "AFL Wins Drug Suppression Case." *Sunday Times*, 30 August 2006. http://www.news.com.au/perthnow/story/0,21598,20304037–500536 1,00.html. Accessed 5 September 2006.

Hemphill, D. 2002. " 'Think It, Talk It, Work It': Violence, Injury and Australian Rules Football." *Sporting Traditions* 19 (1): 17–31.

Holroyd, J. 2007. "AFL Flags Drug Code Review." *Real Footy*, 18 October 2007. http://realfooty.com.au/articles/2007/10/18/1192300914023.html. Accessed 8 November 2007.

Horvath, P. 2006. "Anti-Doping and Human Rights in Sport: The Case of the AFL and the *WADA Code*." *Monash University Law Review* 32 (2): 357–386.

IICGADS (International Intergovernmental Consultative Group on Anti-Doping in Sport). 1999. Sydney Communique. International Intergovernmental Consultative Group on Anti-Doping in Sport. http://www.dcita.gov.au/drugsinsport/communique_17nov.doc. Accessed 26 September 2007.

ISR (Dept. of Industry Science and Resources). 1999a. "TODIS—Foreword." Commonwealth of Australia. http://www.dcita.gov.au/tough_on_drugs/p1.htm. Accessed 24 July 2008.

———. 1999b. "TODIS—Implementing International Best Practice in Drug Testing." Commonwealth of Australia. http://fulltext.ausport.gov.au/fulltext/1999/feddep/tough_on_drugs_in_sport/content.htm. Accessed 25 May 2011.

———. 1999c. "Tough on Drugs in Sport: Australia's Anti-Drugs in Sport Strategy 1999–2000 and Beyond." Commonwealth of Australia. http://fulltext.ausport.gov.au/fulltext/1999/feddep/tough_on_drugs_in_sport/content.htm. Accessed 25 May 2011.

Jeffery, N. 2008. "Performance Drug Fight Stepped Up." *The Australian*, 3 May 2008. http://www.theaustralian.news.com.au/story/0,25197,23636365–5013449,00. html. Accessed 13 February 2009.

Johnson, L. 1997. "Charles Drug Hearing on Thursday." *The Age*, 2 September 1997.

———. 2005. "Drugs Impasse Costs AFL $1.5m." *The Age*, 1 July 2005.

Kelly, J. 2008. "Fans Line Up to Blast AFL's Drug Policy." *Herald Sun*, 22 January 2008. http://www.news.com.au/heraldsun/story/0,21985,23087790–2862,00.html. Accessed 22 January 2008.

Kidd, B., Edelman, R., and Brownell, S. 2001. "Comparative Analysis of Doping Scandals: Canada, Russia, and China." In *Doping in Elite Sport The Politics of Drugs in the Olympic Movement*, edited by Wilson, W. and Derse, E., 153–188. Champgaign, IL: Human Kinetics.

Kogay, P., and Read, B. 2006. "Refusing to Name, Shame Is Confusing." *The Australian*, 1 September 2006. http://www.theaustralian.news.com.au/story/0,20867,20319507–2722,00.html. Accessed 4 September 2006.

Lalor, P. 2007. "Healthy Dose of Sense on Drug Row." *The Australian*, 15 September 2007. http://www.theaustralian.news.com.au/story/0,25197,22420227–5013576,00.html. Accessed 18 September 2007.

Lane, S. 2005a. "Canberra and AFL in a Clash of the Codes." 12 June 2005.

———. 2006a. "Brown Backs Steroid Use." *The Age*, 13 August 2006. http://www.realfooty.theage.com.au/articles/2006/08/12/1154803147220.html. Accessed 14 August 2006.

———. 2006b. "Malthouse Takes Aim at AFL." *Sunday Age*, 12 March 2006.

Lane, T. 2005b. "AFL's Brave Drug Stand." *The Age*, 2 July 2005.

Linnell, G. 1995. *Football Ltd: The Inside Story of the AFL*. Sydney: Pan Macmillan Australia.

Linnell, S. 1997. "Eagle Caught Out by Flu Medication." *The Age*, 1 September 1997.

———. 1998. "League Vows Swift Action on Drug Offences." *The Age*, 5 March 1998.

Macintyre, S. 2011. "AFL Boss Andrew Demetriou: 'We Are Tyring to Control as Much as We Can Control.'" *The Conversation*, 15 August 2011. http://theconversation.edu.au/afl-boss-andrew-demetriou-we-are-trying-to-control-as-much-as-we-can-control-281. Accessed 16 August 2011.

Magdalinski, T. 2000. "The Reinvention of Australia for the Sydney 2000 Olympic Games." *The International Journal of the History of Sport* 17 (2–3): 305–322.

Magnay, J. 2006. "Government Gets Tough on AFL Over Secrecy Surrounding Drug-Testing Policy." *The Sydney Morning Herald*, 8 September 2006. http://www.smh.com.au/news/afl/government-gets-tough-on-afl-over-secrecy-surrounding-drugtestingpolicy/2006/09/07/1157222264974.html. Accessed 8 September 2006.

———. 2008. "Baggaley Faces Drugs Charges in Two States." *The Sydney Morning Herald*, 2 May 2008. http://www.smh.com.au/news/sport/baggaley-faces-drugs-charges-in-two-states/2008/05/01/1209235055647.html. Accessed 13 February 2009.

Masters, R. 2004. "Drugs Chiefs Hold Secret Powwow Over Latest Trends." *The Sydney Morning Herald*, 10 December 2004. http://www.smh.com.au/news/Sport/Drugs-chiefs-hold-secret-powwow-over-latest-trends/2004/12/09/1102182429497.html?oneclick=true. Accessed 19 February 2007.

———. 2007. "Party Drugs and Footballers—The Cloud on the Horizon That Worries Kemp." *The Sydney Morning Herald*, 10 February 2007. http://www.smh.com.au/news/sport/party-drugs-and-footballers—the-cloud-on-the-horizon-that-worrieskemp/2007/02/09/1170524302699.html. Accessed 12 February 2007.

McAsey, J. 2007. "AFL Not Trying in Fight on Drugs." *The Australian*, 4 August 2007. http://www.theaustralian.news.com.au/story/0,25197,22185322–2722,00.html. Accessed 6 August 2007.

McKay, J. 1986. "Hegemony, the State and Australian Sport." In *Power Play*, edited by Lawrence, G. and Rowe, D., 115–135. Sydney: Hale and Iremonger.

McKay, J., and Roderick, M. 2010. " 'Lay Down Sally': Media Narratives of Failure in Australian Sport." *Journal of Australian Studies* 34 (3): 295–315.

McKay, S. 1996. "Famine Threatens a Footy Feast; Football's Boom Times." *The Age*, 9 September 1996.

McNicol, A. 2011. "Failed Drug Tests Down." AFL.com.au, 22 June 2011. http://www. afl.com.au/news/newsarticle/tabid/208/newsid/116819/default.aspx. Accessed 13 July 2011.

Mendes, P. (2001) "Social Conservatism vs Harm Minimisation: John Howard on Illicit Drugs," *Journal of Economic and Social Policy* 6 (1), Article 2. Available at: http://epubs.scu.edu.au/jesp/vol6/iss1/2

Munckton, S. 2010. "Fresh Hysteria on Drugs and Sport." *Green Left Weekly* 851.

Murphy, P. 2006. "Drug Use at a Peak: AFL Star." *The Australian*, 31 March 2006.

Murphy, T. 1997. "Last Week in the AFL. . . . AFL Round 22, Weekly Wrapup." Footy.com.au, 1 September 1997. http://www.footy.com.au/dags/97/wrapup/wrapup_r22.html. Accessed 30 January 2008.

Nadel, D. 1998a. "Colour, Corporations and Commissioners, 1976–1985." In *More Than a Game: An Unauthorised History of Australian Rules Football*, edited by Hess, R. and Stewart, B., 200–224. Melbourne: Melbourne University Press.

———. 1998b. "The League Goes National, 1986–1997." In *More Than a Game: An Unauthorised History of Australian Rules Football*, edited by Hess, R. and Stewart, B., 225–255. Carlton: Melbourne University Press.

Nicholson, M. 2006. "Moving the Goalposts: Change and Challenge in a Competitive Football Market." In *Football Fever: Moving the Goalposts*, edited by Nicholson, M., Stewart, B. and Hess, R., 1–10. Hawthorne, Vic: Maribyrnong Press.

Nixon, R. 1992. "Apartheid on the Run: The South African Sports Boycott." *Transition* 58: 68–88.

Opie, H. 2004. "Drugs in Sport and the Law—Moral Authority, Diversity and the Pursuit of Excellence." *Marquette Sports Law Review* 14: 267–277.

Parham, E. 2008. "Australian and the World Anti-Doping Code 1999–2008." World Anti-Doping Agency. http://www.wada-ama.org/rtecontent/document/Australia_and_the_World_Anti_Doping_Code_1999_2008.pdf. Accessed 2 April 2009.

Pascoe, R. 1995. *The Winter Game: the Complete History of Australian Football*. Port Melbourne: Reed Books Australia.

———. 1997. "The AFL 1996 Centenary Celebrations." *Australian Historical Studies* 28 (108): 113–117.

Phelan, J. 2008. "Illicit Drugs Policy Revamped." Australian Football League, 28 August 2008. http://afl.com.au/News/NEWSARTICLE/tabid/208/Default.aspx?newsId=6651. Accessed 29 August 2008.

Pierik, J. 2006. "Footy's Going to Pot: Rhys-Jones Says AFL a Drugs Playground." *The Mercury*, 5 April 2006.

Ralph, J. 2008. "AFL Clubs Happy with Drug Code Changes." *Herald Sun*, 29 August 2008. http://www.news.com.au/heraldsun/sport/afl/story/0,26576,24258903-19742,00.html. Accessed 2 September 2008.

Rielly, S. 1998. "Spectre of Another AFL Drug Scandal." *The Age*, 8 May 1998.

Roach, G. 2006. "So Certain Senior AFL Players Say They Have No Confidence in the League's Own Anti-Doping System." *The Advertiser*, 18 March 2006.

Schwartz, L., and Connolly, R. 1997. "New Claims of Steroid Use in AFL." *Sunday Age*, 31 August 1997.

Senate Standing Committee on Environment, Recreation and the Arts. 1989. *Drugs in Sport: Interim Report*. Canberra: Commonwealth of Australia.

———. 1990. *Drugs in Sport, Second Report*. Canberra: Commonwealth of Australia.

Senator The Hon Rod Kemp. 2005. Media Release: AFL to Become WADA Code Compliant. Canberra: Australian Government. http://parlinfo.aph.gov.au/par lInfo/download/media/pressrel/8OPG6/upload_binary/8opg63.pdf;fileType=appl ication%2Fpdf#search=%22kemp%20AFL%20pressrel%22. Accessed 4 February 2011.

Slattery, G. 2007. "The Drug Story You Haven't Read, Heard or Seen." *AFL Record* (Melbourne, Aust) (Aug 31–Sept 2): 6–7.

Smith, P. 2006a. "AFL Must Choose Between Welfare of Player and Game." *The Australian*, 16 August 2006. http://www.theaustralian.news.com.au/ story/0,20867,20142944–12270,00.html. Accessed 16 August 2006.

———. 2006b. "Appeasement Policy a Failure." *The Australian*, July 25 2006.

———. 2008. "Contaminated by Its Own Drug Code." *The Australian*, 6 September 2008. http://www.theaustralian.news.com.au/story/0,25197,24301252– 5013459,00.html. Accessed 11 September 2008.

———. 2010. "AFL Drugs Code Must Protect the Sick." *The Australian*, 4 September 2010. http://www.theaustralian.com.au/news/sport/afl-drugs-code-must-protect-the-sick/story-e6frg7t6–122591403199. Accessed 15 February 2011.

Stevens, M. 2004. "Denial Led to Angwin Sacking." *The Daily Telegraph*, 8 April 2004.

Stevens, M., and Barrett, D. 2004. "Carlton Crisis Blue Bust Carlton Board Investigates Norman, Angwin Breach." *Herald Sun*, 7 April 2004.

Stevens, M., Phillips, S., and Cunningham, M. 2004. "It's All Over for Blackened Blue Angwin Sacked Over Drug Use." *The Mercury*, 8 April 2004.

Stewart, B. 2006. "The World Anti-Doping Agency and the Australian Football League: The Irresistible Force Bludgeons the Immoveable Object." In *Football Fever: Moving the Goalposts*, edited by Nicholson, M., Stewart, B. and Hess, R., 107–114. Hawthorne, VIC: Maribyrnong Press.

———. 2007. "Drugs in Australian Sport: A Brief History." *Sporting Traditions* 23 (2): 65–78.

Stewart, B., Dickson, G., and Smith, A. 2008. "Drug Use in the Australian Football League: a Critical Survey." *Sporting Traditions* 25 (1): 57–74.

Stewart, B., Nicholson, M., and Dickson, G. 2005. "The Australian Football Leagues' Recent Progress: A Study in Cartel Conduct and Monopoly Power." *Sport Management Review* (Melbourne, Aust) 8 (2): 95–117.

Stewart, B., Nicholson, M., Smith, A., and Westerbeek, H. 2004. *Australian Sport: Better by Design?: The Evolution of Australian Sport Policy*. London: Routledge.

Stoddart, B. 1986. *Saturday Afternoon Fever: Sport in the Australian Culture*. London: Angus and Robertson.

Timms, D. 2002. "Koops in Clear, Finally." *Herald Sun*. 30 April 2002.

Tonts, M., and Atherley, K. 2010. "Competitive Sport and the Construction of Place Identity in Rural Australia." *Sport in Society* 13 (3): 381–398.

Toohey, K. 2010. "Post-Sydney 2000 Australia: A Potential Clash of Aspirations Between Recreational and Elite Sport." *The International Journal of the History of Sport* 27 (16):2 766–2779.

Toohey, K., and Taylor, T. 2009. "Sport in Australia: 'Worth a Shout.'" *Sport in Society* 12 (7): 837–841.

Walter, B. 2007. "My 14 Years of Drugs: Joey." *The Age*, League HQ, 31 August 2007. http://www.brisbanetimes.com.au/news/sport/my-14-years-of-drugs-joey/2007/ 08/30/1188067339383.html. Accessed 4 September 2014.

Warner, M. 2011. "Six AFL Players Fail Illicit Drug Tests in 2010." *Herald Sun*, 22 June 2011. http://www.heraldsun.com.au/ipad/six-afl-players-fail-illicit-drug-tests-in-2010/story-fn6bfkm6–122607996800. Accessed 28 July 2011.

Weber, M. 1969. *Economy and Society*. 2 vols. Berkeley: University of California Press.

Whitham, J. 2010. "Failed Drugs Tests Falling." AFL.com.au, 13 May 2010. http://www.afl.com.au/news/newsarticle/tabid/208/newsid/94185/default.aspx. Accessed 13 July 2011.

———. 2011. "AFL's $1.25 Billion Broadcast Deal." Australian Football League, 28 April 2011. http://www.afl.com.au/news/newsarticle/tabid/208/newsid/112560/default.aspx. Accessed 16 August 2011.

Wilson, J. 2006a. "Drugs Trio Fight to Stay Anonymous." *Herald Sun*, 22 May 2006.

———. 2006b. "Kennett Raises Heat on Drugs." *Herald Sun*, 4 April 2006.

———.2006c. "Stop Protecting the Cheats: Gosper." *The Australian*, 1 September 2006. http://www.theaustralian.news.com.au/story/0,20867,20320923–23211,00.html. Accessed 4 September 2006.

Wilson, R. 2006d. "AFL Failing Everyone in War against Drugs." *The Advertiser*, 2 September 2006.

———. 2006e. "Name Names and End AFL Drug Farce." *The Advertiser*, 1 April 2006.

———. 2007. "A Sorry Situation." *The Daily Telegraph*, 20 October 2007. http://www.news.com.au/dailytelegraph/story/0,22049,22614222–5006065,00.html. Accessed 31 December 2007.

Wuthnow, R., Hunter, J., Bergesen, A., and Kurzweil, E. 1984. *Cultural Analysis*. London: Routledge.

5   Mediating Legitimacy and Moral Panics

> ... what is this debate ... all about? I'd submit it's about paternalism and control. A few luddites and prudes have ... induced a full-blown moral panic over ... substances that ... have attracted the ire of ... people who have made it their job to tell us what is and isn't good for us.
>
> (Balko 2008, *Reason Online*)

Socio-historical examinations, such as those discussed in previous chapters using the IOC, WADA and the AFL as case studies, explored changing attitudes to drug use in sport over time and examined interactions between organizations in the context of anti-doping regulation. The transfer of authority for anti-doping regulation from the IOC to WADA can be conceptualized as driven by a crisis of legitimacy, contributing to doping as an institutionalized moral panic. Importantly, WADA is not a regulatory body. Nevertheless, it has created an overarching framework that governments have employed to control funding to sporting bodies. This raises questions of governance and control, as financial benefits and international prestige, including participation in Olympic competition, becomes increasingly dependent upon implementation of WADC-aligned anti-doping policies. At the same time, however, the creation of WADA presents SGBs with opportunities to restore legitimacy by being seen to be 'doing the right thing' by implementing WADA-aligned anti-doping policies and control measures in order to protect their particular sporting community.

I considered these issues in the Australian national context using the AFL and its interactions with the Australian federal government. The media played a central role in that debate and provided a forum where stakeholder groups made and challenged claims to legitimacy. Media reports also discussed drugs in Australian football in a manner consistent with the construction of a moral panic. That case study not only demonstrated the multi-dimensional and complex nature of legitimacy, but also pointed to a relationship between legitimacy and a moral panic. Here I investigate that relationship more explicitly by focusing on the media as a site where claims to legitimacy are made, and contested, in a moral panic. The moral panic model formulated by Goode and Ben-Yehuda (2009) provides a valuable theoretical tool to consider media coverage of doping. However, in the particular case of drugs in sport, the multi-dimensional nature of legitimacy and the complex interactions between organizational actors require a modification to that model. Goode and Ben-Yehuda also acknowledge that moral panics can take diverse forms that produce different effects with different outcomes under particular circumstances. I use a legitimacy-inspired modified moral panic model to show that constructions of doping reflect the interests of elite SGBs.

Goode and Ben-Yehuda suggest that a Weberian perspective can be applied to moral panic theory. They focus on the changing nature of foundations of authority in modern society and the "routinization of charisma" (Goode and Ben-Yehuda 2009, 246). From this perspective, obedience stems from the charisma of leaders rather than traditional forms of authority, such as that inherited by birth or through bureaucracy. The "excitement" of a moral panic is similar to the charisma of leaders, which is also volatile and unstable. In this context, charismatic leaders may be more successful in transforming initial expressions of concern into a moral panic. Like "charismatic leaders," Goode and Ben-Yehuda (2009, 246) state, "some moral panics are, almost unwittingly, more successful in routinizing the demands for action that are generated during these relatively brief episodes of collective excitement." This approach usefully sharpens the analysis of moral panics to look at whether they leave an institutional legacy of 'doing something' about the problematic behavior. My aim in this book is to demonstrate that Weber's concept of legitimacy can enhance understandings of efforts by elite groups to maintain authority in some moral panics.

Considering legitimacy is useful, as it analytically captures power relationships between organizations and the way these shape debates. Although privileged, elite groups cannot take for granted claims to the moral authority or legitimacy in order to 'pull the strings.' Rather, these groups must, at least to a certain extent, work to generate and maintain support for an institutional response to a specific problem that is of particular concern (Beamish 2009), which is a central feature of a moral panic. Members of the public are also not passive, easily manipulated recipients of information (Goode and Ben-Yehuda 2009), but filter messages, including those from the mass media, through complex social networks and knowledge frameworks (Reiner 2007). Further, the diversity of stakeholders in modern life means that there are different notions of legitimacy operating in communities (Pakulski 1986; Suchman 1995). This means that dominant groups cannot take claims to legitimacy for granted. Rather, maintaining support, and thus compliance, with regulatory frameworks, such as anti-doping regulation, requires ongoing consensus-making work between and amongst a range of diverse stakeholders.

Next, I outline the moral panic criteria and key aspects of the social theory underpinning analysis of a moral panic formulated by Goode and Ben-Yehuda and my modifications to that model. Drawing on the debate around doping, that discussion is followed by a review of media reports structured around the modified moral panic criteria.

MORAL PANIC THEORY AND CRITERIA

In Chapter 1 of this book I discussed the moral panic criteria listed in Goode and Ben-Yehuda's (2009) model. In summary, those criteria are consensus, concern, hostility, disproportionality and volatility. These are useful tools with which to identify a moral panic. Earlier I also outlined the social theories underpinning Goode and Ben-Yehuda's moral panic analysis, which are the grassroots theory, interest-group theory and the elite-engineered moral panic theory, this last being the approach modified and used in this book. I commence by modifying consensus to consensus-making in order to capture the multi-dimensional nature of legitimacy, which is illustrated by considering the doping debate as an elites-engineered institutionalized moral panic.

Consensus to Consensus-Making

Goode and Ben-Yehuda (2009) note that consensus in a moral panic not only includes generating agreement that an issue threatens the social order from a range of social actors but also extends to include support for particular solutions to that problem. However, consensus can be fractured, as not all groups will agree on the causes, consequences or solutions to the threat presented by a particular issue or group (Garland 2008). Although useful, consensus does not capture the complex interactions and potential conflicts among dominant groups or the role of legitimacy in the context of contemporary social debates. In the case of doping as a moral panic, 'consensus-making' more accurately reflects the interactive processes and negotiated power relationships between dominant groups, such as WADA, elite SGBs, governments as well as the media.

Consensus-making is more appropriate in the debate over PEDs, as it incorporates a range of elite stakeholder groups. These groups have diverse interests and use anti-doping policies to achieve specific outcomes and objectives that are relevant to their sporting community. For example, the AFL used anti-drugs policies as part of a regulatory framework to protect the commercial viability of Australian football and develop the game, which was linked to grassroots participation. The Australian federal government took a strong anti-doping stance to maintain their international status and linked drug-free sport to community well-being (Chapter 4, this volume). Added to this, elite SGBs and governments are not the only stakeholders in modern sport. Athletes, coaches and publics, amongst others, are also stakeholders with a vested interest in sport. SGBs must generate support from these groups for the legitimacy of particular institutional responses to PEDs, as we saw in the case of the AFL and the Australian government.

The media featured heavily in that debate, highlighting Goode and Ben-Yehuda's (2009, 90) description of the media as the "beating heart" of a moral panic capable of influencing elite groups and public opinion. Media reports also provide a forum for challenges to the legitimacy of elite SGBs. Consequently, claim-makers seek to build support, or generate consensus, from the media as another key institutional actor in the doping debate. Consensus-making more accurately describes different elite groups' use of the media to present and maintain concern over doping and generate hostility toward PED-using 'folk devils' who are perceived to threaten social stability and to posit their regulatory solutions as legitimate responses to the issue.

Concern and Hostility

A successful moral panic, explain Goode and Ben-Yehuda (2009), includes public concern that an issue threatens social order as well as a deviant group, a 'folk devil,' identified as threatening community values and against whom community concern and hostility are directed. The media are an integral part of this process. Using melodramatic language to describe the deviant group and the consequences for social well-being, media reports can fan the flames of public concern (Cohen 2002). This also concerns processes of inclusion and exclusion, as identifying the threatening group creates a division between respectable members of society and the "bad guys, undesirables, outsiders, criminals, the underworld, disreputable folk" (Goode and Ben-Yehuda 2009, 38). Media reports point to the agents capable of 'policing' community boundaries by introducing measures to restore order and safeguard community values (Erikson 1966). There are implications here for the legitimacy of claim-makers. A perceived failure to implement necessary and effective regulatory mechanisms to identify, catch or control deviants can create a crisis of legitimacy. For example, media reports criticized the AFL's illicit drug policy as "lame" (Wilson 2006b, *The Advertiser*) and as "tacit approval of recreational drug abuse" (Wilson 2006a, *The Advertiser*). Not only do these types of claims exaggerate the extent and consequences of deviant behavior, contributing to concern and hostility, they also point to the moral panic criterion of disproportionality.

Disproportionality

Exaggerated claims of the extent of deviant behavior fall into Goode and Ben-Yehuda's (2009) moral panic criterion of disproportionality. This criterion describes the belief of a community, or sections of a community, that a larger number of deviant individuals are engaged in the problematic behavior than actually exist. Further, the 'danger' associated with these exaggerated claims is usually not as significant as those posed by other social issues that are more harmful. Exaggerated claims stimulate community concern and hostility based on constructions of the problem as widespread, ongoing and demanding action. This can take the form of a specific institutional response, which can also lead to strengthening existing connections with agents of social control or the incorporation of other agents of control, such as law enforcement authorities (Cohen 2002; Goode and Ben-Yehuda 2009).

In the context of the doping debate, WADA and other elite sporting authorities construct PED use as a growing problem that not only threatens elite sport, but also broader community well-being. WADA is presented as the problem-specific institutional solution, which brings in other law enforcement groups, such as Interpol, in order to effectively curb the spread of the dangerous behavior (Chapter 3, this volume). However, a problem-specific institutional response also provides a basis for evaluations of claims to legitimacy, as claim-makers must maintain support for the legitimacy and authority of that response. This is important because concern and hostility and the associated volatility of a moral panic tend to subside over time.

Volatility

Describing moral panics as volatile refers to the fact that the 'fever pitch' of concern or hostility generated during a moral panic tends to wane over time. This has led some to describe moral panics as "fadlike" (Goode and Ben-Yehuda 2009, 41). However, Goode and Ben-Yehuda also note that, irrespective of the potentially short-lived nature of some moral panics, others leave a significant institutional legacy (see also Cohen 2002; Chapter 1, this volume). The challenge for the generators of these moral panics is to maintain public and media attention over time. There are implications here for claim-makers' legitimacy. The tendency for the initial momentum of a moral panic to subside means that claims to legitimacy cannot be taken for granted. Rather, dominant groups must vigorously work to maintain support for their particular institutional solution to an issue of specific concern. In terms of the doping debate as a moral panic, the task for WADA is to demonstrate that their anti-doping approach catches 'cheats' while contending that continued doping events show that the need for WADA to protect sport remains necessary. This also means that WADA must engage in consensus-making work to maintain support for their legitimacy and moral authority as the institution responsible for the global harmonization of anti-doping frameworks.

The moral panic criteria formulated by Goode and Ben-Yehuda (2009) provides a valuable tool that can be used to consider whether a phenomenon constitutes a moral panic, including doping in sport. To capture the complex interactions between elite stakeholders in the doping debate, I modify that model by expanding consensus to consensus-making, which is also an important criterion for investigating doping as an elite-engineered moral panic or, as I elaborate, an elites-engineered panic.

Elite-Engineered to Elites-Engineered

Goode and Ben-Yehuda (2009) point out that the traditional elite-engineered theory argues that elite groups drive a moral panic. This theory is underpinned by the argument that elites frequently and "intimately interact" with one another and, with interests in common, seek to protect those interests (Goode and Ben-Yehuda 2009, 52–53). In their analysis of mugging in 1970s Britain as an elite-engineered moral panic, Hall et al. (1978) argued that elite groups "orchestrate hegemony." In that instance, elite groups sought to convince the population that criminal elements were the 'problem' in order to deflect attention from a crisis in British capitalism. For Goode and Ben-Yehuda (2009, 66), the claim that elite groups orchestrate a moral panic is "strictly comic book fare" that underplays the active role of other social agents, such as the media and the public. While acknowledging Goode and Ben-Yehuda's point, an elite-engineered theory usefully identifies what might be at stake for dominant groups in a moral panic. However, one difficulty with an elite-engineered approach is that it neglects the diversity of interests and power relationships amongst and between elite groups. A more effective way in which to capture the competing needs of elite groups in the context of PEDs as an institutionalized moral panic is to shift to an 'elites-engineered' theory. This subtle modification to the traditional elite-engineered view highlights the multifaceted aspect of legitimacy influenced by complex relationships between and amongst different elite stakeholders. It also aligns with the significance of consensus-making.

THE MEDIA REVIEW

To illustrate the value of the modified moral panic criteria outlined above, and as the media play a central role in a moral panic, I use a review of media reports of doping and institutional responses to doping. Like the interviews I report in the next chapter, the media review formed part of the multi-dimensional research design used in my doctoral research. The principal data sources for this review consisted of online reports concerning doping and anti-doping responses from international media agencies, with data collection taking place between mid-2006 and mid-2009, generating a data set of over 10,000 articles. I searched these sources using standardized 'Google Alerts' and combinations of search strings with phrases including 'doping,' 'performance-enhancing drugs,' 'World Anti-Doping Agency,' and 'International Olympic Committee.' I located additional material using keywords in databases, such as Australian Public Affairs, Australian Public Affairs Information Service, JSTOR and ProQuest, among others.

The increasingly interdependent nature of the modern media, with information regularly exchanged between wire services and newspapers, complicates data collection. Although increasing the speed with which news flows to the public, this encourages "a parrot-like character in which the various media segments tend to reproduce rather than examine one another's views" (Knopf 1970, 21). To overcome unnecessary article duplication and produce a data set that could be more easily analyzed, I sorted the data by publisher and limited inclusion to publishers with 15 or more articles. This resulted in a data set of 571 articles, as listed in Table 5.1. I acknowledge that these are relatively arbitrary distinctions, however, they reflect the limited resources available to a doctoral candidate in terms of data analysis. Nevertheless, in light of the findings presented below, it is unlikely that using other distinctions would result in any modification to the claim that the doping debate constitutes an institutionalized moral panic.

I explored the reports gathered for descriptions of PED use as problematic behavior engaged in by deviant individuals requiring action to resolve. This included phrases, or a moral panic inventory (Cohen 2002), such as the 'fight against doping,' anti-doping as a 'war' or 'battle' and 'cheats' or 'drug cheats.' Searching media reports for these keywords also reflects the influence of Goode and Ben-Yehuda's moral panic criteria of concern and hostility. These criteria require the identification of 'folk devils' responsible for behavior that threatens social order and provides a focus for collective action.

There were a number of articles (190) with headlines that used phrases from the moral panic inventory but that did not contain any of those phrases in the content. Such headlines nevertheless influence the way that audiences

Table 5.1 Online Media Data Sources (n=571)

Publisher	Number of Articles	Publisher	Number of Articles
Agence France-Presse	59	*Los Angeles Times*	25
BBC	44	*Reuters*	39
Bloomberg	16	*Telegraph*	48
CBC	20	*The Guardian*	60
China View	27	*The New York Times*	52
Deutsche Welle	15	*Times Online*	28
International Herald Tribune	99	*USA Today*	39
Total			**571**

receive information (Ericson, Baranek and Chan 1991). As Parenti (1986, 223) notes, these types of headlines not only "mislead anyone who skims a page without reading the story, they can create the dominant slant on a story, establishing a mind-set that influences how we read the story's text." These types of articles also provided insight into whether the debate over doping are constructed as a moral panic. This 'headline only' group of articles included those that Rowe (1992) describes as 'hard news' and that reported details of athletes and substances in doping events (for example, see "Acrobatic Gymnast Okulova Banned for Doping Offense" in AP 2007a, *International Herald Tribune*). Also included in this group were articles with headlines that implied PED use was a growing problem, with doping 'cheats' threatening the sporting community. Such headlines included "Drug Taking is Rife in Golf, Claims Player" (Kelso 2007, *The Guardian*), "WADA Chief Pound Says Key Players Fear Doping Problem" (*Reuters* 2007) or "Drugs in Sport: Cheats Go to Great Lengths" (Knight 2008, *Telegraph*). These types of headlines suggest a moral panic, with claims that generate concern over doping as a significant issue, focusing attention on PED-using cheats.

To identify groups active in the debate, media reports were examined for statements made by stakeholders and summaries presented by reporters. For instance, a *Reuters South Africa* article reports the IAAF President's insistence that everything possible is being done to win the battle against drug cheats. In the same article the IAAF President is directly quoted as saying: "There are cheats out there but we are doing everything we can to catch them" (Himmer 2007). The direct quote of the IAAF President is an instance of an elite SGB's use of phrases from the moral panic inventory, while the reporter's reference to 'drug cheat' illustrates the media's use of those terms. The context surrounding phrases from the moral panic inventory is also important because the way that issues are categorized as well as how those categories are used to tell stories serve specific functions (Flick 2002; Silverman 2001). In this case, the issue was whether the function of those 'stories' is the construction of doping as an elites-engineered moral panic to protect the legitimacy of elite SGBs.

My use of media reports draws on Williams's (2006, 116) investigation of media representations of sexual assault cases in the AFL. She examined media coverage to "question whether, and how, a folk devil may have been created." I used a media review to examine whether media sources, and SGBs' use of the media, construct doping as a 'moral panic' that creates a PED-using 'folk devil' to restore or maintain the status quo (Cohen 2002; Goode and Ben-Yehuda 2009). Using my modified version of Goode and Ben-Yehuda's (2009) moral panic model, I examined media reports for statements that highlighted the harm or danger that PED-using athletes presented to the social order. These types of reports provide opportunities for expressions of support for an institutional response, such as WADA. This is beneficial to SGBs, as it helps them to enhance their own legitimacy.

However, and as I have noted throughout this book, this also raises issues of governance and control, as SGBs are required to implement WADC-aligned anti-doping policies for inclusion in Olympic competition and access to government funding.

Also of interest here is the context surrounding athletes' use of moral panic words. This is significant, as athletes are often relegated to the edges the debate, based on SGBs' assumptions that athletes' interests correspond with their own. Independent athletes associations are rare (Houlihan 2004). For example, a group of Olympic athletes, including Mark Tewksbury, Dawn Fraser and Zola Bud amongst others, launched Olympic Advocates Together Honorably (OATH) in 1999 to campaign for athletes' rights. The organization experienced financial collapse within two years (Athletes-CAN 1999; Houlihan 2004; OATH 1999a, 1999b). As Houlihan (2004, 421–422) notes:

> Sport policy is generally made for, or on behalf of, athletes, rarely in consultation with athletes, and almost never in partnership with athletes. In the UK, with the exception of professional football and, to a lesser extent, professional cricket, rugby union and rugby league, there are few sports where athletes have an organized and independent voice.

However, "talk about athletes permeates our newspapers, magazines, television programs and the internet," where athletes' lives are "described, held accountable and evaluated" (Lamont-Mills and Christensen 2008, 251–252). The media play an important role in this process, Paccagnella and Grove (1997, 180) explain, with high profile athletes "continuously. . . scrutinized because of their exposure in the visual and print media. Our knowledge and perceptions of these sport stars are shaped by their constant presence in the media." As well as athletes' personal characteristics and behavior, a significant area of interest for sports consumers is whether the way in which athletes achieve success complies with culturally defined norms. This includes classifications of PED use as unacceptable (Fairchild 1989; Paccagnella and Grove 1997). Consequently, the media reports were examined for athletes' responses to allegations of PED use and their 'stories' of doping. This is an important area of investigation for this book because, as Hoberman (1992, 101) explains: "This conflict, with sports bureaucrats and journalists arrayed against the athletes who practice doping and attempt to avoid detection, is the visible core of the 'doping problem' in high-performance sport."

Although athletes are key stakeholders in modern sport, the anti-doping framework centers on regulating these individuals irrespective of whether or not PED use has been alleged or proven to have taken place. In other words, the current anti-doping approach assumes that all athletes are potential 'folk devils.' The danger that this presents to the stability of sport necessitates, and legitimates, strict surveillance. Accordingly, I examined media reports to explore how athletes discussed doping, either in terms of accusations of PED use made against them or in relation to their views on the current anti-doping framework.

THE WAR ON DRUGS IN SPORT—A MORAL PANIC AND ORGANIZATIONAL LEGITIMACY

Goode and Ben-Yehuda (2009) note that each application of a moral panic framework to a social phenomenon reveals something new. In the consideration of the doping debate discussed in this book, I present a review of media reports to demonstrate the role of legitimacy in the creation of PEDs as a moral panic situated within an elites-engineered moral panic theory. Commencing with consensus-making, I illustrate how media reports are used by a range of stakeholders to construct doping as a moral panic with PED-using 'folk devils' as well as to support, and contest, organizational claims to legitimacy.

Consensus-Making

The media, elite SGBs and stakeholders, including athletes, discuss PEDs in a way that suggests broad consensus that doping threatens sport and is a global issue requiring a concerted, harmonized effort to resolve. According to an IOC spokesman: "The fight against doping in sport is a daily battle, which must be fought in concert by the sports authorities, sports teams, athletes and coaches, and governments" (AP 2007f, *International Herald Tribune*). Athletes also indicated that anti-doping required a concerted effort by 'clean' athletes. For example, 2004 Olympic women's 100 meter silver medalist Lauryn Williams stated: "It's not our mess, but as people passionate about the sport and competing . . . it's our responsibility to clean it up . . . " (in Perez 2008, *USA Today*). Governments described doping as an "ever-present specter" (Bond 2007, *Telegraph*), emphasizing the view that the danger from doping was widespread and permanent (Bowen 2007, *Deutsche Welle*). Anti-doping authorities expressed similar views. For example, a member of Germany's National Anti-Doping Agency (NADA) stated: "Everybody has accepted that there is a problem in sport, not only in cycling" (Amies 2007, *Deutsche Welle*).

As well as stressing the extent of doping, media reports pointed to the need for an effective institutional response, namely WADA, with "global efforts to combat doping in sport" underpinned by an improved WADC as the "core document" that has "fine-tune[d] provisions . . . to strengthen global efforts against doping in sport . . . " (Xinhua 2007, *China View*). Other reports generate consensus not only regarding the "magnitude" of the problem, but also point to the appropriate institutional solution:

. . . it's time for Selig [Commissioner for Major League Baseball] and Fehr [Executive Director of the Major League Baseball Players Association] to wave the white flag . . . allow a big-time, independent group with knowledge of the international complexities of the issue to take over the . . . job of MLB drug testing. (Brennan 2007, *USA Today*)

This language generates support for the claim that sport is endangered. Similarly, Germany's Interior Minister stated that doping destroys "the value of sport. . . . Its credibility, its function as a provider of role models and its approval by the public are being put on the test" (*Deutsche Welle* 2007b). Doping, or allegations of doping, "taints the image of sport that is facing a crisis of public confidence" (Broadbent 2008, *Times Online*). For sporting authorities that are "mandated to set the terms and conditions for participation" (Vasciannie 2006), ongoing doping events leading to any crisis of public confidence clearly have implications for claims to organizational legitimacy.

Goode and Ben-Yehuda (2009) note that in a moral panic the media provide an important site for claim-makers to construct issues as problematic based on the threat which the deviant behavior presents to social order. In support of this, articles about PEDs both framed and provided a vehicle for claim-makers to present doping as an issue of concern not only for international elite sport, but also for the amateur sporting community. Doping, argued former WADA Chairman Richard Pound, "is like alcoholism," and "unless people involved realize there is a problem, it's impossible to have a cure." The article goes on to report that there remains a "pressing need to . . . investigate doping in amateur sports," citing Pound's warning that the global community needs to realize "how serious this problem is, and how important it is to . . . turn it around" (*CBC News* 2007). This report supports the moral panic criterion of consensus, where dominant groups present issues as a danger to social order and the importance of community support for a strong anti-doping response. By associating doping with alcoholism, it emphasizes the pervasiveness of the issue.

More specifically, linking doping to a social issue about which audiences may already hold preconceived ideas as problematic contributes to receptive views of progressively more "repressive, tough . . . policy proposals" (Pritchard and Hughes 1997, 49). There is evidence of this in the media reports, with a range of social actors describing doping using a "language of war" (Foster 2001, 181), such as anti-doping authorities that talk about "getting tough" and "expanding the arsenal of weapons" while WADA wages a war against the "drug cheats" (Hemphill 2008, 3). This highlights the 'righteousness' of the anti-doping campaign, which claims to reflect broader community concerns to protect sport for the 'clean' honest athletes (Hemphill 2008). The moral danger presented by doping also creates opportunities to promote the necessity of an institutional, regulatory response.

For example, IOC President Jacques Rogge described drug-free sport as "Utopia" and that it would be "naive to believe that no-one will take drugs" because with "400 million people practicing sport . . . there are not 400 million saints . . . Cheating is embedded in human nature . . . doping is to sport what criminality is to society," which will "always need cops and judges and prisons and jails and rules and regulations" (cited in AFP 2008c). As well as justifying a strong institutional and regulatory response to doping, this comment demonstrates the moral panic criterion of consensus-making by elite groups as they work to maintain support for such an approach.

There is also evidence of consensus-making in comments made by former WADA President John Fahey reported in the media. Fahey argued that the "extremely important" anti-doping efforts of WADA "must succeed" in order to maintain the stability and survival of sport and values popularly associated with it: "Otherwise, I think sport will wither and probably die if we can't get integrity back into it by fair play" (AP 2007c, *International Herald Tribune*). According to WADA, the elimination of doping is essential to protect the very essence of sport. This is best accomplished by applying the ever-increasing store of anti-doping knowledge and enforcement practices that WADA is accumulating. Fahey stresses the importance of this task in order to restore public confidence and "return sport to its very essence." Any failure to do so not only risks losing "part of the world as we've known it" but also that "the public will desert any sport . . . that they are not satisfied has integrity. . . . We are smarter than we used to be and . . . our investigations are becoming effective" (WADA President John Fahey in AFP 2008d). Fahey's consistent reference to 'us' and 'we' provides evidence of consensus-making not only that doping is an ongoing and widespread issue, but also that it requires a concerted and strong institutional response. Further, although claiming that anti-doping "investigations are becoming effective," the continued threat doping presents to "part of the world as we've known it" amplifies, and justifies, the need for WADA's continued efforts. The suggestion that the value and integrity of sport is under attack highlights the need for institutional action to 'combat' drugs in sport.

This review of media reports demonstrates that elite SGBs actively work to generate agreement that doping is problematic behavior. There is also evidence of consensus-making in WADA's efforts to generate support for their actions as the necessary anti-doping response. However, a moral panic will not emerge without a level of public concern. For a successful moral panic, claim-makers must focus public concern on a group identified as the 'folk devil,' which can then be controlled using a particular institutional framework.

Concern and Hostility

A moral panic builds on the fear that a particular behavior or specific group threatens not only the well-being but also the fundamental values of society

(Baerveldt, Bunkers, de Winter and Kooistra 1998; Goode and Ben-Yehuda 1994). The media play an important role in this process. The question here is whether there is evidence in the media reports indicating that stakeholders use the media to make claims that doping is dangerous behavior threatening the integrity of sport as well as any claims linking 'clean' sport to broader social welfare.

The media reports reviewed provided evidence that elite claim-makers generate concern around doping as threatening the integrity of sport. For example, one media report stated that "IOC President, Jacques Rogge . . . sees doping for what it is: Fraud that threatens sport's credibility" (Farquhar 2008, *BBC Sport*). WADA uses media reports to present doping as deviant behavior engaged in by individuals lacking moral integrity, placing sport in danger of losing support from the public and sponsors. One media report describes part of WADA's task as "providing the answers as it seeks to promote clean sport," going on to cite WADA President John Fahey as stating that this includes a requirement to "penetrate the world with the message that only idiots involve themselves in doping." The report continues by noting that "Fahey . . . has warned that sports tainted by doping are at risk of 'moral bankruptcy' and could turn viewers and sponsors away" (cited in Beck 2008, *Reuters*). These comments demonstrate that the debate over doping can be conceptualized as a moral panic, with elite groups generating concern that deviant individuals, described as "idiots," are threatening the sporting community. They also highlight that although couched as defending values popularly associated with 'clean sport,' a concern to protect more instrumental objectives, such as the commercial returns integral to modern sport, underpins the debate.

Stakeholders' use of media reports to manufacture concern over doping incorporated claims that PEDs are a danger to the wider community, including as a public health issue that increasingly threatens youth. Media reports cited WADA's claims that doping was a "global scourge" threatening "public health" and an issue of particular concern because "illicit use" of PEDs spreads into "schools and neighborhoods" (Saraceno 2007, *USA Today*). This creates a sense of urgency, suggesting the danger is close to the audience's immediate social environment (von Hoffman 1985, 10; Chapter 1, this volume). For example, rather than "lurking in some back alley to buy from some pusher," young people "need only sit down at their PC—and they are" (Saraceno 2007, *USA Today*). These constructs provided opportunities for stakeholder-generated media reports to maintain a public focus on, and support for, preferred anti-doping initiatives.

WADA used the media to emphasize that the "public are sick and tired of cheats" and to position WADA's efforts as meeting community expectations regarding drug-free sport, with "enormous" public support for anti-doping initiatives (WADA President John Fahey in Kelso 2008, *The Guardian*). Nevertheless, in the same report WADA goes on to claim that the danger remains, which means that "we have to inculcate" youth into an appropriate values-based approach to sport, namely to play "within the rules," including "fair play." Referring to the 2008 Beijing Olympics, WADA argues that this also creates an obligation for government action to "weed out the cheats. . . . If they make it to Beijing . . . we have every reason to have greater confidence in . . . detection of . . . cheats than . . . any previous Games" (WADA President John Fahey in Kelso 2008, *The Guardian*). These comments illustrate the moral panic criterion of concern and also identify a folk devil, or 'cheat,' who provides a focus for collective action. Exaggerated claims of the extent of doping, such as that PED use has spread into 'schools and neighborhoods,' illustrate the criterion of disproportionality. This also constructs a 'vulnerable' population—youth—that needs defending. These media comments defend the moral values 'popularly' associated with sport, such as 'fair play,' and suggest that the education of young people regarding the importance of 'playing within the rules' is an important element of the anti-drugs campaign. These types of comments highlight the role of consensus toward values such as fair play in conjunction with rules and regulations that 'detect cheats' in securing legitimacy for anti-doping frameworks.

Media reports presenting WADA's regulatory approach as enjoying public support suggest that it has built positive perceptions of legitimacy, and that its anti-doping efforts meet community expectations. Bolstering this view, WADA used media reports to claim that the 'public has warmed up' to the anti-doping campaign. Associating PED use with 'health risks' and links to 'organized crime' that threaten social order, WADA emphasizes the need for a strong regulatory response. In this respect, WADA points to "a new perspective" on the part of "public authorities," one that links "cheating" with "people—including organized crime" as well as "trafficking and selling and distribution of . . . substances." This is a significant problem because, as WADA goes on to state, "it's not just a whole bunch of . . . athletes . . . it's millions and millions of kids unsupervised with stuff that they can buy on the internet" (WADA Chairman Richard Pound, cited in *IHT* 2007b). The extent of this problem, argued WADA, justifies "governments and law enforcement agencies, like Interpol and the FBI, to support the battle against doping rings and suppliers" (Whittle 2008, *International Herald Tribune*). Constructing anti-doping efforts as a battle necessarily implies the existence of an 'enemy,' or 'folk devil,' responsible for the threat and deviant behavior. Identifying those responsible for the threatening behavior normalizes expressions of hostility toward those individuals (Goode and Ben-Yehuda 1994). Claims that 'millions and millions of kids' are exposed to PED use constructs doping as a dangerous problem, including the potential for youth to be manipulated by criminal groups and cybercrime.

While this indicates support for the moral panic criterion of disproportionality, discussed below, these types of media reports also provide opportunities to focus public concern, creating boundaries between 'clean' athletes juxtaposed against PED-using folk devils. In this discourse, PED use constitutes a 'scandal' that represents a lack of morality on the part of doping athletes. It places transgressing individuals outside the 'clean' and respectable community. For example: " 'Doping is unacceptable, a social crime,' Ljungqvist said in Tuesday's *Times* newspaper" (Herman 2007, *The Guardian*). This illustrates Hier et al.'s (2011, 263) point that moral panic discourses can include "defensive group reactions" that emphasize the harm to the social order posed by "irresponsible" others who fail to engage in individual risk management by avoiding PED use. The moral value attached to 'clean' participation reinforces the boundary between 'us'—those who participate within the rules—and the deviant and dangerous 'other.' According to WADA, the "fight against doping is a living exercise" requiring "unwavering vigilance" and "willingness to tackle those people who are the sociopaths of sport—they will always be there" (WADA Chairman Richard Pound, cited in *BBC Sport 2007*). Describing PED-using athletes as 'sociopaths of sport' creates an ever-present folk devil against whom to direct collective action. These types of media reports that often contrast 'clean' athletes with PED-using athletes contribute to public perception that those who are not doping are in the minority:

> It is a gloomy scenario, given the widespread concern about drugs in sport and athletics in particular. Kelly Sotherton, the Briton who finished third in the heptathlon at the World Championships in Osaka, Japan, in August, said that there was suspicion on every podium. (Broadbent 2007, *Times Online*)

These media constructions bring athletes into the frontline of the doping war. Some athletes stress the importance of identifying PED-using 'cheats' to maintain the integrity of sport as well as emphasizing that they participate 'clean.' Some examples generate an atmosphere of pharmacological 'McCarthyism.' For instance, United States sprint star Allyson Felix stated that she would "definitely inform on cheats" and expressed her confidence in the "advanced" testing regime. She went on to admit that although public suspicion of a "great performance" was "undeniable," that was "unfortunate because the clean athletes are out there working hard every single day . . . we have to pay for the poor decisions that other athletes have made" (in Slater 2008, *BBC Sport*). Emphasizing that athletes are on the frontline of the war against drugs in sport, United States Olympic swimmer Dara Torres remarked that "you can't look someone in the eye and say, 'I'm not taking drugs.' . . . You have to take action. I've really tried everything I possibly can to take action and prove that I'm clean" (in Goffa 2008, *Los Angeles Times*). In contrast with cheating 'folk devils,' these types of reports create a counter-image of clean athletes as 'folk heroes.' More specifically, they act to maintain concern over doping as a significant problem and focus attention on the necessity of an effective and firm anti-doping regulatory framework to protect 'clean' athletes and their right to 'fair' competition.

It is also important to underpin this with a discussion of how media reports provide athletes and other members of the sporting community with opportunities to broaden the debate beyond a focus on the individual athlete. For example, professional cyclist Jörg Jaksche described his experiences while working for the Telekom cycling team as his "crash course," including being given a "shot of EPO in my room." According to Jaksche, "I did what I had to do to be better in my job" and in order to keep up with other cyclists because "everyone is doing it. . . . You live in a parallel world in cycling. The team leadership knew everything. It was a fully installed system" (in *Deutsche Welle* 2007c). Other internal stakeholders also point to the influence of structural pressures, such as the status attached to winning performances and monetary incentives, on athletes' decisions to dope. For example:

> . . . They are not so much trying to cheat as they are trying to get the most out of their bodies. And the carrot held out, the gold medals and big money, drives them to push their bodies. (Mark Sisson, former marathon runner and triathlete who has also been Executive Director of the US Triathlon Federation and Chairman of the International Triathlon Union, in Dwyer 2008, *Los Angeles Times*)

While highlighting structural pressures as factors influencing PED use, media reports nevertheless construe doping as deviant behavior that requires strong regulation and control. WADA, underpinned by the WADC, is presented as the primary mechanism to accomplish this task. According to WADA President John Fahey, as well as requiring "enormous energy and commitment, conviction," this is a "fight we must win" and that with "new weaponry to WADA" in the form of a "new [Anti-Doping] Code, to progress and reinvigorate this fight . . . we all have to remind ourselves that this is a worldwide effort and keep the W in WADA" (in AFP 2007a). Support for WADA, through the WADC, to regulate against PED use is also evident in media comments made by government stakeholders. For example, the Dutch Health Secretary praised the role of the WADC in "ensuring that [doping] is combated and punished in the same way everywhere in the world" (*International Herald Tribune* 2007a). Comments such as this focus public concern on doping as a 'fight' that requires a 'worldwide effort' and that positions WADA as the good weapon.

A moral panic includes constructions of deviant behavior that maintain public concern, identify the deviant group and suggest to the public a solution to the problem. As the review of media reports presented here has shown, the moral panic criteria of concern and hostility are evident in the doping debate. Key institutional stakeholders, including the media, WADA, SGBs and governments all use media reports to build concern that doping is widespread, ongoing and requires action to resolve. Media reports constructing PED-using athletes as 'cheats' or 'idiots' that threaten sport and present a public health danger to the community not only generate concern but also provide a focus for anti-doping action. Although media reports provide some space for athletes to 'fight back' against constructions implying that all athletes should be viewed with suspicion as potential PED-using 'folk devils,' these reports nevertheless support the need for a strong regulatory response and position WADA as the necessary solution. The moral panic criterion of disproportionality illuminates the way that dominant groups stimulate public concern and hostility toward deviant individuals and maintain support for their institutional solution.

Disproportionality

Goode and Ben-Yehuda's (2009) criterion of disproportionality refers to a community's view that a larger number of individuals than actually exist are engaged in deviant behavior. The point is not that the particular behavior does not exist; in fact there generally is some measurable level of "damage" caused by the particular social problem (Jones, McFalls and Gallagher 1989, 342). Rather, the important point is the exaggeration of the extent of the problem, which is used to highlight the necessity of an institutional response and associated enforcement practices (Jones et al. 1989). As I noted earlier in this book, in a moral panic statistics are often used to persuade audiences not only to illustrate the extent of the problem but also the efficacy of solutions to the deviant behavior (e.g., see also Best 2002; Chapter 1, this volume). In the debate over drugs in sport, quantification of PED use performs an important function in terms of enhancing claims to moral authority and legitimacy. For example, media reports cited figures of the number of positive tests from the 2008 Beijing Olympics to support claims that anti-doping efforts are succeeding, despite the ongoing nature of the problem, because "with less than a dozen positive cases compared to 26 at Athens . . . the Beijing Games were held up by the IOC as proof that they were winning the war on drugs" (AFP 2008b). This promotes the efforts, and thus the legitimacy of the IOC, in the 'war on drugs.' Further, as the IOC and all Olympic participants are required to be WADC-compliant, it enhances perceptions of WADA's legitimacy and moral authority to regulate the Olympic sporting community.

Reports such as the one just cited demonstrate the efficacy of the anti-doping framework and boost claims to legitimacy by elite SGBs, including WADA and the IOC, by using drugs testing results, such as small numbers of positive tests. Other anti-doping organizational actors, such as NADAs, also report drugs testing statistics in the media. Germany's NADA, for instance, "published figures showing that 62 of the 8196, or 0.7 per cent, of the doping tests it ran in 2006 were positive. Most of the controls were done in track and field sports. The numbers were essentially unchanged since 2005" (*Deutsche Welle* 2007a). These types of reports and the statistical details provided suggest that the claims of some stakeholders that doping is a 'global scourge' appear to be exaggerated. Further, appeals to small numbers of adverse results can also challenge organizational claims to legitimacy, particularly those based on assertions that PED use is a growing issue that threatens public health more broadly, such as WADA. This is because data can be used by interest-groups in order to influence the debate either to support existing policies or criticize a group as failing to address the issue.

Illustrating this point, Burnside (2007) reported on the debate between WADA and the American National Hockey League (NHL) regarding claims of shortcomings in the NHL testing policy. Burnside reported that there had been only one positive test from 3,000 random tests on NHL players over a period of less than two seasons. Revealing that discourses around drug testing results reflect contested claims to legitimacy as much as any indication of the "state of the game, and the role of performance-enhancing drugs in it," he points out that from the perspective of the NHL and its players, these "results reinforce the commonly held belief in hockey . . . that the NHL did not and does not have a problem." However, he says, for others who believe the "league's policy is like Swiss cheese in the number of loopholes it provides, the results mean nothing." This demonstrates that claims to legitimacy, including those reliant on testing statistics, cannot be taken for granted but are contested by other elite claim-makers with vested interests in the debate.

Nevertheless, claim-makers in the doping debate call on statistical data as well as 'socially accredited experts' (Becker 1963) to stress the widespread nature of doping. Experts such as Dr. Gary Wadler, Chairman of WADA's Prohibited List and Methods Sub-Committee (WADA September 2009), are cited to emphasize that doping is a 'silent epidemic' threatening youth. Reporting on the 2007 Monitoring the Future[1] survey data that "2.2% of high school seniors" had used steroids "at least once," a media report suggested that, because this was simply a survey rather than testing results, that percentage was "likely low" (Brennan 2008, *USA Today*). Compared to WADA's 2007 Olympic testing results, which revealed testing results of 1.93% for all banned substances, the report cites Wadler as stating that the survey data was not "insignificant" but revealed a "silent epidemic" (Brennan 2008, *USA Today*). From a moral panic perspective, this report suggests that doping will contaminate society, and particularly youth, 'unless something is done' (Cohen 2002). As well as indicating PED use as a growing problem, the use of statistics also illustrates that negotiated power relationships between organizations and contested claims to legitimacy need to be considered as part of the moral panic surrounding the doping debate.

Using Wadler as an authoritative WADA representative, media reports called the legitimacy of other sporting organizations, such as Major League Baseball (MLB), into question because of their failure to implement adequate anti-doping policies. For example, Wadler is reported as describing baseball's management as "out of their league" and indicating that professional sport, including baseball, needed to "come to the same place

[as] the Olympics" rather than "trying to . . . silence the crisis . . . " (in Brennan 2007, *USA Today*). In contrast, the report enhances the status and legitimacy of the IOC by positioning it as committed to and active in anti-doping. The consequence for other elite SGBs, should they fail to implement WADC-aligned policies, is potential exclusion from the Olympic program (IOC 2013; Chapters 2 and 3, this volume). This also highlights the continued significance of the IOC as a central actor in the debate over doping. For example:

> "We suspect there is substantial noncompliance by many . . . international federations," Dick Pound told the International Olympic Committee assembly. "If a sport or a national Olympic committee is not code compliant, the sport in particular cannot remain on the program of the Olympic Games." (AP 2007h, *International Herald Tribune*)

This also highlights the requirement for SGBs to align anti-doping policies under the broad framework of the WADC, which effectively operates as an enforcement mechanism not only to regulate PED-using athletes but also to govern and control SGBs. Although individual SGBs are responsible for punishing deviance in their sporting community, these disciplinary mechanisms must fall into line with those outlined by the WADC (Chapter 3, this volume). A spokesperson from UK Sport points out: "Punishment is down to the individual sport's governing body. They all have to operate within the parameters of the World Anti-Doping Code, so they have to follow the rules of the sport" (*BBC Berkshire* 2007). However, media reports also point to the possibility for tensions to arise between WADA and other SGBs. The media generally support the WADC as "far more detailed and sophisticated" (Macur 2007, *New York Times*) than SGBs' policies and consequently present it as the necessary mechanism to address the problem of drugs in sport. For example, the WADC is described as: "the central set of drug-testing rules across all sports and countries" (*BBC Sport* 2007) that "takes precedent over the doping controls of an individual sporting federation" (AP 2007d, *International Herald Tribune*). At the same time, however, this implicitly hints at the potential for controversy over governance and control in the doping debate.

These potential tensions emphasize the significance of consensus-making in maintaining concern and focusing concern and hostility toward deviant individuals in addition to the issue of legitimacy of an institutional response. From this perspective, WADA and other elite claim-makers in the doping debate used media reports to maintain its institutional support, to argue for increased disciplinary measures and to incorporate other agents of social control to catch 'cheats.' These measures are justified on the basis that drug-using athletes continue to "skirt the system" and that " 'there will always be drugs that are undetectable' . . . [Pound] said, using the track star Marion Jones as an example of an athlete who . . . was caught only when law enforcement intervened" (Macur 2007, *New York Times*). Incorporating other enforcement agencies is described as the "necessary and inevitable evolution . . . in the fight against doping" (Pound in *CBC Sports* 2007b). Not only do media reports provide space to bolster claims to legitimacy by dominant groups, they also support claim-makers' calls for harsh measures of control. For example, one article reported that "the chairman of the IOC's medical commission Professor Arne Ljungqvist said the Government should make doping a criminal offence. He said stringent measures should be put in place to make sure London 2012 is a clean Games" (Herman 2007, *The Guardian*). Similarly, and referring to the fact that Marion Jones was "tested 160 times" but "never caught," WADA representative David Howman warned that despite conducting "hundreds of tests . . . you still miss some cheaters," which emphasizes not only the need to "use more than one weapon" but also calls on "governments to stop those who traffic and those who possess doping substances" (Howman in Bright 2007, *Telegraph*).

These types of comments fall within a moral panic framework that constructs doping as an ongoing problem requiring innovative, and stricter, methods of social control. Incorporating other agents of social control and calls to criminalize doping offenses illustrate the 'widening the net' process (Cohen 2002; Møller 2009). This perpetuates the view that PED use is a growing problem, adding to concern over doping and directing attention to a PED-using folk devil who is the subject of increasingly tough regulation. Media reports provide evidence in support of the moral panic criterion of disproportionality, with suggestions that a large number of individuals are engaged in deviant behavior contributing to the generation of concern and focusing attention on PED-using folk devils. Claims that a significant number of individuals are using PEDs similarly point to the need for an institutional response and provide opportunities to highlight the efficacy of WADA's policy framework. As we have seen, claim-makers in the doping debate, including WADA, elite SGBs and the media all use statistics and low positive test results to stress the success of the current anti-doping approach. However, it is important to note, as Cohen (2002, xii) points out: "The slide towards moral panic rhetoric depends less on the sheer volume of cases, than a cognitive shift from 'how could it happen in a place like this?' to 'it could happen anyplace.'" The notion that the deviant behavior 'could happen anyplace' is important in maintaining the momentum, or volatility, associated with a moral panic.

Volatility

Goode and Ben-Yehuda (2009) refer to the moral panic criterion of volatility as the difficulty of focusing concern and attention, or the momentum of a moral panic over time. Maintaining public attention is complicated by the fact that social problems, including doping, exist in complex policy and social environments. The competing demands from a range of stakeholder groups in these arenas mean that not all claims for attention are successful (Best 1990; Hilgartner and Bosk 1988; Houlihan 2009). Anti-doping claim-makers also face the problem of promoting the success of anti-doping campaigns while maintaining concern that doping 'could happen anyplace.' WADA must convince the community that doping remains a problem while demonstrating that the WADC is effective, worthwhile and legitimate, thereby warranting continued support.

Measuring the success of anti-doping efforts on the basis of "no major busts in MLB or the Olympics" has the potential to create a situation where "it's easy for people to ignore that the problem exists" (Brennan 2008, *USA Today*). Using the media and socially accredited experts such as Dr. Gary Wadler, WADA highlights the danger of "doping fatigue" as attention to doping slips "off the radar screen of public concern" (cited in Brennan 2008, *USA Today*). To overcome 'doping fatigue,' PED use is constructed as a problem not only for elite sport but one that, without significant action, including from the public as stakeholders in the modern sporting context, also threatens the social order more broadly. For example, a media report cites WADA president Richard Pound as stating that "the biggest challenge is to make sure the public understands this is a real problem" and one that, as the report states, "if left unchecked," risks "younger amateur athletes" believing that PED use is necessary in order to match the performances of athletes at higher competitive levels (*CBC Sports* 2007a). These reports generate concern and focus attention on PED use as dangerous behavior threatening community well-being and particularly vulnerable 'younger' athletes. This also provides opportunities for claim-makers, including elite SGBs such as the IOC, to use the media to boost claims to legitimacy based on the idea that their anti-doping efforts are effective. For example, after the 2008 Beijing Olympics, IOC representatives stated that they were "convinced our (anti-doping) efforts have borne fruit. . . . Even if doping will never be resolved . . . we are more credible than ever and it is more difficult for athletes to use drugs" (IOC President Jacque Rogge in Nebehay 2008, *Reuters*).

Similarly, WADA positions the organization as the institutional solution to restore order and stability to the elite sporting community. As former WADA President John Fahey noted, in the "relatively brief" time since it was established, WADA evolved from "an urgent response to a crisis in sport" into a collaborative "global network of committed sports, government authorities and individuals working . . . to protect athlete health and the integrity of sport," serving as the "independent international body responsible for coordinating and monitoring the global fight against doping . . . " (WADA 2008). Describing WADA as an "urgent response to a crisis in sport" responsible for "coordinating and monitoring the global fight against doping" fit neatly into an elites-engineered institutionalized moral panic framework. Advocating WADA's success in returning stability to elite sport presents other stakeholders with opportunities to restore perceptions of their legitimacy based on a commitment to WADA's anti-doping model. It emphasizes the significance of a regulatory response to address deviance, suggesting that the "normative order is legitimate, official agents of social control are necessary" (Sanders 1990, 7). Individuals may still decide to operate outside the moral boundaries of the group and 'cheat,' but they will 'eventually' be caught and punished appropriately:

> The doping admission by five-time Olympic medalist Marion Jones is good for sport because it shows that drug cheats eventually get caught, IOC president Jacques Rogge said in a French newspaper interview Monday. (AP 2007e, *International Herald Tribune*)

Media reports point to the eventual admission of systematic doping by Marion Jones, who consistently denied PED use over a number of years (Robinson 2007), as an example of the widespread nature of doping. Although not erupting suddenly as a volatile part of the moral panic, the report implies that 'folk devils' are always present with the potential to emerge at any time. This generates concern over doping and contributes to the necessity of a strong institutional response, notwithstanding the fact that Jones was not 'caught' by anti-doping authorities (AFP 2008a; AP 2007g). However, the position of the media as powerful agents of social control also enables criticism and challenges to the version of events postulated by moral panic claim-makers. For example, while testing procedures and developments in testing technology are primary elements used to attest to the efficacy of the WADC framework, these are not without their critics. The media provides a forum where other groups, including some elite athletes, criticize the anti-doping framework:

> "This is not a battle for or against doping, because we all are against doping. It a battle against the system which does not respect the fundamental rights of individuals," Kashechkin's lawyer . . . said Friday. (AP 2007b, *International Herald Tribune*)
> . . . anti-doping controls have nothing to do with equality. Those who want to dope manage it without any problem . . . anti-doping tests are for nothing, if only to waste money and time. (2005 World Cup champion skier Bode Miller, cited in AFP 2007b)

These comments further highlight the multi-dimensional aspect of legitimacy in the doping debate. The issue raised here is not a lack of consensus, concern or hostility toward doping and doping athletes or the necessity of anti-doping regulations. Rather, the problem concerns the definition of the situation, in particular, athletes' rights to fair and equitable treatment. These types of comments indicate support for Donovan et al.'s (2002) point that perceptions of legitimacy are important for anti-doping compliance. Media reports reveal tensions between organizational stakeholders and lead other claim-makers, such as athletes, to challenge WADA's practices, if not its legitimacy.

The media also provide sites where other elite SGBs criticize WADA while seeking to promote their commitment to doping and maintain their moral authority to control their particular sporting community, as in the case of the AFL (see Chapter 4, this volume). Other SGBs have also questioned whether the WADC is suitable for all sporting contexts. For example, at the 2007 Third World Conference on Doping in Sport, the International Hockey Federation (IHF), International Basketball Federation (FIBA) and FIFA 'strongly objected' to changes to the WADC sought by WADA. As one IHF Council member stated: "The one-size fits all approach does not work. . . . My fear is that we will leave . . . with a code carved in stone without some dialogue . . . and a team unable to deliver on it" (AP 2007d, *International Herald Tribune*). Sports governing bodies are careful here not to dispute the need for an institutional anti-doping response or anti-doping regulations. Rather, the point of contention is SGBs' unwillingness to surrender their moral authority and legitimacy to WADA and the WADC as the control mechanism for their sporting community. At the same time, SGBs must carefully negotiate between their independence and their acquiescence in global doping regulation.

Notwithstanding SGBs' efforts to maintain their moral authority and legitimacy, media reports tend to emphasize WADA and the WADC as the appropriate, successful and necessary mechanisms with which to address the problem of drugs in sport. Further, WADA uses media reports to question the legitimacy of SGBs in the field of anti-doping, suggesting that widespread non-compliance with WADA's regulatory framework contributes to increasing PED use. Framing the issue as a worldwide 'problem' opens opportunities to stress the importance of overarching institutional solutions and highlights tensions between organizational actors in the debate:

> Doping . . . worldwide is on the rise because sports governance officials are unwilling or ill-equipped to enforce rules, according to the World Anti-Doping Agency . . . "It will get worse before it gets better," . . . president of the agency said . . . "We are trying to defeat a 21st century problem with 19th century organizations" (Lysaght 2007, *Bloomberg. com*).

WADA used media reports to construct doping not only as the "greatest ethical threat sport has ever known" and as "so pervasive" that it constitutes a "grave" public health risk but also to question the commitment of other organizational actors and position the WADC as a necessary part of the solution (Xinhua 2007, *China View*). For example, the WADA president is reported as stating that to "bolster" efforts to "battle the scourge of doping" it was "incumbent" upon sports authorities as well as governments to approve "refinements to the . . . Code" (Xinhua 2007, *China View*). Reports positioning WADA as the institutional solution to doping and the adoption of a WADC-aligned policy approach as 'incumbent' upon other stakeholders highlights the tensions between WADA and SGBs. For example, referring to the National Football League's (NFL) reluctance to bring their policies into line with WADA's standards, Wadler, as a WADA representative, stated: "They need to get into the end zone, which is with WADA. . . . That's the ultimate place where they need to be" (in Weisman 2007, *USA Today*), and "These are steps in the right direction but they fall short. . . . They need to adopt the world anti-doping code as their standard" (in Kuriloff 2007, *Bloomberg.com*). The implication here is that a failure by SGBs to adopt WADC-based policies questions their commitment to anti-doping with implications for perceptions of their legitimacy and moral authority.

The examples cited throughout this chapter demonstrate that media reports provide opportunities to construct WADA as the necessary institution to restore stability to sport. Media reports also provide an effective vehicle for the articulation of stakeholder claims that construct PEDs as a moral panic and a danger to social order. In addition, media reports illustrate an elites-engineered moral panic, with the contested nature of claims to legitimacy and power relationships between organizations forming an important part of the debate.

CONCLUSION

Media reports and claim-makers' use of the media reveal the value of the criteria presented in Goode and Ben-Yehuda's (2009) moral panic model. As I have shown in this chapter, media reports demonstrate consensus that doping is deviant behavior necessitating measures of social control. These reports provide opportunities for claim-makers to fan public concern over doping and focus hostility on doping athletes as 'folk devils.' Contributing to public concern are exaggerated claims that construct doping as widespread, with the potential to threaten the social order, public health and youth. These types of constructions enable WADA, and other SGBs, to emphasize and justify a strong regulatory response.

The media reports reviewed here also provide support for modification of the moral panic criterion of consensus to consensus-making. In the case of PEDs, consensus-making more effectively captures the complex interactions between diverse claim-makers in the doping debate, which are underpinned by contested claims to legitimacy. The centrality of legitimacy in the doping debate can also be effectively explored using an elites-engineered moral panic theory, which highlights the negotiated power relationships between SGBs and WADA. From this perspective, WADA seeks to maintain their legitimacy and moral authority as the institution responsible for coordinating and harmonizing anti-doping regulation while managing the competing interests of a range of other claim-makers. An important part of this process is WADA's use of the media to reinforce its legitimacy and moral authority. However, as dominant stakeholder groups in the modern sporting context, elite SGBs also enjoy privileged media access that provides them with opportunities to challenge and reassert claims to legitimacy. Consequently, while using the media to enhance their legitimacy by demonstrating support for WADA, elite SGBs sought to balance this with efforts to maintain the authority to govern and control their particular sporting communities.

Elaborating on Goode and Ben-Yehuda's model, the evidence presented here demonstrates that doping represents an elites-engineered institutionalized moral panic driven by the concerns of elite SGBs to maintain legitimacy and moral authority. Goode and Ben-Yehuda's model provides a useful analytical tool with which to examine the debate over drugs in sport. The next chapter continues this process, using qualitative interviews to investigate perceptions of the legitimacy and moral authority of WADA and the WADC as applied by national sporting organizations in Australia. This approach shifts from a 'top down' focus on the media and other organizational actors to consider legitimacy from a 'bottom up' perspective of the grassroots sporting community in Australia.

NOTE

1 The Monitoring the Future survey studies the "behaviors, attitudes and values of American secondary school students, college students and young adults" and is funded by research grants from the National institute on Drug Abuse, conducted by the Survey Research Center in the Institute for Social Research at the University of Michigan (Monitoring the Future 2015).

REFERENCES

AFP (Agence France-Presse). 2007a. Australia's Fahey elected president of sport's anti-doping agency. *Agence France-Presse.* 17 November 2007. http://afp.google.com/article/ALeqM5jms8Y1dYmsURzqwC6s5dmFaFrs7A. Accessed 27 December 2007.

———. 2007b. "Bode Miller Sticks to His Doping Guns." Agence France-Presse, 19 November 2007. http://afp.google.com/article/ALeqM5g-luyognmO5KxsemfBtw WQ0GcDBQ. Accessed 20 November 2007.

———. 2008a. "Disgraced Sprinter Jones Teports to Jail." 7 March 2008. Agence France-Presse, http://afp.google.com/article/ALeqM5j45h2TXIPAcsLvMwWvwl DUeXuKVQ. Accessed 16 February 2009.

———. 2008b. "IOC Chief Expects More Drugs Shame from Beijing." Agence France-Presse, 9 November 2008. http://afp.google.com/article/ALeqM5j89X DQwfkqtT0M7RAksVyuWIvKpw. Accessed 24 November 2008.

———. 2008c. "Rogge Sees Long Battle Against Drugs in Sport." Agence France-Presse, 26 November 2008. http://www.google.com/hostednews/afp/article/ALe qM5iFeba6tA3yRuLeXufCktJ5K6c6fQ. Accessed 27 November 2008.

———. 2008d. "WADA Chief Warns Sports to Beat Drugs or Face Irrelevance." Agence France-Presse, 7 August 2008. http://afp.google.com/article/ALeqM5his pSXtLzWuSeW6IVKIYQLUgzzfA. Accessed 19 August 2009.

Amies, N. 2007. "Soccer Powers to Increase Bundesliga Doping Controls." *Deutsche Welle*, 10 August 2007. http://www.dw-world.de/dw/article/0,2144, 2733276,00.html. Accessed 14 August 2007.

AP (Associated Press). 2007a. "Acrobatic Gymnast Okulova Banned for Doping Offense." *International Herald Tribune*, 27 November 2007. http://www. iht.com/articles/ap/2007/11/27/sports/EU-SPT-GYM-Doping-Okulova.php. Accessed 29 November 2007.

———. 2007b. "Court Case Involving Fired Astana Rider Will Challenge World Doping System." *International Herald Tribune*, 2 November 2007. http://www. iht.com/articles/ap/2007/11/02/sports/EU-SPT-CYC-Kashechkin-Doping.php. Accessed 19 December 2007.

———. 2007c. "Doping Conference Overshadowed by Uncertainty Over Election of WADA President." *International Herald Tribune*, 15 November 2007. http:// www.iht.com/articles/ap/2007/11/15/sports/EU-SPT-Doping-Conference.php. Accessed 12 December 2008.

———. 2007d. "FIFA Leads Team-Sport Criticism of WADA's New Anti-Doping Code." *International Herald Tribune*, 16 November 2007. http://www.iht.com/ articles/ap/2007/11/16/sports/EU-SPT-Doping-WADA-Code.php. Accessed 11 December 2007.

———. 2007e. "IOC President Says Marion Jones Doping Admission 'Good Thing' for Sport." *International Herald Tribune*, 15 October 2007. http://www.iht. com/articles/ap/2007/10/15/sports/EU-SPT-OLY-Rogge-Jones.php. Accessed 17 January 2008.

———. 2007f. "IOC: Recent Doping Busts at Tour de France Show Shift in Attitude Against Cheaters." *Winnipeg Free Press*, 26 July 2007. http://www.winnipeg freepress.com/historic/32338974.html. Accessed 27 July 2007.

———. 2007g. "Marion Jones Pleads Guilty." Associated Press, 8 October 2007. http:// ap.google.com/article/ALeqM5jUq0dOf2wXE-ySJWjMfV_pDxwfVQD8S3AB18. Accessed 10 October 2007.

———. 2007h. "WADA Chief Warns Lax Doping Rules Could Cost Slot in Olympics." *International Herald Tribune*, 6 July 2007. http://www.iht.com/articles/ ap/2007/07/06/sports/LA-SPT-OLY-IOC-Doping.php. Accessed 16 July 2007.

AthletesCAN. 1999. "Athletes CAN Supports OATH—Olympic Advocates Together Honorably." AthletesCAN: The Association of Canada's National Team Athletes. http://www.athletescan.com/Content/News/News Archives/Archives 1999/ 990316OATH.asp. Accessed 20 February 2007.

Baerveldt, C., Bunkers, H., de Winter, M., and Kooistra, J. 1998. "Assessing a Moral Panic Relating to Crime and Drugs Policy in the Netherlands: Towards a Testable Theory." *Crime, Law and Social Change* 29 (1): 31–47.

Balko, R. 2008. "Should We Allow Performance Enhancing Drugs in Sports?" *Reason Online*, 23 January 2008. http://reason.com/news/show/124577.html. Accessed 24 December 2008.

BBC Berkshire. 2007. "Drugs testing: Q & A." BBC Berkshire, 7 June 2007. http://www.bbc.co.uk/berkshire/content/articles/2007/05/10/speedway_ wada_070510_feature.shtml. Accessed 7 June 2007.

BBC Sport. 2007. "The Fight Against Drugs in Sport." *BBC Sport*, 17 November 2007. http://news.bbc.co.uk/sport2/hi/other_sports/7099845.stm. Accessed 6 March 2008.

Beamish, R. 2009. "Steroids, Symbolism and Morality: The Construction of a Social Problem and Its Unintended Consequences." In *Elite Sport, Doping and Public Health*, edited by Moller, V., McNamee, M. and Dimeo, P., 55–73. Odense: University of Southern Denmark.

Beck, L. 2008. "Athletes Learn Risks, Rules at Anti-Doping Centre." *Reuters*, 10 August 2008. http://www.reuters.com/article/GCA-Olympics/idUSPEK24374 20080810?sp=true. Accessed 25 August 2009.

Becker, H. S. 1963. *Outsiders*. New York: Free Press.

Best, J. 1990. *Threatened Children: Rhetoric and Concern about Child-Victims*. Chicago: University Press of Chicago.

———. 2002. "Monster Hype." *Education Next* Summer: 51–55.

Bond, D. 2007. "Shake-Up in Fight Against British Drug Cheats." *Telegraph*, 5 December 2007. http://www.telegraph.co.uk/sport/main.jhtml;jsessionid=F1EQ FKL0UXANHQFIQMFCFGGAVCBQYIV0?xml=/sport/2007/12/05/sofron105. xml. Accessed 12 December 2007.

Bowen, K. 2007. "Mass Doping Is Now the Order of the Day." Deutsche Welle, 24 May 2007. http://www.dw-world.de/dw/article/0,2144,2556989,00.html. Accessed 15 June 2007.

Brennan, C. 2007. "A Call for Baseball to Toughen Drug Testing." *USA Today*, May 2007. http://www.usatoday.com/sports/columnist/brennan/2007–05–02-brennan-baseball-drug-testing_N.htm. Accessed 5 June 2007.

———. 2008. "Enough about the BCS; Why Aren't we Focusing on Doping?" *USA Today*, 21 November 2008. http://www.usatoday.com/sports/columnist/ brennan/2008–11–19-Christine_N.htm. Accessed 24 November 2008.

Bright, R. 2007. "Doping Tests for Cycling to Increase." *Telegraph*, 23 October 2007. http://www.telegraph.co.uk/sport/main.jhtml?xml=/sport/2007/10/23/ socycl123.xml. Accessed 4 December 2007.

Broadbent, R. 2007. "Britain's Drug Test Pioneer Still Chasing Place on Front Line in War against Cheats." Times Online, 21 November 2007. http://www.timesonline.co.uk/ tol/sport/more_sport/athletics/article2910302.ece. Accessed 27 December 2007.

———. 2008. "Maurice Greene Accused of Being Drugs Cheat." *Times Online*, 14 April 2008. http://www.timesonline.co.uk/tol/sport/more_sport/athletics/arti cle3739937.ece. Accessed 14 April 2008.

Burnside, S. 2007. "Debate Over NHL's Drug-Testing Policy Rages On." *ESPN*, 6 August 2007. http://sports.espn.go.com/nhl/columns/story?columnist=burnside_ scott&id=296370. Accessed 8 August 2007.

CBC News. 2007. "Pound Quits World Anti-Doping Agency." *CBC*, 18 September 2007. http://www.cbc.ca/canada/montreal/story/2007/09/18/qc-pound0918. html. Accessed 20 September 2007.

CBC Sports. 2007a. "WADA's Pound Calls for More Awareness on Public Health Problems Posed by Doping." *CBC*, 13 May 2007. http://www.cbc.ca/cp/ sports/070513/s051347A.html. Accessed 25 May 2007.

———. 2007b. "World Anti-Doping Agency Boss Applauds U.S. Moves Against Doping Underground." *CBC*, 12 March 2007. http://www.cbc.ca/cp/sports/070312/ s031227A.html. Accessed 13 March 2007.

Cohen, S. 2002. Folk devils and moral panics: the creation of the Mods and Rockers 3rd ed. Abingdon, Oxon, New York: Routledge.

Deutsche Welle. 2007a. "German Cabinet Pushes New Anti-Doping Law." *Deutsche Welle*, 8 March 2007. http://www.dw-world.de/dw/article/0,2144,2377262,00. html. Accessed 9 March 2007.

———. 2007b. "German Government Probes Doping Scandal." *Deutsche Welle*, 30 May 2007. http://www.dw-world.de/dw/article/0,2144,2569575,00.html. Accessed 31 May 2007.

———. 2007c. "German Rider Admits to Doping from Notorious Spanish Doctor." *Deutsche Welle*, 30 June 2007. http://www.dw-world.de/dw/article/0,2144, 2652273,00.html. Accessed 5 July 2007.

Donovan, R. J., Egger, G., Kapernick, V., and Mendoza, J. 2002. "A Conceptual Framework for Achieving Performance Enhancing Drug Compliance in Sport." *Sports Medicine* 32 (4): 269–284.

Dwyer, B. 2008. "Olympic Drug Cheats Still Ahead of the Cops." *Los Angeles Times*, 1 August 2008. http://articles.latimes.com/2008/aug/01/sports/sp-olydwyredrugs. Accessed 14 August 2008.

Ericson, R. V, Baranek, P. M., and Chan, J. B. L. 1991. *Representing Order*. Toronto: University of Toronto Press.

Erikson, K. T. 1966. *Wayward Puritans: A Study in the Sociology of Deviance*. New York: John Wiley and Sons.

Fairchild, D. 1989. "Sport Abjection: Steroids and the Uglification of the Athlete." *Journal of the Philosophy of Sport* XVI: 74–88.

Farquhar, G. 2008. "IOC Steps Up War on Dopers." *BBC Sport*, 8 October 2008. http://www.bbc.co.uk/blogs/olympics/2008/10/ioc_steps_up_war_on_dopers.html. Accessed 10 October 2008.

Flick, U. 2002. *An Introduction to Qualitative Research*. London: Sage Publications.

Foster, K. 2001. "The Discourses of Doping: Law and Regulation in the War Against Drugs." In *Drugs and Doping in Sport: Socio-Legal Perspectives*, edited by O'Leary, J., 181–203. London: Cavenidsh Publishing.

Garland, D. 2008. "On the Concept of Moral Panic." *Crime Media Culture* 4 (1): 9–31.

Goffa, D. 2008. "Drug Questions Dog Dara." *Los Angeles Times*, 12 July 2008. http://latimesblogs.latimes.com/olympics_blog/2008/07/drug-questions.html. Accessed 30 September 2008.

Goode, E., and Ben-Yehuda, N. 1994. "Moral Panics: Culture, Politics and Social Construction." *Annual Review of Sociology* 20 (3): 149–171.

———. 2009. *Moral Panics: The Social Construction of Deviance*. Chichester, West Sussex: Wiley-Blackwell Publishing.

Hall, S., Critcher, C., Jefferson, J., Clarke, J., and Roberts, B. 1978. *Policing the Crisis: Mugging, the State, and Law and Order*. London: The MacMillan Press.

Hemphill, D. 2008. "War on Drugs in Sport." *Bulletin of Sport and Culture* 29: 3–4.

Herman, M. 2007. "IOC calls on Britain to criminalise doping." *The Guardian*, 24 July 2007. http://sport.guardian.co.uk/breakingnews/feedstory/0,,-6801161,00.html. Accessed 26 July 2007.

Hier, S., Lett, D., Walby, K., and Smith, A. 2011. "Beyond Folk Devil Resistance: Linking Moral Panic and Moral Regulation." *Criminology and Criminal Justice* 11 (3): 259–276.

Hilgartner, S., and Bosk, C. L. 1988. "The Rise and Fall of Social Problems: A Public Arenas Model." *The American Journal of Sociology* 94 (1): 53–78.

Himmer, A. 2007. "IAAF Wants Tougher Bans for Doping." *Reuters Africa*, 23 August 2007. http://africa.reuters.com/sport/news/usnBAN331064.html. Accessed 6 September 2007.

Hoberman, J. 1992. *Mortal Engines: The Science of Performance and the Dehumanisation of Sport*. New Jersey: The Blackburn Press.

Houlihan, B. 2004. "Civil Rights, Doping Control and the World Anti-Doping Code." *Sport in Society* 7 (3): 420–437.

———. 2009. "Doping, Public Health and the Generalisation of Interests." In *Elite Sport, Doping and Public Health*, edited by Moller, V., McNamee, M. and Dimeo, P., 41–54. Odense: University Press of Southern Denmark.

International Herald Tribune. 2007a. "Dutch Secretary of Health Advocates Removal of Recreational Drugs from Anti-Doping Code." *International Herald Tribune*, 12 February 2007. http://www.iht.com/articles/ap/2007/02/12/sports/EU-SPT-Netherlands-Anti-Doping-Code.php. Accessed 14 February 2007.

———. 2007b. "World Anti-Doping Head Sees Progress as Term Nears End." *International Herald Tribune*, 13 May 2007. http://www.iht.com/articles/ap/2007/05/14/sports/NA-SPT-WADA-Pound.php. Accessed 25 May 2007.

IOC (International Olympic Committee). 2013. "Olympic Charter." International Olympic Committee. http://www.olympic.org/Documents/olympic_charter_en.pdf. Accessed 9 January 2015.

Jones, B. J., McFalls, J. A., and Gallagher, B. J. 1989. "Toward a Unified Model for Social Problems." *Journal of the Theory of Social Behavior* 19 (3): 337–356.

Kelso, P. 2007. "Drug Taking Is Rife in Golf, Claims Player." *The Guardian*, 19 July 2007. http://www.guardian.co.uk/frontpage/story/0,,2129777,00.html. Accessed 20 July 2007.

———. 2008. "War on Drugs Will Never Be Won, Says Anti-Doping Chief." *The Guardian*, 28 February 2008. http://www.guardian.co.uk/sport/2008/feb/28/ath letics.sport. Accessed 17 April 2009.

Knight, T. 2008. "Drugs in Sport: Cheats Go to Great Lengths." *Telegraph*, 23 June 2008. http://www.telegraph.co.uk/sport/othersports/drugsinsport/2303890/ Drugs-in-sport-Cheats-go-to-great-lengths.html. Accessed 19 February 2009.

Knopf, T. A. 1970. "Media Myths on Violence." *Columbia Journalism Review* 9 (1): 17–25.

Kuriloff, A. 2007. "NFL, Players to Increase Drug Testing By 40 Percent." *Bloomberg.com*, 24 January 2007. http://www.bloomberg.com/apps/news?pid=206010 79&sid=aYHjeRMj4cUc&refer=home. Accessed 29 January 2007.

Lamont-Mills, A., and Christensen, S. 2008. "'I Have Never Taken Performance Enhancing Drugs and I Never Will': Drug Discourse in the Shane Warne Case." *Scandinavian Journal of Medicine and Science in Sports* 18 (2): 250–258.

Lysaght, B. 2007. "Athlete Doping Incidents Are Rising, Enforcement Chief Says." *Bloomberg.com*, 1 November 2007. http://www.bloomberg.com/apps/news? pid=20601079&sid=a.CY1pwYDddg&refer=home. Accessed 9 December 2008.

Macur, J. 2007. "Doping Officials Question Baseball's Policy on Drugs." *The New York Times*, 17 November 2007. http://www.nytimes.com/2007/11/17/sports/ baseball/17madrid.html?ref=sports. Accessed 26 December 2007.

Møller, V. 2009. "Conceptual Confusion and the Anti-Doping Campaign in Denmark." In *Elite Sport, Doping and Public Health*, edited by Moller, V., McNamee, M. and Dimeo, P., 13–28. Odense: University Press of Southern Denmark.

Monitoring the Future. 2015. "Monitoring the Future: A Continuing Study of American Youth." The Regents of the University of Michigan. http://monitor ingthefuture.org/. Accessed 26 June 2015.

Nebehay, S. 2008. "Rogge Says IOC More Credible on Doping since Beijing." *Reuters*, 30 September 2008. http://www.reuters.com/article/sportsNews/idUS TRE48T4OE2008093. Accessed 24 October 2008.

OATH. 1999a. "First Ever Olympic Athlete Sponsored Symposium on IOC Reform Convenes in New York." Olympic Advocates Together Honourably. http://www. prnewswire.com/cgi-bin/stories.pl?ACCT=104&STORY=/www/story/06–11– 1999/0000961706&EDATE=. Accessed 20 July 2006.

———. 1999b. "Olympic Advocates Launch International organization to Renew Olympic Spirit." Olympic Advocates Together Honourably. http://www.prnews wire.co.uk/cgi/news/release?id=13026. Accessed 20 July 2006.

Paccagnella, M., and Grove, R. J. 1997. "Drugs, Sex, and Crime in Sport: An Australian Perspective." *Journal of Sport and Social Issues* 21 (2): 179–188.

Pakulski, J. 1986. "Legitimacy and Mass Compliance: Reflections on Max Weber and Soviet-Type Societies." *British Journal of Political Science* 16 (1): 35–56.

Parenti, M. 1986. *Inventing Reality*. New York: St. Martin's Press.

Perez, A. J. 2008. "Poll: Doping Questions Cloud Americans' View of Games." *USA Today*, 31 July 2008. http://www.usatoday.com/sports/olympics/beijing/2008–0 7-31-poll-doping-cover_N.htm. Accessed 14 August 2009.

Pritchard, D., and Hughes, K. D. 1997. "Patterns of Deviance in Crime News." *Journal of Communication* 47 (3): 49–67.

Reiner, R. 2007. "Media-Made Criminality: The Representation of Crime in the Mass Media." In *The Oxford Handbook of Criminology*, edited by Maguire, M., Morgan, R. and Reiner, R., 302–337. Oxford, UK: Oxford University Press.

Reuters. 2007. "WADA Chief Pound Says Key Players Fear Doping Problem." *Reuters UK*, 22 July 2007. http://uk.reuters.com/article/UK_GOLF/idUKL2202 024320070722?pageNumber=. Accessed 24 July 2007.

Robinson, S. 2007. "Drugs in Sport: A Cure Worse Than the Disease?" *International Journal of Sports Science and Coaching* 2 (4): 363–368.

Rowe, D. 1992. "Modes of Sports Writing." In *Journalism and Popular Culture*, edited by Dahlgren, P. and Sparks, C., 96–112. London: Sage.

Sanders, C.R. 1990. " 'A Lot of People Like It': The Relationship Between Deviance and Popular Culture." In *Marginal Conventions: Popular Culture, Mass Media and Social Deviance*, edited by Sanders, C.R., 3–13. Bowling Green, OH: Bowling Green State University Popular Press.

Saraceno, J. 2007. "For a Real Drug Deterrent, Start Naming Names." *USA Today*, 26 September 2007. http://www.usatoday.com/sports/columnist/saraceno/2007–09–25-drugs-feds_N.htm. Accessed 27 September 2007.

Silverman, D. 2001. *Interpreting Qualitative Data: Methods for Analysing Talk, Text and Interaction.* London: Sage.

Slater, M. 2008. "US Stars Lead Anti-Doping Battle." BBC Sport, 6 May 2008. http://news.bbc.co.uk/sport2/hi/olympics/athletics/7384365.stm. Accessed 11 May 2008.

Suchman, M.C. 1995. "Managing Legitimacy: Strategic and Institutional Approaches." *The Academy of Management Review* 20 (3): 571–610.

Vasciannie, S. 2006. "As Fast As a Drug." *Jamaica Gleaner*, 7 August 2006. http://www.jamaica-gleaner.com/gleaner/20060807/cleisure/cleisure2.html. Accessed 7 August 2006.

von Hoffman, N. 1985. "The Press: Pack of Fools. Killer Bees, Missing Kids, and Other Phoney Stories." *The New Republic* 3681: 9–11.

WADA (World Anti-Doping Agency). 2008. "President's Welcome Message." World Anti-Doping Agency. http://www.wada-ama.org/en/dynamic.ch2?pageCategory.id=25. Accessed 9 January 2008.

———. 2009 (September). "Governance—List Working Committees." World Anti-Doping Agency. http://www.wada-ama.org/en/dynamic.ch2?pageCategory.id=31. Accessed 1 September 2009.

Weisman, L. 2007. "Anti-Doping Agency Assails NFL Policy, Despite Changes." *USA Today*, 25 January 2007. http://www.usatoday.com/sports/football/nfl/2007–01–25-nfl-testing_x.htm. Accessed 5 February 2007.

Whittle, J. 2008. "The World Anti-Doping Agency's Diplomatic New Chief." *International Herald Tribune*, 29 February 2008. http://www.iht.com/articles/2008/02/29/sports/DRUGS.php. Accessed 13 April 2008.

Williams, A. 2006. "Football Folk Devils: Changes in Newspaper Representation of Sexual Assault Cases in the Australian Football League." In *Making Histories, Making Memories the Construction of Australian Sporting Identities*, edited by Hess, R., 115–138. Melbourne: Australian Society for Sports History.

Wilson, R. 2006a. "AFL Failing Everyone in War Against Drugs." *The Advertiser*, 2 September 2006.

———. 2006b. "Name Names and End AFL Drug Farce." *The Advertiser*, 1 April 2006.

Xinhua. 2007. "WADA to Revise Anti-Doping Code." *China View*, 14 November 2007. http://news.xinhuanet.com/english/2007–11/15/content_7077921.htm. Accessed 26 December 2007.

6 Legitimacy, Doping and the Grassroots Sporting Community

I think there's a cultural change there as well, that certainly in the sport as a whole, I think people believe that we're actively working to reduce taking of illegal substances. And that may serve as a deterrent to some practices. I think the national sporting organizations certainly can't be seen to be turning a blind eye to anything these days. I think they must feel that they're accountable.

(Interview 141082)

The debate over PEDs in sport can be conceptualized as a socially constructed moral panic driven by elite sporting organizations' concerns to restore or maintain perceptions of organizational legitimacy. In other words, the doping debate constitutes an elites-engineered, institutionalized, moral panic. The creation of WADA provided a case study of legitimacy based on a normative rational-legal framework (the WADC) underpinned by values encapsulated in the spirit of sport statement (Chapter 3, this volume). From that perspective, WADA represented a specific response to doping as a serious problem threatening sport. While implementing WADA-aligned policies provides opportunities for sporting organizations to enhance their legitimacy, this also challenges their authority to govern their particular sporting communities. This highlights the multifaceted nature of legitimacy and reveals that organizational power relationships are complicit in framing the doping debate.

The importance of legitimacy in the doping debate was evident in the debate surrounding the AFL's anti-drugs in sport policies (Chapter 4, this volume). As well as highlighting the multi-dimensional nature of legitimacy, this revealed the way that different claim-makers in the doping debate use anti-doping policies to achieve diverse objectives. That discussion illustrated the role of the media as a forum where stakeholders made and challenged claims to legitimacy. A review of media reports, examined through the lens of a modified version of Goode and Ben-Yehuda's (2009) moral panic criteria, demonstrated that the actions of WADA can be conceptualized as an institutionalized response to a moral panic. The evidence presented fulfilled the moral panic criteria and also demonstrated the validity of the modified criterion of consensus-making within an elites-engineered theory.

Here the focus returns to legitimacy. Rather than a 'top-down' institutional view, I take a 'bottom-up' approach to explore the views of another key stakeholder in modern sport, namely members of the Australian grassroots sporting community. Legitimacy rests on organizations' ability to implement 'proper procedures' that are accepted by communities and that define appropriate conduct for the group (Ericson et al. 1991; Habermas 1976; Wuthnow et al. 1984). As Schneider (2000) points out in her discussion of the IOC, legitimacy and moral authority, founded on public support, are linked to commercial viability. This also applies to sporting organizations. To secure financial resources generated by public support, such as revenue from match attendances as well as access to government funding, sporting organizations are also reliant on public perceptions that their sport is 'clean' (Bette and Schimank 2001). A further motivating factor is a concern to increase participation rates, including grassroots development programs that are necessary to grow the game (Chapter 4, this volume). This places pressure on SGBs to maintain public perceptions that anti-doping efforts are effective.

I used qualitative interviews to gauge the perceptions of members of the Australian grassroots sporting community, which enabled me to take account of the evaluative subjective nature of legitimacy. The value of using interviews in conjunction with surveys is supported by Anshel (1991), who notes that in his research "a personal interview . . . allowed for greater probing of certain responses to gain further understanding of the issues under discussion. Thus, the interviewer could ask for specific examples or for clarification of responses." The interviews that I report here formed part of my doctoral research, conducted throughout 2007 and 2008. Contact with the interviewees resulted from a quantitative e-survey that, as part of the multi-dimensional research design used in my doctoral work, I sent to 22 Australian NSOs and sporting organizations for distribution to their members (see Appendix 6.1 for further details regarding this research methodology). The e-survey included provision for individuals to confidentially supply their contact details to arrange an interview. Most interviewees resulted from an invitation in the e-survey, although a small number (five) resulted from interviewee's introductions to others in their sporting community.

There were a total of 28 interviews, with four female and 24 male interviewees that identified as athletes, administrators, coaches and officials at club level, team managers, sporting event promoters and parents of athletes. They also identified their minimum current level of sporting activity as club level (see Appendix 6.2). Determining interviewees' levels of participation demonstrates that their expressed views were based on their experiences and knowledge of the current anti-doping model as applied by their sporting organization. In other words, interviewees did not simply engage in recreational sport but had some awareness of their obligations under their sporting organizations' regulatory frameworks.

The data discussed here show that members of the grassroots sporting community are divided in their views of the legitimacy of sporting organizations, although a clear majority indicated that these groups face a crisis.[1] This division in the data illustrates the dynamic and contested nature of legitimacy. Further, this is useful for consideration of doping as a moral panic, highlighting the value of consensus-making as a moral panic criterion and the important role of community concern in the generation of a moral panic. However, it is important to note that the small number of cases that comprise the sample means that the data cannot be generalized beyond this book. Nevertheless, although the data do not enable any claims that sporting organizations face crises of legitimacy, the data do show that a number of issues tend to have a negative effect on the attitudes of the interviewees toward SGBs' legitimacy.

In Australia, SGBs are classified as National Sporting Organizations (NSOs), and this terminology is used to describe organizations for the interviews. This classification follows the ABS (2001) definition of Sports and Physical Recreation Administrative Organizations, which describes these as "units" that are "mainly engaged in the administration and/or control of sports or physical recreation disciplines and/or groups of clubs. These units may be responsible for the policies, rules and regulations governing the conduct of an individual sporting or physical recreation discipline, or may distribute funding to affiliated member organizations." The phrase 'grassroots sports community' indicates organized club level sport, distinguished from participation in recreational sporting activities. As Cantelon (2005, 84) notes, "high performance" sport is not restricted to elite or Olympic participation and includes "elite minor league competition in the local community."

Targeting organized club level sport is relevant to the goals of this book, as participation at that level requires that individuals obtain a license from their NSO, which includes agreeing to comply with WADA and WADC-based policies. Although several interviewees were parents of children and young people involved in elite sports and thus had a sound knowledge of the processes and athletes' compliance requirements, at their personal level of participation, most of my interviewees were unlikely to be subject to testing. Nevertheless, their sporting involvement is dependent upon compliance with a WADA-based anti-doping framework as stipulated by their club license. Thus, their perceptions of the system have implications for the legitimacy of the current anti-doping model as applied by Australian NSOs as well as for WADA more broadly.

SPORTING ORGANIZATIONS AND LEGITIMACY

The interviews are segregated into three key areas that were chosen based on their association with fundamental aspects of WADA's anti-doping approach as stipulated in the WADC. As such they provide a framework against which to evaluate perceptions of claims to legitimacy by WADA and NSOs. The first key area is 'Information and Education' and concerns perceptions of NSOs' provision of information and education about permissible substances, including the role of values in the WADC that also underpin anti-doping education. The second key area considers the role of testing and sanctions in the current framework, including perceptions of the scientific accuracy of testing as well as equity and consistency of sanctions. The third key area explores perceptions of factors influencing athletes' doping decisions, and particularly the strict liability principle and NSOs' responsibility to athletes.

Information and Education

Education in anti-doping has a historical foundation, as demonstrated by the IOC's focus on education to change athletes' behavior. A key goal for WADA is developing anti-doping education programs and distributing anti-doping information (WADA 2009). For example, WADA (2007) states that, together with deterrence and research, over the "long term education plays a central role in the creation of a true anti-doping culture" and that this includes "athletes, as well as their coaches, doctors, trainers, agents, and parents, about the dangers of doping and its consequences." WADA claims to be "dedicated" to facilitating the distribution of anti-doping information and education to ensure "worldwide compliance with the Code" (WADA 2006). This preventative educational anti-doping strategy includes building a WADA-aligned values system, which WADA argues is important because athletes' decisions to use PEDs do not result simply from a lack of information. Rather, these individuals are, according to WADA's website, "fully aware of the necessary factual information" regarding doping (WADA 2009). In contrast, individuals that choose not to dope often do so because of their "personal convictions, of which the foundation is a strong values system. A preventive education program aimed at values development will ensure that young people, athletes and athlete support personnel have reasons to decide to avoid doping and to stick to that decision" (WADA 2009).

WADA's emphasis on the WADC underpinned by values-based education constitutes a measure against which to gauge perceptions of legitimacy. The shared norms and values said to underpin the WADC, and that are central to WADA's anti-doping campaign, are that doping is a risk to athletes' health, is unfair to non-doping athletes, provides a bad role model for youth, is increasingly a public health issue, is morally wrong and is against the 'spirit of sport' (WADA 2015; Chapter 3, this volume). In a deterrence-based anti-doping framework that includes testing and sanctions, education is also important for perceptions of NSO legitimacy. To be effective, and enjoy legitimacy, such a policy requires that individuals are educated regarding the rules and their obligations under that scheme. Added to this, NSO licensing requirements stipulate that their members comply with testing and sanctions, which implies that individuals need knowledge of their obligations under that framework.

All interviewees indicated their awareness that they are subject to anti-doping regulations under the terms of their club licenses and are willing to comply with those requirements. As one interviewee pointed out: "Well, you do need to know because from club level upwards you can be tested" (Interview 140933–2). Another interviewee stated: "I'm a license holder so ASADA can walk in now and even though I haven't . . . race[d] for three years I still have to submit to a drug test, which is fine. I've got a license so I subscribe to that" (Interview 141050). Overall, the interviewees indicated that NSOs are providing information on anti-doping rules and regulations. As this interviewee said: "I would view that the avowed or articulated anti-doping position that's the talk, the walk seems to be consistent with that" (Interview 140961). Expressions by the interviewees that NSOs did provide anti-doping information can be interpreted as reinforcing perceptions of legitimacy among NSO members. For example: "It validates my assumption that [sport] bodies actually are doing something about it . . . certainly at an international level I think they're doing something about it" (Interview 140995).

Although most interviewees had some knowledge of their NSOs' anti-doping requirements, nearly half felt that information and educational material was not easily accessible or distributed effectively to the grassroots sporting community. One interviewee who held positive views of NSOs' legitimacy and felt that information was provided also noted that finding information was not difficult for those involved in administration or coaching. At issue for this interviewee was their NSOs' failure to distribute that information more broadly, with information "only really known by those people who have had exposure to that communication" (Interview 141082). For other interviewees a failure to use or improve existing delivery methods, such as newsletters or websites, to distribute anti-doping information affected their perceptions of NSO legitimacy. For example, one interviewee who held positive views of NSO legitimacy nevertheless indicated:

> . . . if they can email out a newsletter at regular intervals . . . what's the harm in putting in some information in there? . . . if they did provide that sort of information on a regular sort of basis then it would give me the impression that they were really on top of it and they were really trying to overcome drug abuse from an early stage. (Interview 140902)

Another interviewee described their NSO's website as "a nightmare . . . a really shit website" (Interview 001). For this interviewee, such a problem could be easily overcome, as in "this day and age you can make great websites which are really easy to get around." Another interviewee felt that a more structural approach was necessary to effectively distribute anti-doping information. This interviewee suggested that rather than simply sending a newsletter that "somebody could just . . . throw it away," NSOs should engage more proactively by linking anti-doping initiatives to clubs' "licensing renewal, that they've got to have talked about doping and any other thing that may have come up. But that doesn't happen" (Interview 002). In other words, even those who had a positive view of their NSO felt that more action is required to ensure that information reaches various levels of the sporting community. This included providing information in an easy to understand format. As one interviewee critical of NSO legitimacy stated:

> If they provide it to the clubs, nationwide, it's no good providing it to the national body or to the state bodies. It can come through them, but they need to say this must go to every [sport] Club in Australia. It must. Because what happens is if the national body gets it, they'll pop it on their website. Well, that's only good for those people that visit that website, that have access to Internet, and that can take a drug policy that's on the Internet and say we understand that. (Interview 141410)

This comment reveals how the failure to provide anti-doping information in an easily understood format detracts from its usefulness. This issue was seen as particularly important for those engaged in junior sport, as one interviewee critical of NSOs' legitimacy indicated:

> So unless the kid gets on the websites, and let's be honest, a word that's that long [spreads arms out wide], in [sport], they can't read it, they certainly can't spell it, they certainly don't have a clue what it stands for. And they wouldn't know whether it's in butter menthols or cough medicine. (Interview 141050)

Some interviewees who indicated doubts regarding NSOs' legitimacy pointed out that while holding a sporting license indicated agreement with anti-doping policy, the lack of an accompanying "educational process" left the policy "open for you to interpret" (Interview 140995). For these interviewees, without an educational process, NSOs lack legitimacy and authority to implement testing protocols and impose sanctions. One interviewee with negative views of NSOs' legitimacy pointed out that despite the provision of educational material, these needed to be supported by " . . . resources for the education. And I think without the education, you can't impose the penalties" (Interview 141131). Other interviewees shared this view. As one commented: "I mean if you're going to do drug testing you have to do drug education . . . so people are aware what their responsibilities are as well as what the risks are and the damages and everything else that go with it" (Interview 140933–2). These comments are representative of attitudes held across the group of interviewees and highlight the subjective evaluative aspect of legitimacy. The interview data show a clear expectation by interviewees that NSOs could make more efficient use of existing delivery methods to provide anti-doping information, including a more effective educational process. The perception that NSOs devoted insufficient attention to this area had the potential to create negative attitudes toward NSOs' legitimacy, including their authority to impose testing protocols and sanctions.

Information and Education: Focus on Elite Competition

There was also a feeling that NSOs maintain a narrow focus on elite sport rather than incorporating the grassroots community. Interviewees, regardless of whether they indicated positive or negative perceptions of NSOs' legitimacy, shared the view that these organizations should incorporate the grassroots community in anti-doping education. For example, one interviewee who felt NSOs faced a crisis of legitimacy stated: "I'm sure for the elite sports . . . they would be well aware of what they can or can't do. . . . But at the level I compete at, I'm not aware of what I can and can't do and then what are the penalties" (Interview 141574). Another interviewee who was supportive of NSOs indicated that anti-doping education "doesn't happen until they're at that [elite] level" (Interview 141082). This corresponds with other findings in the existing literature.

Gucciardi et al. (2011) suggest that educational programs addressing PED use should target a range of groups, including coaches, parents and athletes and note that educational initiatives "may be more beneficial for younger athletes in their formative years" (Gucciardi et al. 2011; see also Petroczi and Aidman 2008; Striegel et al. 2002; Turner and McCrory 2003). Mazanov et al. (2010) also point to the value of more targeted educational initiatives. They write that, based on interviews with athletes, coaches and other support personnel, there may be "natural intervention points" for educational initiatives. These may include transitions in athletes' sporting career path, such as in and out of sponsorship arrangements or potential team selection or de-selection. While focused on elite athletes, they suggest that "periods of behavioral instability around transitions between stable career states . . . might provoke the temptation to dope" (Mazanov et al. 2010, 109). Although noting that more research is required into whether career transitions lead to doping, the implication is that earlier provision of education may assist athletes in managing stressful transition periods. This literature indicates a level of support for the view of some interviewees, as shown here, that an educational approach inclusive of the grassroots sporting community is important for building an elite anti-doping culture.

However, there was division amongst the interviewees regarding whether grassroots education would affect athletes' doping behavior. Some expressed the view that education at the grassroots level played an important role in building an anti-doping culture in elite sport. As one interviewee noted: "If you educate, you train, and you teach . . . if you start at grassroots level then it's going to follow you through, as long as you keep education, yes, definitely" (Interview 141015). Others appreciated the value of increased grassroots education but doubted it would affect individuals' doping behavior. One interviewee was critical of NSOs' legitimacy but emphasized personal responsibility: "you can do as much education as you want, but they're a human being they're still going to make a decision whether they want to do that or not" (Interview 140991). Overall interviewees were divided in their views regarding whether provision of anti-doping information and education would alter athletes' behavior.

The research results indicate that most NSOs *are* distributing and making anti-doping information available. My interviewees identified a range of delivery methods, such as NSOs' websites, information sessions (including through clubs, seminars or orientation programs at government-funded sporting institutes) and coaching courses. In this way most of the grassroots sporting community members interviewed indicated they were generally aware of anti-doping information. Individuals who felt they received information and education were slightly less likely to be critical of NSOs' legitimacy, with interviewees who felt they did not receive anti-doping information and education tending to express more negative views toward the legitimacy of NSOs.

Information and Education: WADA and the WADC—Rules, Values and Legitimacy

WADA claims that adopting the WADC is essential for sporting organizations' integrity and credibility (Pound 2007). As I have shown throughout this book, legitimacy can be based on a 'system of rational norms' grounded in shared norms and values (Weber 1969). The legitimacy of the WADC as a rational-legal regulatory framework is underpinned by a values-based component, which is that doping contravenes the values encapsulated in the spirit of sport (WADA 2015) as well as concern for athletes' rights to engage in fair competition. This corresponds with Donovan et al.'s (2002) legitimacy criteria, which includes perceptions that anti-doping laws are morally right and fair.

Interviewees were divided in their views of a values-based regulatory approach to anti-doping, although there were slightly more expressions of support for anti-doping laws and regulation than critical views of the framework. On the positive front, one interviewee indicated that the foundation for anti-doping sanctions was "morally and ethically correct" (Interview 140995). Another interviewee who was supportive of NSOs' legitimacy stated:

> So, by focusing on that moral, ethical side of things you might be encouraging the athletes to think about not only the effect it has physically on themselves but also the impact it will have on the sport. . . . I think it probably would improve the legitimacy because it's showing the world that the country is in line with the international standard . . . you would hope that the international standard would be the best one and the one to follow. So if a national sporting organization can show the world basically that it's adopting the same policies, it has the same

standards then you would like to think that it's definitely something to aspire to. (Interview 140902)

Other interviewees felt that a values-based regulatory approach was problematic. Comments from these interviewees emphasized the importance of consistently applying all aspects of an anti-doping framework to enhance perceptions of legitimacy. One interviewee critical of NSOs' legitimacy noted that: "Oh, it would depend on what that moral-based framework was, because it doesn't seem to be consistent. It's certainly not consistent across let's say the football codes in Australia" (Interview 141455). Another interviewee with negative views of NSOs' legitimacy commented that the WADC "cuts it in a perfect world if you can start again and get ten little Johnnys, all from similar backgrounds whose parents have said, Johnny be a good boy. But the world's not that simplistic is it?" (Interview 141050).

The majority of interviewees tended to identify the need for a rules-based approach along with a values-based foundation. One interviewee, although pointing out that "rules were rules," recognized the complementary role of values and rules: "Well, you got me, because you need that values-based underpinning to discourage people from trying to push the limits all the time . . . otherwise everyone's going to be at 4.99 per cent of the 5 per cent limit . . . which is not really what you want" (Interview 140986). More strongly, another interviewee emphasized the need for a rules-based approach even while admitting that values:

> Makes it look friendlier on the surface, but it's not going to deter dopers. Cheaters are cheaters and they don't care about other people. . . . I don't think it's got any effectiveness in terms of deterring people from doping. Penalties I think are the best deterrent. But it's risk/benefit. At the moment benefits are huge. The risks have to be huge too. (Interview 141530)

This interviewee felt that "self-greed" would invariably "overrule any sort of moral." Although there is some division amongst interviewees, the majority tended to support a combination of rules and values as an effective way to approach anti-doping regulation. This suggests that there is support from the grassroots sporting community for a rules and values-based framework such as the WADC. Attitudes toward NSO legitimacy are enhanced by the view that those organizations are adopting such an approach. The interview data suggests that, in the Australian context, NSOs have successfully generated and maintained support for a WADA-aligned anti-doping model.

The Current Framework: Testing, Sanctions and Legitimacy

Donovan et al. (2002) have suggested anti-doping compliance is more likely if anti-doping authorities enjoy the moral authority and legitimacy to impose testing protocols and sanctions. Accordingly, in this topic area

I investigated interviewees' attitudes toward NSO legitimacy in relation to these procedural elements. Of interest here is whether interviewees view testing as sufficiently accurate, whether sanctions are applied equitably and if this had any impact on their attitudes toward NSOs and WADA. Issues of fairness and equity are important in the context of the severe penalties under the strict liability principle that holds athletes responsible for any banned substances found in their body (Chapter 3, this volume).

The Current Framework: Testing and Legitimacy

Although all interviewees supported the necessity of testing, some felt that testing technology failed to keep pace with doping practices or were skeptical of administrative processes. One interviewee critical of NSOs' legitimacy felt the technology "lagged behind . . . the latest either performance-enhancing drugs or methodology of administering that drug" (Interview 140961). For another interviewee supportive of NSOs' legitimacy, the fact that "200 tests went missing after the Beijing Games" (Interview 140902) created doubt over administrative procedures. The results, which were all negative, were later located with the error attributed to a "communication problem" (AP 2008; Magnay 2008). Other interviewees felt that NSOs should be more accountable and transparent when positive drug tests did occur. As one interviewee who was critical of the legitimacy of NSOs stated: "And if the person's caught let everybody know, don't put it in the closet, don't sweep it under the carpet . . . put it out for everyone to see" (Interview 141121). Other interviewees who were critical of NSOs' legitimacy nevertheless indicated their support for the accuracy of testing as well as the procedural elements of testing protocols:

> I have no concerns about the accuracy. I'm a scientist so the testing's the testing. In fact the testing's probably more generous in its limits than it could be because they're trying to minimize the false positives. So there's a buffer there and I'm sure there are people who get away with it all the time because they're on that margin. (Interview 141530)

> I think, well my perspective is that with the testing, the testing is great. I have no issues with the way they do it or the way they did it in my day. (Interview 141036)

Although a majority supported the necessity of anti-doping measures, interviewees were divided in their views of testing technology and administrative procedures. This suggests that sporting organizations and anti-doping authorities need to ensure these elements of the anti-doping framework are operating efficiently in order to create, and maintain, positive attitudes toward their legitimacy.

Testing and Legitimacy: Focus on Elite Competition

Similarly to comments regarding the provision of information and education, a majority of interviewees stressed the importance of including grassroots sport in the testing framework. The view here was that increased testing, or raising community awareness of testing, in grassroots sport would assist in developing clean elite sport. This was a view shared by interviewees who indicated negative views of NSOs' legitimacy and those who did not. For example, one interviewee who was supportive of the legitimacy of NSOs indicated: "the way to improve is actually to get physically in place seeing people getting tested at the grassroots level" (Interview 140933). Another interviewee with a negative view of NSOs' legitimacy stressed: "you can never stop the testing. . . . It has to be in their face, every club should have a drug tester . . . if you win a club title you've got to pee in the bottle" (Interview 141049). A perceived NSO bias toward testing only at elite levels had the potential to adversely affect attitudes of interviewees toward NSOs' legitimacy. One interviewee was supportive of NSOs' legitimacy but their comment is representative of other interviewees' views:

> . . . considering we don't see testing for the people further down the field or for the younger athletes. Their focus is definitely on the elite athletes, whether that's a budgetary thing, whether they just don't have the funding to test as widely as they would like . . . or with the junior athletes whether there's ethical issues. . . . But if there were no restrictions then I think it would be good to see it occur at a wider range. (Interview 140902)

While acknowledging that testing is "expensive and time consuming" (Interview 142013), the consequence of a lack of testing, or simply increased awareness around testing, at non-elite levels of sport can create negative views of NSOs' legitimacy.

Rather than expanding testing to include non-elite competition, which was acknowledged as impractical, an option identified by some interviewees was raising the visibility and awareness of testing. Highlighting the value of a 'bottom-up' educational approach, interviewees proposed initiatives to increase awareness of the testing framework, including opportunities at larger competitive sporting events for individuals to ask questions or obtain information on the anti-doping framework. Suggestions ranged from a 'Drug Education Pro-Shop' to banners or signage at club meets. For example, one interviewee with a son involved in elite sport suggested putting resources into "a tent with a stand and all your brochures and information that you can pick up . . . educating people and why not?" (Interview 141410). Another interviewee who was supportive of NSOs' legitimacy also indicated that increased visibility regarding testing would enhance views of NSOs' legitimacy:

> It also creates, I think, more avenues so people go if I want more information, or not sure about stuff, maybe I can go and ask them because they distribute stuff in this area, whereas, well, no, they don't, yeah, never hear anything from them. (Interview 141082)

Some interviewees suggested that a greater NSO focus on raising awareness of testing in non-elite sport has the potential to influence individuals'
decisions to avoid PED use. As one interviewee said: "the kid that might
be on the brink, he might be an A grade and I might just take this so I can
win for my Dad, will go oh hang on I might get tested" (Interview 140933).
Interviewees identified NSOs as responsible for implementing programs that
increased visibility or generated awareness of anti-doping at the grassroots
level. As one interviewee stated: "The sport should do that . . . whatever
sport it is their governing body should" (Interview 140933–2). Interviewees also recognized the financial constraints facing NSOs, which highlight
the government's responsibility in creating an anti-doping culture based on
a strong foundation at non-elite levels. As these interviewees with critical
views of NSOs' legitimacy stated:

> Mainly because I can't see [NSO] turning around and saying oh we're
> going to get ourselves a person from ASADA to monitor this situation
> because we just couldn't . . . afford it . . . and testing obviously would
> cost a lot of money and some sports don't want to test. I believe it falls
> back to the government. (Interview 142013)

> I'm not sure what the average cost of a drug test is but from what
> I gather it's not insubstantial. So I think you would try to have as much
> faith as you could if it was government backed rather than Association
> backed. So having ASADA . . . I think that's a positive thing because
> that's an independent body outside the organizations. So I think that
> gives a lot more weight. (Interview 140951)

These comments illustrate that there is support for a government backed and
appropriately funded testing body independent of NSOs, such as ASADA in
Australia. The comments also reflect the point that the commercially driven
nature of modern sport creates a situation where entrusting drug testing to
NSOs is problematic (Connor 2009; Voy 1991). This is relevant to perceptions of NSO legitimacy where claims by sporting bodies to be adequately
and openly testing are met with skepticism, as one interviewee stated:

> To answer your question another way, the teams are now doing
> self-testing which is simply the most ridiculous thing I've ever heard in
> my entire life. Well, we own the team! Or we can do whatever we like
> with the results. Yes, and it's very, very, you know, I like your morality
> and you're going to stick it on a website. So what? How do you know if
> it's right or wrong? So, the teams putting a fence around it themselves,
> they're doing that because the sponsors are running a mile. They're put-
> ting that in as part of their sponsor pitch. (Interview 141050)

These comments suggest that interviewees' attitudes were influenced by their
perceptions of the actions and efforts of NSOs regarding testing, including

administrative processes and the scientific accuracy of testing. For some interviewees, NSOs' failure to stay ahead of doping practices, poor administration and a focus on elite sport rather than raising grassroots awareness of testing procedures as well as a concern to protect commercial and sponsor interests resulted in negative views of NSOs' anti-doping efforts.

The Current Framework: Sanctions and Legitimacy

A slight majority of interviewees expressed the view that NSOs' application of sanctions was inconsistent and 'soft,' which raised doubts over NSOs' commitment to dealing with PEDs. Although some sporting bodies were seen as "trying to improve," other organizations, such as the AFL and rugby league, "do it very poorly. They're not consistent . . . I think they just paid lip service, this is a process we have to do, let's just do it" (Interview 141257). Another interviewee stated: " . . . you take the footballers; they get three goes at it apparently. It should be the same for everyone. If you're a sportsperson and . . . you're earning money from that sport . . . there should be only one rule for everyone and not change" (Interview 002). Other interviewees criticized the AFL's three strikes policy in comparison to severity of penalties attached to doping offenses in other sports, such as cycling. Interviewees both critical and supportive of NSO legitimacy held this view, as indicated by these representative quotes:

> I think someone like the AFL; I think their policy is a complete joke. The three strikes business is ridiculous. I don't know any other sport, I'm not that well informed either, but certainly in cycling you don't get three strikes. One test for a positive for a recreational substance even out of competition can land you with a ban. I think the AFL needs to lift their game. Particularly given the nature of the organization, three strikes I think sends a bad message. (Interview 141530)

> It drives me nuts seeing football codes just having their own rules and believing that they're keeping the fight up against the dopers in their sport. It's an absolute joke, and the head of the AFL his comments on their three strike . . . just makes a mockery of the whole anti-doping process. (Interview 141155)

> And when you were asking about the inconsistency and fairness again? Same kind of punishment for the same kind of issue . . . if Tom over there took that drug he should get a 12-month ban and so should Peter over there if he did the same thing. Not have someone have 12 months, someone have three months, which I know that does happen too. (Interview 001)

Interviewees had clear expectations that all NSOs should implement anti-doping policies that applied consistent sanctions. As the interview comments indicate, inconsistent application of sanctions and lack of fairness adversely influence attitudes toward the legitimacy of NSOs.

Although not enabling any statements that NSOs face a crisis of legitimacy, the data reveals a clear division in views toward Australian NSOs' anti-doping efforts regarding testing and sanctions. Despite division in the views expressed by interviewees, their responses stress the importance of a bottom-up approach that includes grassroots sport. As well as highlighting education as a key part of creating an anti-doping culture, interviewees suggested initiatives to raise community awareness and visibility of the testing framework. Underpinning these suggestions were the views of the majority of interviewees that creating and maintaining 'clean' elite competition required a strong foundation in grassroots sport. Interviewees were also divided in views over whether NSOs consistently and equitably applied sanctions. Although slight, a majority of interviewees felt that sanctions were applied inconsistently among NSOs, some of whom were not sufficiently strict. Nevertheless, there were clear expectations that consistent application of sanctions should constitute part of NSOs' regulatory approach to doping. The interview results suggest that legitimacy of anti-drugs policies, in sport as elsewhere, appears to rest on perceptions that all elements of those policies form a cohesive and mutually supportive framework, including the elements that link education to testing (Battin et al. 2008; Donovan et al. 2002).

Athletes and PEDs: Strict Liability

The current anti-doping framework is based on deterrence and sanctions and, under the strict liability principle, holds athletes ultimately responsible for doping (Chapter 3, this volume). However, some research suggests a lack of support for such an inflexible criterion. For example, DrugScope (2004, 21) note that a strict liability approach may lead to a situation that "many people will find hard to reconcile with their sense of natural justice." As well as perceptions of the strict liability principle, I asked interviewees whether they felt that groups, other than athletes, were responsible for preventing drug use. Also of interest was whether the identification of external pressures as influencing athletes' doping decisions translated into qualifications of support for WADA's strict liability principle. As well as trying to gauge perceptions of NSOs' legitimacy based on this approach, this line of inquiry was underpinned by claims in the literature that the "public begins to recognize that to a great extent athletes are pushed into doping by structural constraints . . . as well as by temptations and pressures from inside as well as outside sports. That is why athletes cannot be blamed alone for their transgressions" (Bette and Schimank 2001, 51; see also Breivik et al. 2009).

The majority of interviewees supported strict liability with only two individuals indicating a lack of support for such an approach. One majority interviewee stated that "the encumbrances of what you do" as a professional athlete included strict liability and individual accountability "for what I do, what I say, where I go, what I eat" (Interview 141574). More significantly, if the goal of stakeholder groups in sport (including athletes) is to "clean up sport," which is "what WADA's trying to do," then athletes "must expect that this is going to come with it" (Interview 141155). In other words, it is not an unreasonable expectation that athletes are subjected to tough regulatory measures, such as strict liability, to achieve and maintain clean sport. Nevertheless, while interviewees supported individual accountability, there were indications of misgivings over strict liability. NSOs were perceived as failing to provide appropriate support to athletes who might take PEDs and failing to investigate factors that might contribute to those decisions. For example:

> You are treated like you're invincible and you're a superstar and that the whole world revolves around you. But if that starts crashing down, where do you go? At the end of the day it is your own responsibility. You shouldn't be propping these people up for making their own personal choices. . . . But they make those choices for a reason and we don't seem to try and find out what the reason is and then say well if it's psychological, medical or physical, there's nothing there to help them. (Interview 140995)

> I've always maintained that the philosophy of the administrators and everything else around that is that they jump off a sinking ship as soon as the bloody torpedo hits. They abandon the athlete, they abandon ship, and then all of a sudden the investigation goes on and then it all goes quiet again. (Interview 141036)

These comments suggest that some interviewees felt that NSOs could do more to help athletes develop skills to cope with structural pressures that may affect doping behavior. For these interviewees, this adversely affected their attitudes toward NSOs' legitimacy. Other interviewees were uncertain over whether greater NSO involvement and provision of structural support would impact on individuals' choices to use PEDs. As one interviewee stated: "I don't think that would really affect the use of drugs in sport, it may affect the retention of participants in sport" (Interview 141082). This is nevertheless an important point, as maintaining participation rates is important for the ongoing commercial viability and development of sporting codes. For example, the AFL's anti-drugs in sport policies included an educational, rehabilitative and counseling component that, in part, aimed to enhance the popular appeal of the code (Chapter 4, this volume). The interview data show that the majority of interviewees supported strict liability but were divided in their views of whether greater structural support for athletes would change doping behavior.

The interviews also explored interviewees' views on whether the pressure to perform or team pressure might play a role in terms of drug use in sport. Described as the 'sport ethic,' team pressure is not unique to elite sport but "operates at various levels of sport, from local gyms to the locker rooms of professional sport teams" (Coakley 2007, 185). There is evidence of the influence of the 'sport ethic' in the interview data. One interview participant recalled their personal experience in elite sport: "all routines of normality are excluded, you're not allowed to work. If you're seen to be working you're not seen to be dedicated . . . unless you're totally engrossed in this then forget it" (Interview 141036). Supporting this view, another interviewee with a background in elite sport said: "the mentality out there is unless you're winning . . . you haven't made it in sport" (Interview 141109). For this interviewee, such an attitude "breeds the drug culture." Other interviewees involved in elite sport pointed out that not all athletes take drugs to win. Rather, for some athletes, PEDs provide an "insurance policy . . . my contract is worth $100,000 a year and I need to perform at a certain level 120 times a year, therefore to do that I need to do this as an insurance policy" (Interview 141050).

These views of some interviewees resonate with comments of former professional athletes. For example, Paul Kimmage (1998) a former *domestique* with the RMO cycling team in the Tour de France, wrote of his experience with the pressure to use PEDs. According to Kimmage, meeting the performance expectations of team managers was essential for riders to secure ongoing employment. Failure to meet those expectations created a situation where:

> I felt like abandoning a hundred times . . . I couldn't, for I felt my survival as a professional rider depended on getting to Paris . . . at the end of the season the weak men would be sacked and new blood brought in . . . I had a contract for two years so I was assured of my place for 1987, but already I was thinking ahead to 1988. . . . In a year's time, Thévenet [team director] would remember not that I had finished the Tour on my hands and knees but that I'd finished. (Kimmage 1998, 93)

Athletes' efforts to meet these types of expectations may lead to 'over-conformity' to the sport ethic and contribute to a situation where:

> . . . as long as some athletes are willing to take performance-enhancing substances to gain the edge they need to continue playing at the highest possible level of competence, others will conclude that they also must use similar substances to stay competitive at that level, even if it's against their better judgment. (Coakley 2007, 185)

Nevertheless, the majority of interviewees in this research indicated their support for strict liability and felt that individual athletes must bear the responsibility and consequences for their decisions to use PEDs. At the same time, however, interviewees also indicated that strict liability places a responsibility upon NSOs to ensure that other components of the anti-doping system operate efficiently and equitably. This illustrates the evaluative and subjective nature of legitimacy and the importance of ensuring that policy approaches meet and support community expectations.

Ensuring that policy frameworks operate consistently and efficiently in order to meet community expectations is particularly important in terms of the application of the strict liability principle. Half of the interviewees stressed that all procedural elements of the anti-doping framework needed to operate efficiently if the strict liability principle was to work. For example, one interviewee stated that strict liability lacked legitimacy without accurate testing: "the processes and controls . . . have been proven on a number of occasions to be flawed. How do you apply strict liability to an individual when third parties can stuff up the process?" (Interview 140995). Another element identified as essential for legitimate application of strict liability included due process similar to "reasonable doubt" (Interview 141109) in a legal setting. An "occupational health and safety approach" was also mentioned (Interview 141131).

Athletes and PEDs: Strict Liability, the Grassroots Community and Education

Although the majority felt athletes should be responsible for using PEDs, for some interviewees legitimate application of strict liability meant greater incorporation of the grassroots community through increased anti-doping education and raising awareness of testing protocols. Failure to do so meant that there was a potential that strict liability could infringe on athletes' rights. As this interviewee stated:

> So I think that certainly before the punishment is dished out there needs to be proof of guilt. That it is the person took the choice to . . . take it. Yeah, definitely again back to . . . education . . . making them aware of the consequences if they do get caught taking it and they are guilty of taking it well this is what's going to happen. (Interview 001)

The role of education, including greater education at the grassroots level, was a consistent theme in the data. However, the discussion surrounding strict liability broadened the role of education beyond the scope of anti-doping to include programs that develop a range of skills for 'life after sport.' Hardie et al. (2010) conducted research in Australian cycling that supports this view. Their interviews noted the tension between entering into cycling as an all-consuming, but relatively short-lived, profession and a "certain rhetoric" where:

> Professional cycling was seen as the 'be all and end all,' eclipsing any thought of longer term security or contingency plans should something go wrong. That rhetoric contained within it a suggestion that, with enough commitment to cycling, one might never need to work again . . . many of the interview participants not only recognized this as an

unrealistic expectation but actively critiqued it and were, even in the earlier phases of their careers, concerned about life post-cycling. (Hardie et al. 2010, 23)

Some of my interviewees with a background in elite sport expressed similar views of the 'all encompassing' nature of elite sport. Hardie et al. (2010, 23) found that irrespective of the amount of hard work or athletes' commitment to their sport, at some point they faced a transition into the conventional workforce where their professional cycling credentials would not be recognized. They noted that, for Australian cyclists, there is a lack of viable 'second' career options for athletes when they leave their sport. These were issues raised by some of my interviewees as an important area for NSOs to address, across a range of sports and not limited to cycling.

A slight majority of interviewees felt that NSOs should assist athletes in developing skills for life after their sporting careers. Interviewees acknowledged that "as part of their job," NSOs are obligated to "look after the interests of their sport" (Interview 141574). This interviewee went on to state that NSOs should "realize that it's in the best interest of their sport to put in place traineeship programs . . . or something that can help them return back into life." These views were not only limited to issues around doping, but also included support for athletes who might find their careers at a sudden end due to injury as well as those individuals "that have come up through the ranks, not made it, but have given 10 years of their life to try" (Interview 141574). Other interviewees supported this view, particularly as not all athletes "end up being a . . . celebrity athlete but you've put your whole life into it up to that point, what's there to do after that?" (Interview 001). For example:

> Now to me I find that very hard to deal with because if coaches or ambassadors of their sport or administrators of their sport are doing this to young bodies and young lives, then what's going to be the outcome for that individual in years to come? The time that you're in a sport or that you're at elite level is a very small window of time. So you've got to think about ultimately how you're going to be in years to come and what you want to do in your life. (Interview 141036)

Some saw a more holistic educational approach, including initiatives such as supporting athletes in attaining academic qualifications, as playing an important role in building an anti-doping culture. As this interviewee stated: "Anyway . . . we pay you based on how many subjects you pass at University. You don't pass we pull the money out. And clearly, in [*sport*] we deal with that lack of education, if they've got what I call an employment alternative the ability to say no [to doping] is infinitely higher" (Interview 141050). These sentiments were underpinned by the view that assisting athletes in developing skills or qualifications applicable outside sport may reduce the pressure to use PEDs as an 'insurance policy' to prolong the financial benefits of a sporting career. In their interviews with elite Australian cyclists, Hardie et al. (2010, 154) also found that education was perceived as "an important means to shifting the anti-doping bell curve."

The data discussed here has shown that interviewees view athletes as primarily responsible for ensuring that sport is PED-free, although there were indications that structural factors associated with modern sport could contribute to PED use by some athletes. This raises the question of whether structural pressures place a responsibility upon NSOs to support athletes and whether this influenced attitudes toward NSOs' legitimacy. Although the majority of interviewees supported the principle of strict liability, views were divided over whether structural factors placed a responsibility upon sporting organizations to provide greater levels of support for athletes and whether this would affect athletes' doping behavior. Divided views illustrate the subjective nature of the concept of legitimacy and the difficult task facing organizations, such as NSOs, in formulating policy approaches to complex issues like drugs in sport that meet diverse community expectations. Nevertheless, the interview comments discussed here have revealed that support for strict liability is dependent on all aspects of the anti-doping framework operating efficiently and consistently. Some interviewees emphasized that strict liability required more inclusive anti-doping education, such as raising awareness of testing protocols at the grassroots level. Some interviewees expanded the role of education to include initiatives that helped athletes develop skills for 'life after sport.' This was based on their belief that providing athletes with opportunities to develop non-sporting based skills removes the pressure to view PED use as a necessary part of their sporting career.

The data discussed here are not meant to be fully representative of views held by members of the Australian grassroots sporting community. Rather, it is indicative of a range of answers and views relating to the issues explored in this book. Overall, these comments emphasize that organizations responsible for sports governance, as well as anti-doping authorities, must actively work to maintain support, including from the grassroots sporting community, for the legitimacy of institutional solutions to doping.

CONCLUSION

Previously in this book, I considered institutional actors in the doping debate using socio-historical case studies and media reports of doping events. Here I have highlighted the evaluative and subjective aspect of legitimacy by taking a 'bottom-up' approach to consider attitudes of members of the grassroots sporting community. To accomplish this task, I used qualitative interviews to discuss three topic areas that represent central elements of WADA's anti-doping campaign. Those areas were values-based anti-doping information and education, including the WADC, testing and sanctions and, finally, views of the strict liability principle. The data revealed division in the attitudes of interviewees. This division is significant as, in addition to emphasizing the subjective aspect of legitimacy, it highlights that any crisis of legitimacy involves conflicting views. This does not undermine the value of the concept of a legitimacy crisis. Crises provide opportunities for organizations, including NSOs, to consider how they can engage in processes of regulatory change that enhance perceptions of their legitimacy. They always provide room for maneuverability and change.

For the interviewees, this progressive change meant ensuring that all elements of anti-doping policies form a mutually supportive and cohesive framework. This incorporated providing anti-doping information and education as well as accurate testing, efficient administrative processes and consistently applied sanctions. Despite divisions in views, the majority of the interviewees tended to support a rules-based regulatory approach underpinned by values, such as the WADC, as an effective anti-doping approach. The interview data revealed that application of such an anti-doping framework enhanced attitudes toward NSO legitimacy. Members of the grassroots sporting community also demonstrated a qualified level of support for the principle of strict liability. While supporting the view that athletes are responsible for their doping decisions, support for strict liability required equitable and efficient operation of all other components of the anti-doping system, such as testing, consistently applied sanctions and greater concern for the post-sport life-chances of individual athletes. This is consistent with the arguments of Battin et al. (2008) and Donovan et al. (2002) that to enjoy legitimacy, anti-drug policies must be coherent, consistent and easily evaluated.

The interview results are also pertinent to considerations of doping as a moral panic. From this perspective, the interview comments show that there is community concern and agreement that doping is problematic behavior requiring action. However, the division in the data emphasizes that claim-makers, namely elite sporting organizations, cannot take the organizational legitimacy and moral authority of anti-doping responses for granted. Rather, these groups must actively work to generate and maintain support for institutional responses to doping as a particular problem threatening sport and the social order. The focus here has been on identifying the empirical characteristics of perceptions of the organizational legitimacy of NSOs at the grassroots level. As Goode and Ben-Yehuda (2009) note, the public cannot be considered dupes ready to consume any claim presented in the media. Claims are filtered through people's life experiences.

NOTE

1   Twenty of the 28 interviewees indicated the view that NSOs face a crisis of legitimacy and five answered in the negative. The remaining interviewees were unsure.

REFERENCES

ABS (Australian Bureau of Statistics). 2001. *4902.0 — Australian Culture and Leisure Classifications, 2001*. Canberra: Australian Bureau of Statistics.

Anshel, M.H. 1991. "A Survey of Elite Athletes on the Perceived Causes of Using Banned Drugs in Sport." *Journal of Sport Behavior* 14: 283–308.

AP (Associated Press). 2008. "IOC: No Missing Test Results from Beijing." *International Herald Tribune*, 16 October 2008. http://www.iht.com/articles/ap/2008/10/16/sports/OLY-IOC-Beijing-Tests.php. Accessed 17 October 2008.

Battin, M.P., Luna, E., Lipman, A.G., Gahlinger, P. M., Rollins, D.E., Roberts, J.C., and Booher, T.L. 2008. *Drugs and Justice: Seeking a Consistent, Coherent, Comprehensive View*. Oxford: Oxford University Press.

Bette, K., and Schimank, U. 2001. "Coping with Doping: Sport Associations Under Organisational Stress." In *Proceedings from the Workshop Research on Doping in Sport*, 51–69. Oslo: The Research Council of Norway. http://web.bi.no/forskning/isforg.nsf/62af2dc31b641632c12566f30039282c/c9d01468d7b9ebe8c1256701 00428c50/$FILE/proceedings%20-%20doping.PDF. Accessed 7 December 2009.

Breivik, G., Hanstad, D.V., and Loland, S. 2009. "Attitudes Towards Use of Performance-Enhancing Substances and Body Modification Techniques. A Comparison Between Elite Athletes and the General Population." *Sport in Society* 12 (6): 737–754.

Cantelon, H. 2005. "Amateurism, High-Performance Sport, and the Olympics." In *Global Olympics: Historical and Sociological Studies of the Modern Games*, edited by Young, K. and Wamsley, K.B., 83–101. Amsterdam: Elsevier AI.

Coakley, Jay J. 2007. *Sports in Society: Issues and Controversies*. Boston: McGraw-Hill Higher Education.

Connor, J. 2009. "Towards a Sociology of Drugs in Sport." *Sport in Society* 12 (3): 327–343.

Donovan, R.J., Egger, G., Kapernick, V., and Mendoza, J. 2002. "A Conceptual Framework for Achieving Performance Enhancing Drug Compliance in Sport." *Sports Medicine* 32 (4): 269–284.

DrugScope. 2004. "The Doping Scandal: A Question for Sport." *Drug Think Series*. DrugScope.

Ericson, R. V, Baranek, P. M., and Chan, J.B.L. 1991. *Representing Order*. Toronto: University of Toronto Press.

Goode, E., and Ben-Yehuda, N. 2009. *Moral Panics: The Social Construction of Deviance*. Chichester, West Sussex: Wiley-Blackwell Publishing.

Gucciardi, D.F., Jalleh, G., and Donovan, R. 2011. "An Examination of the Sport Drug Control Model with Elite Australian Athletes." *Journal of Science and Medicine in Sport* 14 (6): 469–476.

Habermas, J. 1976. *Legitimation Crisis*. London: Heinemann Educational.

Hardie, M., Shilbury, D., Ware, I., and Bozzi, C. 2010. *I Wish I Was Twenty One Now—Beyond Doping in the Australian Peloton*. Waurn Ponds, VIC: Deakin University Faculty of Business and Law.

Kimmage, P. 1998. *Rough Ride: Behind the Wheel with a Pro Cyclist*. London: Yellow Jersey Press.

Magnay, J. 2008. "Missing Test Results Turn Up but WADA Isn't Happy." *The Sydney Morning Herald*, 17 October 2008. http://www.smh.com.au/news/sport/missing-test-results-turn-up-but-wada-isnt-happy/2008/10/16/1223750232514.html. Accessed 17 October 2008.

Mazanov, J., Huybers, T., and Connor, J. 2010. "Qualitative Evidence of a Primary Intervention Point for Elite Athlete Doping." *Journal of Science and Medicine in Sport* 14 (2011): 106–110.

Petroczi, A., and Aidman, E. 2008. "Psychological Drivers in Doping: The Life-Cycle Model of Performance Enhancement." *Substance Abuse Treatment, Prevention, and Policy* 3 (7). Published online 2008 March 2010. doi: 2010.1186/1747-2597X-2003-2007.

Pound, R. W. 2007. "Code Compliance: The Time Is Now." *Play True: An Official Publication of the World Anti-Doping Agency* 2: 1–2.

Schneider, A. 2000. *Olympic Reform, Are We There Yet?* Paper presented at the Bridging Three Centuries, Fifth International Symposium for Olympic Research, University of Western Ontario, London, Ontario, Canada.

Striegel, H., Vollkommer, G., and Dickhuth, H.-H. 2002. "Combating Drug Use in Competitive Sports: An Analysis from the Athletes' Perspective." *Journal of Sports Medicine and Physical Fitness* 42 (3): 354–359.

Turner, M., and McCrory, P. 2003. "Social Drug Policies for Sport." *British Journal of Sports Medicine* 37 (5): 378–379.

Voy, R. 1991. *Drugs, Sport and Politics*. Champaign, IL: Leisure Press.

WADA (World Anti-Doping Agency). 2006. "Chairman's Message." World Anti-Doping Agency.http://www.wada-ama.org/en/dynamic.ch2?pageCategory.id=25. Accessed 5 October 2006.

———. 2007. "Education." World Anti-Doping Agency. http://www.wada-ama.org/rtecontent/document/05_FS_Education_en.pdf. Accessed 2 February 2007.

———. 2009 (October). "Programs—Education, Introduction." World Anti-Doping Agency. http://www.wada-ama.org/en/dynamic.ch2?pageCategory.id=26. Accessed 1 October 2009.

———. 2015. "World Anti-Doping Code 2015." https://wada-main-prod.s3.amazonaws.com/resources/files/wada-2015-world-anti-doping-code.pdf. Accessed 3 September 2014.

Weber, M. 1969. *Economy and Society*. 2 vols. Berkeley: University of California Press.

Wuthnow, R., Hunter, J., Bergesen, A., and Kurzweil, E. 1984. *Cultural Analysis*. London: Routledge.

Conclusion

No folly is more costly than the folly of intolerant idealism. When standards of conduct or morals which are beyond the normal public sentiment of a great community are professed and enforced, the results are invariably evasion, subterfuge, and hypocrisy.

(Winston Churchill, cited in Dawson and McNamee 2009, 183)

In this book I have drawn on the work of Cohen (2002) and elaborated upon by Goode and Ben-Yehuda (2009) to add a Weberian-inspired consideration of legitimacy (Weber 1969) to a moral panic framework. In doing so, I have responded to a question posed by Ben-Yehuda (2009, 2): "But what happens to moral panics in multicultural societies where morality itself is constantly contested and negotiated?" A legitimacy-inspired moral panic model analytically captures the way that power relationships between elite groups influence contemporary debates that are constituted by the competing claims of multiple social actors. I illustrated the value of this approach by applying it to the debate over drugs in sport, which can be viewed as a socially constructed moral panic underpinned by elite SGBs' efforts to maintain their moral authority and legitimacy in the global sporting community.

I began this book with an overview of Weber's concept of legitimacy, highlighting its multi-dimensional and subjective component (Weber 1969). Fundamental to dominant groups' ability to secure, and maintain, compliance with rules and regulations is that their claims to legitimacy are perceived as valid. This is important because it enables those groups to determine, and police, the boundaries of their particular communities. Further, compliance based on a belief in the validity of claims to legitimacy and moral authority is "less costly" than coercive or rewards-based compliance (Matheson 1987, 200). However, in modern societies elite groups' claims to legitimacy cannot be taken for granted but must compete for attention, and thus support, amongst myriad other claims by diverse stakeholders. Amidst these competing claims, a crisis can emerge if dominant groups are perceived to have failed to implement regulatory frameworks, or 'proper procedures' that meet community expectations as well as existing social norms or values (Habermas 1976; Wuthnow et al. 1984). Rather than con-ceptualizing crisis as social disintegration, a more useful view is to see it as signaling the possibility of transformative regulatory change (Andrews 2000; Holton 1987). Such a process enables claim-makers to reinstate or restore their claim to legitimacy by introducing "special agencies" (Weber 1969, 944) to resolve questions of doubt. I further noted the dynamic and multi-dimensional nature of legitimacy, which is influenced by factors and events in the broader social context as well as the particular problems to which it is applied (Suchman 1995). This provided the starting point for my argument that claim-makers must actively work to generate and maintain support for their legitimacy and moral authority in order to avert crises of legitimacy.

Throughout this book I situated legitimacy in a moral panic frame-work. Like legitimacy, successful moral panics require support for insti-tutional solutions presented as necessary for social stability. Goode and Ben-Yehuda (2009) noted that, similarly to legitimacy, broader social fac-tors and socio-historical circumstances influence the forms and effects of a moral panic. The tools postulated in Goode and Ben-Yehuda's model, namely the moral panic criteria of consensus, concern, hostility, dispro-portionality and volatility, provide a useful lens through which to consider contemporary social issues as moral panics. Building on that foundation, I modified Goode and Ben-Yehuda's model to enhance its analytical effi-cacy and applied it to the drugs in sport debate as a particular case study. In the context of the doping debate, the diversity of stakeholders and their contested claims to legitimacy led me to modify the moral panic criterion of consensus to *consensus-making*. In the particular case of drugs in sport, consensus-making more accurately captures the multi-dimensional and con-tested nature of claims to legitimacy. The diversity of stakeholder groups in modern sport and the contested power relationships between these social actors requires a theoretical framework that acknowledges their different interests and objectives. To more effectively consider the way that elite SGBs use the anti-doping debate to enhance or restore their legitimacy, I modi-fied 'elite-engineered' to *'elites-engineered'* moral panic theory. The efficacy of this modified legitimacy-inspired moral panic model was demonstrated using the socio-historical case studies of the IOC, WADA and an Australian sporting organization, namely the AFL.

There are three key themes that emerged from the socio-historical case studies of the IOC (Chapter 2, this volume) and WADA (Chapter 3, this vol-ume). First, the socially contingent nature of the debate over PEDs, includ-ing changing attitudes toward drug use in sport, had implications for the legitimacy of elite SGBs and particularly the IOC. Attitudes toward doping were influenced by broader social factors, such as the political climate of the Cold War and the medicalization of sport as well as shifting concerns over drug use from a health issue to a "moral crisis" (Dimeo 2007, 93; Hoberman 1992). These factors and the deaths of athletes linked to drug use contributed to the necessity for anti-doping regulation (Houlihan 2002; Stokvis 2003). A consequence emerged whereby SGBs' regulatory responses to doping provided a measure against which their legitimacy could be evaluated. This was particularly the case for the legitimacy of the IOC as the guardian of the values and ideals underpinning Olympic competition (Schneider 2000) codified in the *Olympic Charter*. Over the course of the latter half of the twentieth century, despite being in a position of sports leadership, the IOC's legitimacy was challenged by what many perceived to be a lack of effective action in the face of continuing doping scandals.

The second point from the socio-historical case studies of the IOC and WADA was that a crisis of legitimacy for the IOC contributed to a transformation of authority to regulate the elite sporting community. This transformation reflected views that the IOC failed to meet, and support, community expectations of their responsibilities and obligations as guardian of Olympic drug-free sport. The 1998 Tour de France doping scandal, described as a crisis of legitimacy for the IOC (MacAloon 2001), contributed to the creation of WADA. This process was also driven by the more extrinsic, instrumental and globalized nature of modern sport. The amateur ethos of participation was replaced by more commercial imperatives that contributed to and influenced PED use. These structural changes required a new way of 'imagining' (Anderson 1991) the global elite sporting community and placed greater emphasis on codified rules to regulate behavior, including doping. WADA transformed anti-doping authority with a new range of 'proper procedures' (the WADC), which shifted the previous narrow focus on Olympic competition under the IOC, using the *Olympic Charter* and, later, the IOC Medical Code, to incorporate the global sporting community. WADA, as the organization responsible for the globalized harmonization of anti-doping frameworks, set new boundaries around participation for the elite sporting community. Conditions of inclusion or exclusion, or 'athlete citizenship' (Henne 2015), were redefined and regulated by WADA as a 'policing agent' (Erikson 1966), using a rational-legal framework of rules and regulations, including testing procedures and protocols, codified in the WADC.

The third key point from the socio-historical case study of the IOC and WADA was the value of situating legitimacy within a moral panic framework. As for the IOC, doping scandals challenge WADA's claim to legitimacy and create the potential for audiences to lose interest in doping, or as Dr. Gary Wadler described it, to succumb to 'doping fatigue' (Chapter 5, this volume). This means that WADA must actively engage in consensus-making work with a range of diverse stakeholders in order to maintain support for their regulatory approach as successfully catching 'cheats.' Rather than ongoing doping scandals raising questions regarding WADA's legitimacy, the challenge is to construct those events as not only demonstrating the necessity of their strong regulatory approach but also to support increasingly harsh measures to control and prevent the deviant behavior from contaminating wider society. This also raises issues of governance and control as, although support for WADA provides an opportunity for SGBs to enhance perceptions of their legitimacy and commitment to anti-doping, some elite SGBs resist WADA's imposition of authority (see Dvorak et al. 2006). I discussed this tension using a national sporting organization in Australia, namely the Australian Football League (AFL), and their interactions with the Australian federal government as a third socio-historical case study (Chapter 4, this volume).

A key point that emerged here was that elite claim-makers, which are not limited to SGBs, but can also include governments and other anti-doping organizations, manipulate the doping debate to meet outcomes relevant to their community and objectives. The Australian federal government pursued their objective of maintaining their status as a world leader in anti-doping, using policies such as *Tough on Drugs in Sport* and the *Backing Australia's Sporting Ability: A More Active Australia*. As well as supporting WADA's tough on drugs in sport approach, the Australian government linked 'clean' sport to Australia's national identity, strong economic growth, community well-being and healthy lifestyles. These policies were also used by the Australian federal government to frame the anti-drugs in sport approach of other organizations, such as the AFL, as flawed. From this perspective, the Australian government argued that the AFL's insistence on a WADC-aligned ADC together with the separate IDP policy, which focused on player education, rehabilitation and counseling, undermined the government's 'tough on drugs' approach. Further, the AFL's position challenged the authority and legitimacy of WADA as the organization responsible for global harmonization of anti-doping policies using the WADC as formally constituted rules and regulations underpinned by values articulated in the spirit of sport statement.

The AFL, recognizing the potential for drug use in sport, either PEDs or illicit drugs, to negatively affect their legitimacy based on community attitudes toward this issue, introduced anti-drugs policies. The ADC and later IDP formed part of a regulatory framework that addressed a range of issues, such as racial vilification, and provided important mechanisms used to bolster perceptions of the AFL's legitimacy. Importantly, a fundamental concern for the AFL was the role of these policies in enhancing the popularity and commercial viability of Australian football (Stewart 2007; Stewart et al. 2008; Stewart et al. 2005). The ADC and IDP were important mechanisms intended to demonstrate that the AFL met and supported community expectations regarding acceptable behavior, including identifying and sanctioning deviance—in this case drug use in sport (Ericson et al. 1991; Habermas 1976; Wuthnow et al. 1984). The interactions between the AFL and the Australian federal government revealed the wider dimensions of the debate around drugs in sport. This demonstrates that elite groups' contested claims to the legitimacy and moral authority to govern and regulate their particular communities are important and influential elements to consider critically in any analysis of the doping debate.

In that chapter, I also pointed out that the media discussed the AFL's anti-drugs policies in a manner suggesting the construction of a moral panic. Media reports sought to generate public concern that drug use in Australian football was widespread. Some media reports presented the issue as potentially threatening social order more broadly by linking drug use in Australian football to drug addiction in the wider community. These reports focused public concern and hostility by constructing participants in Australian football as 'folk devils,' described as 'lame brains,' requiring tough regulatory control to protect community well-being. This created opportunities for elite claim-makers, such as the Australian federal government and the AFL, to position their respective policy models as the necessarily strong regulatory response most appropriate to address the issue. This moral panic highlighted the contested nature of legitimacy and that organizational power relationships are part of the anti-doping debate. All stakeholder groups used media reports to make claims as well as challenge the claims of others to legitimacy as providers of the most effective solution to control drug use in the Australian sporting community.

I then shifted the focus from legitimacy to explore the doping debate as a moral panic using a review of media reports of doping to consider the media's role in the construction of a moral panic (Chapter 5, this volume). In that chapter, I demonstrated that the doping debate constituted a moral panic that created PED-using 'folk devils.' I presented evidence to show that the media, and elite SGBs, made claims that fulfill Goode and Ben-Yehuda's (2009) criteria, identifying the debate over drugs in sport as a moral panic. The evidence also supported consensus-making as a modified moral panic criterion. The media review demonstrated that elite SGBs, and primarily WADA, use media reports to engage in consensus-making work in support of WADA as the institutional response to doping. Reviewing media reports was also relevant to considerations of legitimacy and, specifically, the way that different elite stakeholders used the media to make and challenge claims to legitimacy. This supports an elites-engineered modified moral panic theory, which illuminated the negotiated power relationships between dominant groups evident in the debate. The case studies and review of media reports examined legitimacy from a 'top-down' perspective of institutional actors in the debate over doping.

Moving away from institutional actors, I then considered legitimacy from the 'bottom-up' perspective of Australian grassroots sporting participants (Chapter 6, this volume). Using qualitative interviews, I explored attitudes toward NSOs' legitimacy by canvassing views on anti-doping information and education, testing and sanctions, WADA and the WADC as well as the strict liability principle. The data showed that across all areas a majority of participants indicated there was a crisis of legitimacy, although they varied in their views over the causes of such a crisis. These interview findings emphasize how claims to legitimacy cannot be taken for granted. Rather, stakeholder groups, in this case Australian NSOs, must actively work to maintain perceptions of legitimacy. This is also relevant to consideration of doping as an institutionalized moral panic. Indications of a crisis of legitimacy and divided views over its causes highlight that elite groups must engage in ongoing consensus-making work to maintain support for institutional responses to PED use, including from the grassroots community.

In this book, I have demonstrated that conceptualizing claims to legitimacy as underpinning the construction of a moral panic helps to shed light upon and explain debates over the contemporary issue of drugs in sport. This challenges discourses and individualistic analysis that tend to ignore broader social factors and focus on the doping behavior of the athlete-user. The dominant approach to drugs in sport regulation also inadequately examines the possibility that there are linkages between SGBs' efforts to maintain legitimacy and the presentation of doping as a moral panic.

IMPLICATIONS AND INFERENCES

A modified moral panic framework incorporating the concept of legitimacy broadens the analysis to examine institutional actors in the doping debate. The value of this multi-dimensional model is that it enables the analysis to move beyond individualistic explanations to place the issue in the social realm (Connor 2009). In modern social life, the legitimacy of dominant groups, in this case sporting organizations, rests on their implementation of rules and regulations to promote social order, including apprehending deviant (doping) individuals. Perceptions that dominant groups have failed to implement 'proper procedures' oriented toward the common good can lead to a crisis of legitimacy (Habermas 1976; Wuthnow et al. 1984). The notion of a crisis of legitimacy is valuable analytically, as it does not necessarily imply institutional paralysis but a myriad of responses from stakeholders who might perceive the issue and the stakes involved differently. For example, not all diverse stakeholder groups in modern sport share the same attitudes or objectives toward the regulation of PED use in sport (e.g., see Hanstad et al. 2010; Kidd et al. 2001). Examination of legitimacy in the context of stakeholder interactions and their impact on the doping debate, as well as anti-doping regulation, is an area under-regarded by the current approaches to drugs in sport. This brings us back to the relevance of situating legitimacy within a moral panic framework, which includes consideration of the media as key institutional actors, in particular, their ability to influence debates and public attitudes.

In terms of claims to legitimacy, this is beneficial for elite groups. Their privileged access to the media opens opportunities to enhance perceptions of their legitimacy as providers of necessary solutions to restore order. The review of media reports showed that elite groups use the media to keep the public's attention focused on the ongoing danger presented by the problematic behavior, in this case doping and PED-using 'folk devils.' These claims support Goode and Ben-Yehuda's (2009) moral panic typology. Further, and similarly to Cohen (2002), Goode and Ben-Yehuda point out that some moral panics leave an institutional legacy that contributes to social change. In these types of moral panic, institutional responses are necessary to address a *specific* issue of *particular* concern (Beamish 2009). In the drugs in sport debate, the specific issue is doping, which is of particular concern because it undermines the integrity of sport, or the 'spirit of sport.' WADA claims legitimacy as the particular institutional response and the most significant claim-maker in the debate over doping as an issue of specific concern and danger, not only to elite sport, but also to public order and stability. These claims do not go uncontested, however, and the media provide a forum for other groups to challenge elite interpretations and to attempt to impose alternative views on the debate. Further, the dynamic social context of modern life includes a tendency for public problems, such as the emergence of new PEDs, to mutate and for the 'fever pitch' of concern or hostility in a moral panic to wane over time.

An effective explanatory model requires a theoretical framework that takes these diverse and complex factors into account. Situating legitimacy within a modified moral panic framework accomplishes this task. The contested nature of claims to legitimacy and the dynamic nature of modern social life support a modified moral panic model that includes consensus-making and elites-engineered theory. Consensus-making is a valuable concept, as claims to legitimacy cannot be taken for granted but require active efforts from elite groups to maintain support for their moral authority and legitimacy amongst a range of competing claims. Elites-engineered moral panic theory brings power relationships and the negotiated nature of interactions among elite groups, such as WADA and SGBs, into the analysis as they make and contest claims to legitimacy. For example, elite SGBs endeavor to remain in control of their sporting community while at the same time enhancing their legitimacy by demonstrating their commitment to a harmonized and globalized approach to anti-doping by supporting WADA.

There is considerable literature on the sociology of sport addressing PEDs and the social construction of such behavior as deviant. An area lacking in attention is the extent to which individuals at the grassroots level support the idea that doping is deviant behavior and perceive SGBs to be committed to addressing the issue. In other words, do individuals perceive these organizations' anti-doping efforts as legitimate? Publics are key stakeholders in the modern sporting context and, as Schneider (2006) notes, are not always in agreement with SGBs' responses to doping. This highlights how claims to legitimacy for any specific institutional response to doping cannot be taken for granted. The interviews emphasized that, to enjoy perceptions of legitimacy, anti-drugs policies, including those used in sport, must be coherent, consistent and easily evaluated (Battin et al. 2008; Donovan et al. 2002). The interviewees had clear expectations of NSOs' responsibilities in relation to anti-doping, and perceptions that NSOs failed to support those expectations affected their views of NSOs' legitimacy. In other words, without ensuring that all elements of the anti-doping framework operate coherently and consistently, NSOs face a potential crisis of legitimacy.

I have not discussed issues such as public anti-doping policy in this book. Nevertheless, the evidence I have presented suggests that NSOs should consider methods and initiatives that will build perceptions of organizational legitimacy at the grassroots level. This speaks directly to concerns over the commercial viability of sporting contexts, which was clearly an issue for the AFL and their introduction of anti-drugs policies. Community expectations that sporting bodies implement strong regulatory frameworks, including rules with a basis in shared values, is relevant here. I discussed this issue using the IOC, where I noted that preserving values associated with (Olympic) sport is important for maintaining legitimacy and community support. Similarly, Schneider (2000, 225) wrote that public perceptions that Olympic values were "mocked" by the actions of the IOC would have negative consequences for the commercial value of the Olympic Games. Consequently, she explains, "preservation of Olympic ideals" constitutes the "best way to preserve the financial success of the Games." These sentiments are no less relevant to other SGBs (see also Bette and Schimank 2001).

Considering the role of legitimacy brings organizational power relationships into the analysis and highlights the dynamic social context in which social problems, such as doping, take place. The idea of a crisis of legitimacy suggests that the manner in which claims to legitimacy are made points to a 'socially situated beholder.' In other words, a 'fully-fledged' crisis is not limited to its impact on social structures but includes a subjective element linked to challenges to "values, ideas and beliefs shared by members of a social group" (Andrews 2000, 226, 250). Further, the diversity of stakeholders in modern life means that there are different notions of how legitimacy operates in particular communities. Given this, and the multi-dimensional nature of legitimacy, any crisis of legitimacy may in fact be unresolvable. Nevertheless, the concept of a crisis of legitimacy is useful as it points to a transformative process of social change, rather than a chaotic process of organizational collapse. The transformative potential of a crisis provides elite groups with opportunities to restore or enhance their claims to legitimacy and moral authority.

The multi-dimensional model presented here has highlighted the value of adapting the moral panic framework to conceptualize contemporary issues, such as the drugs in sport debate. This model helps to identify what interests might be at stake for elite groups in the construction of a moral panic. However, it expands the analysis beyond the somewhat limited observation that economic imperatives or issues of social control motivate elite groups. Rather, situating legitimacy within a moral panic framework demonstrates that elite interests, including the ability to pursue a commercial agenda and maintain control of their particular community, rest on perceptions that their authority is legitimate and valid. In other words, legitimacy is the cornerstone upon which rests the ability of elites to successfully achieve other goals. The model presented in this book contributes to the body of sociological literature by developing and expanding on an existing framework. This provides a mechanism with which to apply a holistic approach to the way debates over contemporary social issues can be conceptualized.

POSTSCRIPT: DRUGS AND CORRUPTION IN AUSTRALIAN SPORT—A CRISIS OF LEGITIMACY

Earlier in this book I discussed the way that interactions between the Australian federal government and the AFL revealed the multi-dimensional nature of legitimacy and the way that different stakeholders manipulate the debate to meet objectives relevant to their particular comminutes. I concluded that discussion by noting that the AFL faced the ongoing challenge of maintaining public support for their legitimacy based on a regulatory framework that meets and supports community expectations toward drug use in sport while also safeguarding athlete welfare. As this book was being finalized, the AFL's legitimacy again came under pressure as a scandal involving alleged inappropriate administration of supplements to players of one AFL club emerged.

In 2013, the Australian Crime Commission (ACC) released a report entitled *Organised Crime and Drugs in Sport New Generation Performance and Image Enhancing Drugs and Organised Criminal Involvement in their use in Professional Sport* (ACC 2013). The report followed a year-long investigation, code-named Project Aperio, and alleged links between sport, organized crime and sports betting. There were significant implications here for the AFL, as doubts emerged around a sports supplement regime administered by the Essendon Football Club that was alleged to have potentially contravened the WADC (although the status of that claim became increasingly unclear as the debate unfolded). Responses to the ACC report from the federal government, elite SGBs and the media provide further evidence that contested claims to legitimacy are important elements to consider critically in the debate around drugs in sport.

Investigations into the issues raised by the ACC report remain before the Australian Courts with much still to play out. As a result, I use the debate as indicative of an elites-engineered moral panic driven by contested claims to legitimacy and do not make any evaluations of the veracity of the claims made, or any moral evaluations of any alleged practices. Rather, the objective is to consider the narratives and discourse that are constructed around these types of events to explore the 'interests' that might be involved and what might be at stake for those groups in the construction of a moral panic (e.g, see Dingelstad et al. 1996). The ACC report included allegations against National Rugby League (NRL) players as well as AFL players

(AAP 2013), however, as I have focused in this book on the AFL's anti-drugs approach, I limit my discussion to that code.

The ACC report was released at a joint media conference with federal government minsters flanked by the CEOs of Australia's main professional sporting codes (Pearlman 2013). The federal Home Affairs Minister, Jason Clare, described the findings of the ACC report as "shocking" and noted that its revelations of conduct across Australian sporting codes would "disgust fans" (Gordon 2013). There are clear implications here for the legitimacy of Australian professional sporting codes, including the AFL, based on perceptions that they failed to meet community expectations toward drug use in sport. Seizing on comments by former ASADA head, Richard Ings, media headlines described the release of the ACC report as the "blackest day in Australian sport." Clearly identifying a 'folk devil,' Ings claimed that the "most troubling" element was that successful, highly paid athletes "have abused the trust of the Australian public" (Clark et al. 2013). International media reports also picked up on the saga, with headlines such as: "'Darkest Day' Down Under as Australian Sport Rocked by Revelations of Drug Taking and Links to Organized Crime" (Pearlman 2013). This media report suggested that faith in Australian sport had been undermined, linking the events to international doping scandals. For example, Anthony Sharwood from *Punch* wrote: "Your favorite sports star and mine . . . your team and my team too—all of them are Lance Armstrong today" (Sharwood 2013). The responses and actions of elite claim-makers to the ACC report demonstrate an elites-engineered moral panic underpinned by a crisis of legitimacy for NSOs in Australian sport.

Claims and counter-claims swirled throughout the media, as accusations were levelled at sporting organizations, anti-doping authorities, club officials as well as club medical officials, sports scientists, coaches and, of course, players. This included the Australian federal government, which at the time was under extreme political stress across a number of areas. Not least of these was leadership contention between then Prime Minister Julia Gillard and federal Minister Kevin Rudd. The Liberal Opposition accused the government of using the ACC report to create a "media circus" in order to divert attention from their "political troubles and leadership tensions" (South Australian Liberal MP Jamie Briggs, in Whinnett 2015). Demonstrating that contested claims to legitimacy are part of the debate, the AFL expressed concern around the Australian government's approach, complaining that the press conference was "severely damaging. . . . The world was told there was some very large issue—underworld—infiltrating sport" and that it "impugned just about every athlete in this country," which was an "unfortunate way to commence that investigation. It damaged lots of very, very good sports, lots of very, very good people" (AFL CEO Demetriou in *The Sunday Telegraph* 2014). There are clearly elements of a moral panic framework here. The issue is constructed as 'very large' with the potential for other dangerous elements, such as the 'underworld,' to 'infiltrate' sport.

The report also hints at the construction of 'folk devils,' as athletes are 'impugned' by the government's handling of the situation.

Nevertheless, the government demonstrated their resolve to take a strong stance against drugs in sport. Also in 2013, the government passed legislation strengthening ASADA's powers to include the "legal right to compel any person it believes to have information about doping practice, or a specific doping breach to give evidence in an interview . . . ASADA would also have the right to compel witnesses to produce documents or other related material" (Lane 2013; Lundy 2013). While intended to close loopholes in anti-doping regulation, and similarly to the updated WADC discussed earlier in this book (Chapter 3, this volume), these provisions illustrate a process whereby regulations tend to tighten around individuals and, from a moral panic perspective, include increasingly harsh measures of social control.

There were also concerns around the joint AFL Tribunal and ASADA investigation that flowed from the ACC report. In particular, the investigation was criticized for taking two years to determine whether or not 34 players at the Essendon Football Club had been administered a banned peptide, Thymosin Beta-4, during the 2012 season (Chalkley-Rhoden 2015a; McGarry 2015). ASADA faced criticism for taking 18 months from announcing their investigation into the Essendon allegations to issue players with 'show causes notices' (Chalkley-Rhoden 2015a). The legitimacy and authority of ASADA was further questioned by Essendon Football Club coach James Hird, who argued that the anti-doping authority had acted outside its powers and lodged an (unsuccessful) legal challenge in the Federal Court (Ryan 2015). Also at issue was the legitimacy of the Essendon Football Club, as their governance frameworks were called into question and subsequently found wanting by an AFL Commission inquiry (AFL 2013, 121). The Essendon Football Club also sought to restore perceptions of its legitimacy by implementing its own internal investigation. The club appointed a well-respected Australian business leader, Dr. Ziggy Switkowski, to examine the governance and management of the 2012 supplement program (AFL 2013; Switkowski 2013). The responses to the ACC report by the AFL and other elite stakeholders in Australian sport demonstrate that elite groups' claims to legitimacy cannot be taken for granted. Further, the response to the 'crisis' by these diverse stakeholders reveals elements of an elites-engineered moral panic as organizations acted to maintain, or restore, organizational legitimacy.

Organizational responses to the ACC report show that, in response to the dangerous behavior and practices of certain 'folk devils,' NSOs sought to implement 'proper procedures' that tightened control around individuals in order to return stability and order to their sporting community. For the AFL, this included strengthening integrity units, which had been established in 2008 in order to monitor gambling and compliance with rules and regulations, including the ADC (AFL 2013). Similarly to earlier claims regarding their anti-drugs policies, the AFL responded to criticism that the integrity units had failed to provide substantial results, arguing that the unit was "a world leader" with a model that was "starting to be followed by other sports internationally" (Browne 2013). Measures to strengthen the AFL's integrity unit included an organizational restructure that saw the creation of a "stand-alone" department within the AFL, namely the Competition Integrity Department (AFL 2013, 113). There was a significant focus on investigations, with former Victorian police Detective Superintendent Gerard Ryan (AAP 2014) and Detective Senior Constable Tony Keane taking up full-time roles (AFL 2013, 113). The AFL 'revamped' the ADC to include "intelligence gathering and investigations," emphasizing that the changes took the ADC "above and beyond that of the World Anti-Doping Code" (AFL 2013, 119). WADA would similarly incorporate a focus on non-analytical investigations together with testing under changes to the 2015 WADC (Chapter 3, this volume). The AFL's strong stance, which went beyond that of WADA at the time, as well as tough sanctions against the Essendon Football Club and some of its senior staff, bolstered the AFL's claims to legitimacy (for a summary of the sanctions, see AFL 2013).

Organizational actors also 'diffused' and 'escalated' their controls in response to claims in the ACC report. For example, the ACC and the AFL agreed to a range of measures, including information sharing by the ACC to inform the AFL of any doping offenses revealed as part of the ongoing ACC investigations. The ACC also agreed to "enhance club registries, in particular regard to sports scientists" (*Sportal.com.au* n/d). This refers to the fact that the ACC report contributed to allegations that sports scientist Stephen Dank, who had worked with the Essendon Football Club in 2012, orchestrated a supplement regime that included injecting Essendon players with inappropriate substances (Chalkley-Rhoden 2015a). From a moral panic perspective, Dank could be conceptualized as a 'folk devil' responsible for contaminating the integrity of the AFL's competition. Claims that the Essendon Football Club, James Hird and others had engaged in conduct that damaged the "integrity of the AFL competition" (AFL 2013, 122) were central elements in the sanctions meted out to those groups and individual actors. However, as a 'folk devil' in the debate, Dank pushed back by using the media to argue that "ASADA fabricated claims . . . to serve its own purposes . . . the thing I've found that's sometimes been comical . . . we're having a due process which has followed no process . . . we've had a process which has been devoid of anything that resembles proper judicial processes" (in Mark 2015). This emphasizes that 'folk devils' are also active social agents that influence debates around contemporary social issues.

However, the AFL worked to strengthen existing relationships with other agencies, such as law enforcement agencies, in order to implement new measures to curb the spread of the dangerous, deviant behavior and thus boost their claims to legitimacy. For example, measures sought by the AFL included providing their integrity unit with access to wiretap results that involved AFL players. The media reported that the AFL had "intensified its lobbying . . . governments to change laws" that currently blocked their access to those sorts of findings (Browne 2013). According to the AFL, these types of changes were necessary because of the "risk of corruption," which meant that it was "vitally important to let sporting bodies work more closely with police and other agencies to protect the integrity of sport" (in Browne 2013). Other media reports described the AFL as "morphing into the Stasi. In the avid pursuit of noble ideals like integrity you can justify to yourself listening in to people's private conversations but then suddenly you're extracting their fingernails and attaching their nether regions to an electricity supply" (Sutherland 2013). The AFL also suggested measures, such as that players be required to submit a "list of all their friends and associates," which would be used as a "reference guide" by AFL integrity officers in order to "consider relationships that could potentially cause problems and need to be monitored" (Gleeson 2013). Although not pursued by the AFL, there are clearly concerns here around players' civil liberties, not limited to their right to privacy.

From a moral panic perspective, they demonstrate the way that in response to a crisis of legitimacy, elite claim-makers can seek to implement controls that are increasingly more strict and that tighten around individuals (Goode and Ben-Yehuda 2009; Weber 1969). Demonstrating that challenges to organizational legitimacy are part of the debate, the report cited above went on to describe the AFL's response as "slightly manic" but "understandable" because it was "shocked and embarrassed" to learn that PEDs were an issue, particularly as only one player had been brought before the AFL Tribunal for PED use, which was "Richmond's Justin Charles in 1997" (Sutherland 2013). This categorization raised doubts over whether the AFL's anti-drugs approach, which had commenced in the 1990s in response to instances of PED use in other sports, were as robust as the organization claimed (Chapter 4, this volume). There were broader implications for the AFL, which as I discussed earlier, had long promoted the success of its anti-doping and illicit drugs frameworks in keeping Australian football 'clean' (see also Robinson 2014).

The brief discussion presented here does not cover all aspects that emerged throughout the controversial period following the release of the ACC report. However, the discussion does emphasize that in any consideration of the debate around doping, the claims and counter-claims of a range of organizational actors must be taken into account. These claims and the actions of elite sporting stakeholders have a significant influence on the debate. Throughout the debate in Australian sport, a number of 'folk devils' were constructed and vigorously pursued. These included organizational 'folk devils' in the form of the Essendon Football Club as well as individuals that bore the brunt of allegations, such as sports scientist Stephen Dank, Essendon Football Club coach James Hird and other support staff at the Essendon Football Club. Of course, the group that faces the ultimate consequences from this event are the 34 past and present Essendon Football Club players that continue to wait for the final outcome of this saga (AAP 2015).

In early 2015, although not returning a not guilty finding, the AFL Tribunal indicated that they "were not comfortably satisfied" that any player had been administered Thymosin Beta 4 (Chalkley-Rhoden 2015b; Whateley 2015). Nevertheless, and demonstrating that organizational claims to legitimacy are part of the debate, WADA has stepped into the ring to appeal the decision (Gleeson 2015; Pierik 2015). Meanwhile, the AFL Anti-Doping Tribunal handed down a lifetime ban against sports scientist Stephen Dank, who responded by stating that he will "leave no stone unturned in pursuing justice," with legal action against the AFL planned (*ABC News* 2015). This debate, its manipulation by elite claim-makers and contestations by other social actors, including a range of so-called 'folk devils,' is yet to be finally played out. Nevertheless, the outline presented here illustrates the importance of considering the way that claim-makers, as well as some 'folk devils,' influence the debate to meet particular objectives relevant to their own personal needs as well as organizational imperatives.

REFERENCES

AAP. 2013. "Sharks Players Warned to Come Forward." ABC News, 7 March 2013. http://www.abc.net.au/news/2013–03–07/sharks-players-warned-to-come-forward/455894. Accessed 12 February 2015.

———. 2014. "Senior Detective Gerard Ryan to Lead Investigations in AFL Integrity Unit." *Herald Sun*, 2 February 2014. http://www.heraldsun.com.au/sport/afl/senior-detective-gerard-ryan-to-lead-investigations-in-afl-integrity-unit/story-fni5f22o-122681609867. Accessed 29 June 2015.

———. 2015. "Essendon Skipper Jobe Watson Says There Is Anxiety at Club Ahead of Landmark AFL Anti-Doping Tribunal Verdics." *ABC News*, 25 March 2105. http://www.abc.net.au/news/2015–03–25/watson-admits-anxiety-at-bombers-ahead-of-tribunal-decision/634720. Accessed 29 June 2015.

ABC News. 2015. "Stephen Dank Handed Lifetime Ban by AFL Anti-Doping Tribunal Following Essendon Supplements Saga." *ABC News*, 26 June 2015. http://www.abc.net.au/news/2015–06–26/stephen-dank-handed-lifetime-ban-from-afl-tribunal/657596. Accessed 29 June 2015.

ACC (Australian Crime Commission). 2013. "Organised Crime and Drugs in Sport." Commonwealth of Australia. https://www.crimecommission.gov.au/sites/default/files/organised-crime-and-drugs-in-sports-feb2013.pdf. Accessed 29 June 2015.

AFL (Australian Football League). 2013. "Annual Report 2013." Australian Football League. http://www.afl.com.au/staticfile/AFL%20Tenant/AFL/Files/Annual%20Report/2013%20AFL%20Annual%20Report.pdf. Accessed 14 February 2015.

Anderson, B. 1991. *Imagined Communities Reflections on the Origin and Spread of Nationalism*. London: Verso.

Andrews, I. 2000. "From a Club to a Corporate Game: The Changing Face of Australian Football 1960–1999." *International Journal of the History of Sport* 17 (2/3): 225–254.

Battin, M. P., Luna, E., Lipman, A. G., Gahlinger, P. M., Rollins, D. E., Roberts, J. C., and Booher, T. L. 2008. *Drugs and Justice: Seeking a Consistent, Coherent, Comprehensive View*. Oxford: Oxford University Press.

Beamish, R. 2009. "Steroids, Symbolism and Morality: The Construction of a Social Problem and Its Unintended Consequences." In *Elite Sport, Doping and Public Health*, edited by Moller, V., McNamee, M. and Dimeo, P., 55–73. Odense: University of Southern Denmark.

Ben-Yehuda, N. 2009. "Moral Panics—36 Years On." *British Journal of Criminology* 49: 1–3.

Bette, K., and Schimank, U. 2001. "Coping with Doping: Sport Associations Under Organisational Stress." In *Proceedings from the Workshop Research on Doping in Sport*, 51–69. Oslo: Research Council of Norway.

Browne, A. 2013. "AFL to Boost Integrity Unit." Australian Football League. http://www.afl.com.au/news/2013–02–14/boost-for-integrity-unit. Accessed 29 June 2015.

Chalkley-Rhoden, S. 2015a. "AFL Anti-Doping Tribunal to Hand Down Decision on Essendon Players Over Supplements Program." *ABC News*, 31 March 2015. http://www.abc.net.au/news/2015–03–25/afl-anti-doping-tribunal-to-hand-down-essendon-decision/634772. Accessed 29 June 2015.

———. 2015b. "Essendon ASADA Investigation: Players into Guilty of Using Banned Peptide, AFL Anti-Doping Tribunal Finds." *ABC News*, 31 March 2015. http://www.abc.net.au/news/2015–03–31/essendon-supplements-afl-anti-doping-tribunal-decision/636100. Accessed 29 June 2015.

Clark, J., Harper, T., and Shackleton, S. 2013. "Ex-ASADA Chairman Richard Ings Says It's 'Blackest Day in Australian Sport' as Scandal Rocks Nation." *The Australian*, 7 February 2013. http://www.theaustralian.com.au/archive/news/ex-asada-chairman-richard-ings-says-its-blackest-day-in-australian-sport-as-scandal-rocks-nation/story-fncagcd8–122657270002. Accessed 29 June 2015.

Cohen, S. 2002. Folk devils and moral panics: the creation of the Mods and Rockers 3rd ed. Abingdon, Oxon, New York: Routledge.

Connor, J. 2009. "Towards a Sociology of Drugs in Sport." *Sport in Society* 12 (3): 327–343.

Dawson, A., and McNamee, M. 2009. "Doctors' Duties and Doping Dilemmas." In *Elite Sport, Doping and Public Health*, edited by Moller, V., McNamee, M. and Dimeo, P., 179–190. Odense: University Press of Southern Denmark.

Dimeo, P. 2007. *A History of Drug Use in Sport 1876–1976: Beyond Good and Evil*. New York: Routledge.

Dingelstad, D., Gosden, R., Martin, B., and Vakas, N. 1996. "The Social Construction of Drug Debates." *Social Science and Medicine* 43 (12): 1829–1838.

Donovan, R. J., Egger, G., Kapernick, V., and Mendoza, J. 2002. "A Conceptual Framework for Achieving Performance Enhancing Drug Compliance in Sport." *Sports Medicine* 32 (4): 269–284.

Dvorak, J., Graf-Baumann, T., D'Hooghe, M., Kirkendall, D., Taennler, H., and Saugy, M. 2006. "FIFA's Approach to Doping in Football." *British Journal of Sports Medicine* 40: 3–12.

Ericson, R. V., Baranek, P. M., and Chan, J. B. L. 1991. *Representing Order*. Toronto: University of Toronto Press.

Erikson, K. T. 1966. *Wayward Puritans: A Study in the Sociology of Deviance*. New York: John Wiley and Sons.

Gleeson, M. 2013. "AFL Considers 'Friends Register' for Player." *The Sydney Morning Herald*, 1 March 2013. http://www.smh.com.au/afl/afl-news/afl-considers-friends-register-for-players-20130228–2f98d.html?skin=text-only. Accessed 29 June 2015.

———. 2015. "WADA Wants Essendon Case Heard in Switzerland." *The Age*, 20 May 2015. http://www.theage.com.au/afl/afl-news/wada-wants-essendon-case-heard-in-switzerland-20150519-gh5ath.html. Accessed 29 June 2015.

Goode, E., and Ben-Yehuda, N. 2009. *Moral Panics: The Social Construction of Deviance*. Chichester, West Sussex: Wiley-Blackwell Publishing.

Gordon, M. 2013. "'This Is the Blackest Day in Australian Sport.'" *The Sydney Morning Herald*, 8 February 2013. http://www.smh.com.au/national/this-is-the-blackest-day-in-australian-sport-20130207-2e1i3.html. Accessed 3 January 2015.

Habermas, J. 1976. *Legitimation Crisis*. London: Heinemann Educational.

Hanstad, Dag Vidar, Skille, E. Å., and Loland, S. 2010. "Harmonization of Anti-Doping Work: Myth or Reality?" *Sport in Society* 13 (2): 418–430.

Henne, K. 2015. *Testing for Athlete Citizenship: Regulating Doping and Sex in Sport*. New Brunswick, NJ: Rutgers University Press.

Hoberman, J. 1992. *Mortal Engines: The Science of Performance and the Dehumanisation of Sport*. New Jersey: Blackburn Press.

Holton, R.J. 1987. "The Idea of Crisis in Modern Society." *The British Journal of Sociology* 38 (4): 502–520.

Houlihan, B. 2002. *Dying to Win*. Strasbourg Cedex: Council of Europe.

Kidd, B., Edelman, R., and Brownell, S. 2001. "Comparative Analysis of Doping Scandals: Canada, Russia, and China." In *Doping in Elite Sport: The Politics of Drugs in the Olympic Movement*, edited by Wilson, W. and Derse, E., 153–188. Champgaign, IL: Human Kinetics.

Lane, S. 2013. "Bill Will Boost Powers of Anti-Doping Agency." *The Age*, 7 February 2013. http://www.theage.com.au/sport/bill-will-boost-powers-of-antidoping-agency-20130206-2dz2v.html—ixzz2KYVBv73s. Accessed 20 April 2015.

MacAloon, J. 2001. "Doping and Moral Authority: Sport Organisations Today." In *Doping in Elite Sport: The Politics of Drugs in the Olympic Movement*, edited by Wilson, W. and Derse, E., 205–224. Champaign, IL: Human Kinetics.

Mark, D. 2015. "Stephen Dank says AFL, ASADA 'constructed' story to incriminate him and Essendon Bombers in supplements saga." ABC News, http://www.abc.net.au/news/2015–02–05/afl-and-asada-constructed-story-to-incriminate-bombers-dank-says/607405. Accessed 15 February 2015.

Matheson, C. 1987. "Weber and the Classification of Forms of Legitimacy." *The British Journal of Sociology* 38 (2): 199–215.

McGarry, A. 2015. "Essendon ASADA Investigation: Tribunal Decision to Reveal Guilt or Innocence of 34 Current and Former Bombers Players." *ABC News*, 31 March 2015. http://www.abc.net.au/news/2015–03–30/day-of-reckoning-arrives-for-essendon/636032. Accessed 29 June 2015.

Pearlman, J. 2013. "'Darkest Day' Down Under as Australian Sport Rocked by Revelations of Drug Taking and Links to Organized Crime." *The Telegraph*, 7 February 2013. http://www.telegraph.co.uk/sport/othersports/drugsinsport/9854446/Darkest-day-Down-Under-as-Australian-sport-rocked-by-revelations-of-drug-taking-and-links-to-organised-crime.html. Accessed 29 June 2015.

Pierik, J. 2015. "Swiss Court Could 'Stike Down' Appeal Against Essendon 34." *The Age*, 27 June 2015. http://www.theage.com.au/afl/afl-news/swiss-court-could-strike-down-appeal-against-essendon-34–20150627-ghz82k.html. Accessed 29 June 2015.

Robinson, M. 2014. "Essendon's Governance Was Shoddy, But ASADA and AFL Have Let Us All Down." *Herald Sun*, 13 August 2014. http://www.heraldsun.com.au/sport/afl/essendons-governance-was-shoddy-but-asada-and-afl-have-let-us-all-down-writes-mark-robinson/story-fni5f0at-1227023438691?nk=2f552dc2dd5169d33ff17b73a46e4bcc. Accessed 17 August 2014.

Ryan, R. 2015. "So Many Questions, So Few Answers." *The New Daily*, 30 January 2015. http://thenewdaily.com.au/sport/2015/01/30/asada-shambles-many-questions-answers/. Accessed 10 February 2015.

Schneider, A. 2000. "Olympic Reform, Are We There Yet?" In *Bridging Three Centuries, Fifth International Symposium for Olympic Research*, 225–232.

——. 2006. "Cultural Nuances: Doping, Cycling and the Tour de France." *Sport in Society* 9 (2): 212–226.

Senator the Hon Kate Lundy. 2013. Media Release: Important New Anti-Doping Powers for ASADA Pass Through Parliament. Australian Government. http://www.asada.gov.au/media/ministerial.html. Accessed 15 April 2015.

Sportal.com.au. n.d. "AFL Beef Up Integrity Unit." *Sportal.com.au*, http://www.sportal.com.au/afl/news/afl-beef-up-integrity-unit/3yrn6ahkxwyh1g6vdsqx4b9sr. Accessed 29 June 2015.

Stewart, B. 2007. "Drugs in Australian Sport: A Brief History." *Sporting Traditions* 23 (2): 65–78.

Stewart, B., Dickson, G., and Smith, A. 2008. "Drug Use in the Australian Football League: a Critical Survey." *Sporting Traditions* 25 (1): 57–74.

Stewart, B., Nicholson, M., and Dickson, G. 2005. "The Australian Football Leagues' Recent Progress: A Study in Cartel Conduct and Monopoly Power." *Sport Management Review* (Melbourne, Aust) 8 (2): 95–117.

Stokvis, R. 2003. "Moral Entrepreneurship and Doping Cultures in Sport." In *ASSR Working Paper Series*, 1–25. Amsterdam School for Social Science Research.

Suchman, M. C. 1995. "Managing Legitimacy: Strategic and Institutional Approaches." *The Academy of Management Review* 20 (3): 571–610.

Sutherland, A. 2013. "Integrity Unit Could Lose Its Integrity." *The Roar*, 3 March 2013. http://www.theroar.com.au/2013/03/03/integrity-unit-could-lose-its-integrity/. Accessed 29 June 2015.

Switkowski, Z. 2013. "Dr. Ziggy Switkowski Report." Essendon Football Club. http://www.essendonfc.com.au/news/2013-05-06/dr-ziggy-switskowski-report. Accessed 12 February 2015.

The Sunday Telegraph. 2014. "ASADA: Australia's Blackest Day in Sport Was a Dark Day for Julia Gillard." *The Sunday Telegraph*, 10 August 2014. http://www.dailytelegraph.com.au/news/opinion/asada-australias-blackest-day-in-sport-was-a-dark-day-for-julia-gillard/story-fni0cwl5-1227018896179.

Weber, M. 1969. *Economy and Society*. 2 vols. Berkeley: University of California Press.

Whateley, G. 2015. "Essendon Players the Only Ones Vindicated by AFL Tribunal Verdict, Gerard Whately Writes." *ABC News*, 1 April 2015. http://www.abc.net.au/news/2015-04-01/only-the-players-vindicated-by-verdict—whateley/636394. Accessed 29 June 2015.

Whinnett, E. 2015. "'Darkest Day in Sport' Now Looks More Like a Political Stunt." *Herald Sun*, 1 April 2015. http://www.heraldsun.com.au/news/victoria/darkest-day-in-sport-now-looks-more-like-a-political-stunt/story-fni0fit3-122728719974. Accessed 29 June 2015.

Wuthnow, R., Hunter, J., Bergesen, A., and Kurzweil, E. 1984. *Cultural Analysis*. London: Routledge.

Appendix 6.1
Interview Research Methodology

In contrast with the media review (Chapter 5, this volume), which considered international sport, the e-survey and later qualitative interviews focused on the Australian sporting context. This means that I am unable to make any generalizations beyond the Australian context. There have been a number of surveys that investigate issues such as perceived prevalence of PED use or factors that may influence athletes' doping behavior. For example, Hanstad and Loland (2009) conducted an electronic survey of athletes' attitudes toward WADA's introduction of new measures of athlete monitoring. Using surveys and interviews, Mugford et al. (1999, 5) conducted research into elite athletes' perceptions of the "effectiveness of the establishment's response to doping cases." However, these surveys do not discuss their findings in the context of perceptions of SGBs' legitimacy.

I applied a specific set of criteria to determine the NSOs to approach for the e-survey. In particular, I identified organizations recognized as NSOs by the ASC and that receive federal government funding through that organization (ASC 2007a). This reflects the Australian federal government's "zero tolerance approach to doping in sport" with access to ASC funding dependent on implementing WADC-compliant policies (Chapter 4, this volume). The *ASC National Sporting Organisation 2006/07 Grants and AIS Allocation* lists 56 sporting groups as receiving ASC coordinated federal government funding (ASC 2007b). The selection criteria were further refined to limit inclusion to NSOs that received a minimum of AUD$1,000,000 in the ASC 2006/07 Grants and AIS Allocation. Sports recognized by the IOC as governed by International Federations or part of the Olympic program were also included (ASC 2007b; IOC 2007). This resulted in a sample of 28 NSOs, including the ASC and the AIS, based on their role in developing Australia's Olympic athletes and the fact that the AIS receives government funds through the ASC. I also approached ASADA, the organization responsible for monitoring NSOs' compliance with the WADC and providing doping-control personnel and anti-doping educational material to NSOs. I included non-Olympic and professional sporting codes, specifically the AFL, football (soccer), rugby league, rugby union, netball, golf and cricket. These groups were included because they receive government funding through the ASC and are consequently required to implement WADA-aligned anti-doping frameworks (ASC 2007b).

In an effort to gauge athletes' perceptions of NSOs' regulatory response to PEDs, I approached a number of Players Associations based on their membership in the Australian Athletes' Alliance (AAA). The AAA advocates on behalf of athletes at the state and national levels and, at that time, represented over 2,000 of Australia's elite and professional athletes. At the time I approached the AAA, they represented athletes from groups including the AFL, cricket, rugby union, rugby league, football (soccer), netball, swimming and, from 2010, professional jockeys (Australian Athletes Alliance 2010; Australian Athletes Association 2007). I selected the AAA because of their stated commitment to providing a unified representative voice on issues concerning athletes, including anti-doping initiatives such as the Australian government's National Anti-Doping Scheme (Australian Athletes Alliance 2008). At the time fieldwork was conducted, the AAA was a newly formed organization with no centrally located administrative structure. Consequently, I approached each individual member association separately. I also contacted associations representing sporting officials connected to sports represented by the AAA, such as the AFL Umpires Association, Professional Footballers' Association Inc. and the Australian Swimmers' Association, amongst others. In cases where these groups were incorporated into the organizational structure of NSOs, I addressed my request to the NSO only.

I approached a total of 47 organizations with a request to distribute the e-survey. These consisted of 28 NSOs from the *ASC National Sporting Organisation 2006/07 Grants and AIS Allocation*, nine Players Associations, and seven Associations representing Umpires/Officials as well as the AIS, ASC and ASADA. Of the organizations approached, 22 agreed to distribute the e-survey (16 NSOs, ASADA, the ASC, two Players Associations and two Umpires/Officials Associations). Three of the 47 organizations (one Players Association and two Umpires/Officials Associations) did not respond and 22 (13 NSOs, four Players Associations and five Umpires/Officials Associations) declined to participate. For some groups, reasons for refusal to participate included being "intensely focused on the [2008] Beijing Olympic Games." Others were reluctant to add to the already time-intensive demands on athletes by anti-doping organizations. For example, one NSO declined to participate on the basis that:

> Athletes have to advise ASADA online everyday of their whereabouts and provide a one-hour time/place where they will be so they can be tested. While athletes can nominate the time, they resent the invasion of privacy and are sick and tired of filling in on-line forms.

Other groups highlighted limited organizational resources, apologizing that their "one man organization" prevented their participation. Nevertheless, there was also strong support for the e-survey based on the fact that it was quick, convenient and cost effective. The e-survey removed the necessity for NSOs and associations to engage in extra administrative work. This was particularly beneficial for smaller NSOs with athletes scattered throughout Australia and internationally. For example, some NSOs simply included a hyperlink to the e-survey in their monthly e-newsletter or on their website. As well as the convenience of sending the e-survey link directly to the NSO or association, this enhanced confidentiality for respondents, with a total of 232 responses received. The e-survey included provision for individuals to confidentially supply their contact details to arrange an interview, with the majority of interviewees resulting from that invitation.

Interviews were conducted in line with the requirements of the Australian National University Human Research Ethics Committee (Protocol: 2007/0192), including interviewees signing an Informed Consent Form to enable the interview to take place. I used open-ended semi-structured interview questions and the key topic areas listed in Chapter 6 of this volume. As demonstrated in other research into drugs in sport, this format enabled me to cover relevant interview topics while avoiding control over the interview or leading respondents in any particular direction (Grogan et al. 2006). Interviews were later transcribed and the data disaggregated into the topic areas, supplemented with unanticipated variables that emerged from the interview data. The value of the interview data for the central focus of this book is that they take account of the evaluative subjective nature of legitimacy.

The choice of interview participants for this thesis was wholly dependent upon the willingness of individuals to participate further in the research following the initial contact through the e-survey. Thirty-three individuals who completed the e-survey indicated their willingness to participate in an interview. However, changes in respondents' circumstances, such as paid work commitments, the hospitalization of one respondent after a serious cycling accident, participants' overseas travel, incorrect contact details and the failure of several participants to attend the prearranged interview reduced the initial sample from 33 to 23. Despite this, I conducted a total of 28 interviews, with four female and 24 male participants, with the five additional interviews resulting from participants' introductions to others in their sporting community (Chapter 6, this volume).

The minimum level of sporting participation for all interview participants was competitive club level sport. However, a number of participants held multiple roles in their sporting community and engaged in multiple sporting contexts. For example, in addition to club level sport, eight also competed in Masters Games events, eight were retired representative or professional athletes, nine were engaged in coaching, five were involved in club administration and one participant had formerly been involved in developing anti-doping policies at the level of Australian State government (see Appendix 6.2). As I explain in Chapter 6 of this book, the phrase 'grassroots sports community' indicates organized club level sport, distinguished from participation in recreational sporting activities. The e-survey, although not reported here, and interviews provided opportunities to consider whether the creation of WADA, in response to doping as a crisis, illustrates an elites-engineered institutionalized moral panic. The point of interest here was whether a level of preexisting community concern that doping is problematic behavior promotes the construction of doping as a moral panic (Chapter 6, this volume).

REFERENCES

ASC (Australian Sports Commission). 2007a. "Australian Sport Directory." Australian Sports Commission. http://www.ausport.gov.au/about/australian_sport_direc tory2/australian_sport_directory?sq_content_src=%2BdXJsPWh0dHAlM0ElM kYlMkZ3ZWJhdXNwb3J0JTJGbWF0cml4X3Nwb3J0ZGlyZWN0b3J5JTJGY XNjc3RhdHVzLmFzcCZhbGw9MQ%3D%3D. Accessed 5 March 2008.
———. 2007b. "NSO 2006/07 Grants and AIS Allocations." Australian Government. http://www.ausport.gov.au/funding/NSO_funding_2006–2007.pdf. Accessed 6 September 2007.
Australian Athletes Alliance. 2008. "Submission to ASADA regarding Amendments to National Anti-Doping (NAD) Scheme." Australian Athletes Association. http://www.ausathletesall.com.au. Accessed 1 September 2015.
———. 2010. "Welcome to Australian Athletes' Alliance." Australian Athletes Alliance. http://www.athletesalliance.org.au/. Accessed 8 August 2010.
Australian Athletes Association. 2007. "AAA Announces Policy Position on Illicit Drugs in Sport." Australian Athletes Association. http://www.pfa.net.au/index. php?id=103&aid=80. Accessed 21 September 2007.
Grogan, S., Shepherd, S., Evans, R., Wright, S., and Hunter, G. 2006. "Experiences of Anabolic Steroid Use In-depth Interviews with Men and Women Body Builders." *Journal of Health Psychology* 11 (6): 845–856.
Hanstad, D.V., and Loland, S. 2009. "Where on Earth Is Michael Rasmussen?— Is an Elite Level Athlete's Duty to Provide Information on Whereabouts Justifiable Anti-Doping Work or an Indefensible Surveillance Regime?" In *Elite Sport, Doping and Public Health*, edited by Moller, V., McNamee, M. and Dimeo, P., 167–177. Odensa: University Press of Southern Denmark.
IOC (International Olympic Committee). 2007. "Recognised Sports." International Olympic Committee. http://www.olympic.org/uk/sports/recognized/index_ uk.asp. Accessed 27 April 2007.
Mugford, S., Mugford, J., and Donnelly, D. 1999. "Social Research Project: Athletes' Motivations for Using or Not Using Performance Enhancing Drugs." Canberra: Australian Sports Drug Agency.

Appendix 6.2
Interview Participants: NSOs, Information & Education (*n*=28)

Interview ID	Crisis of Legitimacy	NSO provides Information	NSO provides Education
141109-R2	No answer	No	No
001	No answer	Yes	No
Sub-Total		1 = No; 1 = Yes	2 = No
140933	No	No answer	No answer
140902	No	No	No
141025	No	Yes	No
141082	No	Yes	No
141155	No	Yes	No
140933-R2	No	Yes	No
Sub-Total	5 = No	1 = No; 4 = Yes	5 = No
141257	Yes	No	No answer
141121	Yes	No answer	No
141574	Yes	No	No
142013	Yes	No	No
002	Yes	No	No
003	Yes	No answer	No answer
Sub-Total	6 = Yes	4 = No	4 = No
140991	Yes	Yes	No answer
Sub-Total	1 = Yes	1 = Yes	0
140951	Yes	Yes	Yes
141036	Yes	Yes	Yes
141049	Yes	Yes	Yes
141050	Yes	Yes	Yes
141455	Yes	Yes	Yes
Sub-Total	5 = Yes	5 = Yes	5 = Yes
140995	Yes	Yes	No
141015	Yes	Yes	No

(Continued)

Interview ID	Crisis of Legitimacy	NSO provides Information	NSO provides Education
141109	Yes	Yes	No
141410	Yes	Yes	No
140961	Yes	Yes	No
140986	Yes	Yes	No
141131	Yes	Yes	No
141530	Yes	Yes	No
Sub-Total	8 = Yes	8 = Yes	8 = No
Totals	5 = No; 20 = Yes	6 = No; 19 = Yes	19 = No; 5 = Yes

Bibliography

3AW Football. 2010. "AFL statement on Travis Tuck." *3AW*, 1 September 2010. http://www.3aw.com.au/blogs/3aw-football-blog/afl-statement-on-travis-tuck/20100901–14frl.html. Accessed 18 February 2011.

AAP. 2006. "Howard Defends 'Tough on Drugs' Policy." *The Sydney Morning Herald*, 4 May 2006. http://www.smh.com.au/news/National/Howard-defends-tough-on-drugs-policy/2006/05/04/1146335863149.html. Accessed 25 May 2011.

———. 2007a. "AFL Letter Defends Drug Policy." *The Age*, 28 March 2007. http://www.theage.com.au/realfooty/news/afl/afl-letter-defends-drug-pol icy/2007/03/27/1174761475630.html. Accessed 10 April 2007.

———. 2007b. "Banned for Life under New Drugs Policy." *The Age*, 6 October 2007. http://www.theage.com.au/news/National/Banned-for-life-under-new-drugs-pol icy/2007/10/06/1191091408100.html. Accessed 21 November 2007.

———. 2007c. "Change AFL Drug Policy, Repeats Brandis." *The Age*, 17 October 2007. http://www.theage.com.au/articles/2007/10/17/1192300834795.html. Accessed 24 October 2007.

———. 2007d. "New Govt to keep Drugs Pressure on AFL." *The Age*, 26 November 2007. http://www.theage.com.au/news/Sport/Swans-looking-at-inhouse-drug-policy/2007/11/26/1196036782057.html. Accessed 27 November 2007.

———. 2009. "Cousins Facing Testing Future." *WWOS.com.au*, 6 January 2009. http://wwos.ninemsn.com.au/article.aspx?id=70694. Accessed 7 January 2009.

———. 2011. "AFL Says Number of Positive Tests for Recreational Drugs Down from 14 in 2009." *The Australian*, 22 June 2011. http://www.theaustralian.com.au/news/sport/afl-says-number-of-positive-tests-for-recreational-drugs-down-from-14-in-2009/story-e6frg7mf-122607988333. Accessed 28 July 2011.

———. 2013. "Sharks Players Warned to come Forward." ABC News, 7 March 2013. http://www.abc.net.au/news/2013–03–07/sharks-players-warned-to-come-forward/455894. Accessed 12 February 2015.

———. 2014. "Senior Detective Gerard Ryan to Lead Investigations in AFL Integrity Unit." *Herald Sun*, 2 February 2014. http://www.heraldsun.com.au/sport/afl/senior-detective-gerard-ryan-to-lead-investigations-in-afl-integrity-unit/story-fni5f22o-122681609867. Accessed 29 June 2015.

———. 2015. "Essendon Skipper Jobe Watson says there is Anxiety at Club ahead of Landmark AFL Anti-Doping Tribunal Verdicts." *ABC News*, 25 March 2015. http://www.abc.net.au/news/2015–03–25/watson-admits-anxiety-at-bombers-ahead-of-tribunal-decision/634720. Accessed 29 June 2015.

AAP, and *ABC News*. 2012. "AFL Applauds Drug Testing Tesults." ABC News, 21 June 2012. http://www.abc.net.au/news/2012–06–21/afl-applaud-drug-testing-results/408404. Accessed 14 February 2015.

ABC and AFP (Agence France-Presse). 2013. "Lance Armstrong: Career Timeline." ABC News, 18 January 2013. http://www.abc.net.au/news/2012–10–22/lance-armstrong-chronology/432796. Accessed 28 March 2015.

ABC News. 2015. "Stephen Dank Handed Lifetime Ban by AFL Anti-Doping Tribunal following Essendon Supplements Saga." *ABC News*, 26 June 2015. http://www.abc.net.au/news/2015–06–26/stephen-dank-handed-lifetime-ban-from-afl-tribunal/657596. Accessed 29 June 2015.

ABC Premium News. 2004. "Carlton Sacks Angwin, Keeps Norman." *ABC Premium News*, 7 April 2004.

———. 2006. "AFL's Drug Policy Flawed: Coaches." *ABC Premium News*, 30 March 2006.

ABC Sport. 2005. "WADA attack AFL over failure to sign code." *ABC Sport*, 1 July 2005. http://www.abc.net.au/sport/content/200507/s1404945.htm. Accessed 29 May 2007.

ABS (Australian Bureau of Statistics). 2001. *4902.0 — Australian Culture and Leisure Classifications, 2001.* Canberra: Australian Bureau of Statistics. http://www.abs.gov.au/Ausstats/abs@.nsf/66f306f503e529a5ca25697e0017661f/13DD5C7E0EED0D3ECA256AB500836615?opendocument. Accessed 21 August 2007.

———. 2006. *8680.0 — Sports and Physical Recreation Services, Australia, 2004–05.* Canberra: Australian Bureau of Statistics,. http://www.abs.gov.au/ausstats/abs@.nsf/ProductDocumentCollection?OpenAgentandproductno=8686.0andissue=2004–0. Accessed 21 May 2010.

———. 2012. "Sport and Recreation: A Statistical Overview, Australia 4156.0." Australian Bureau of Statistics. http://www.ausstats.abs.gov.au/ausstats/subscriber.nsf/0/6E28777ED2896A2BCA257AD9000E2FC5/$File/41560_2012.pdf. Accessed 17 February 2015.

ACC (Australian Crime Commission). 2013. *Organised Crime and Drugs in Sport.* Commonwealth of Australia. https://www.crimecommission.gov.au/sites/default/files/organised-crime-and-drugs-in-sports-feb2013.pdf. Accessed 29 June 2015.

AFL (Australian Football League). 2006. "Australian Football Anti-Doping Code January 2006." AFL Official Web page. Australian Football League. http://www.aflpa.com.au/media/Anti-DopJan06.pdf. Accessed 7 March 2006.

———. 2007. "Illicit Drugs Policy." Australian Football League. http://afl.com.au/Portals/0/afl_docs/afl_hq/Policies/Illicit Drugs Policy Feb 2007.pdf. Accessed 13 June 2008.

———. 2009. "2008 Illicit Drugs Policy results." Australian Football League. http://www.afl.com.au/news/newsarticle/tabid/208/newsid/77745/default.aspx. Accessed 29 May 2009.

———. 2013a. "AFL / AFLPA Amendments to AFL Illicit Drugs Policy (IDP) / Release of 2012 Testing Results." Australian Football League. http://www.afl.com.au/news/2013–05–16/afl-aflpa-amendments-to-afl-illicit-drugs-policy-idp-release-of-2012-testing-results. Accessed 14 February 2015.

———. 2013b. Annual Report 2013. Australian Football League. http://www.afl.com.au/staticfile/AFLTenant/AFL/Files/AnnualReport/2013AFLAnnualReport.pdf. Accessed 14 February 2015

———. 2014a. "2014 Toyota AFL Premiership Season Fixture Released." Australian Football League. http://www.afl.com.au/news/2014–10–30/max-4-words. Accessed 14 February 2015.

———. 2014b. "AFL CEO Gillon McLachlan Thanks AFL Supporters." Australian Football League. http://www.afl.com.au/news/2014–09–29/afl-ceo-gillon-mclachlan-thanks-afl-supporters. Accessed 14 February 2015.

AFL (Australian Football League), and AFLPA (Australian Football League Players' Association). 2008. "AFL Players Say 'No' To Drugs." Australian Football League and Australian Football League Players' Association. http://www.afl.com.au/Portals/0/afl_docs/AFLPlayersSayNoToDrugs.pdf. Accessed 12 January 2009.

AFLPA (Australian Football League Players' Association). 2008. "AFL Players and the AFL have a Simple Message: Say NO to Drugs." Australian Football League Players' Association. http://www.afl.com.au/Default.aspx?tabid=1221. Accessed 29 August 2008.

AFP (Agence France-Presse). 2007a. "Australia's Fahey Elected President of Sport's Anti-Doping Agency." Agence France-Presse, 17 November 2007. http://afp.google.com/article/ALeqM5jms8Y1dYmsURzqwC6s5dmFaFrs7A. Accessed 27 December 2007.

———. 2007b. "Bode Miller Sticks to his Doping Guns." Agence France-Presse, 19 November 2007. http://afp.google.com/article/ALeqM5g-luyognmO5KxsemfBtwWQ0GcDBQ. Accessed 20 November 2007.

———. 2008a. "Disgraced Sprinter Jones Reports to Jail." Agence France-Presse, 7 March 2008. http://afp.google.com/article/ALeqM5j45h2TXIPAcsLvMwWvwl-DUeXuKVQ. Accessed16 February 2009.

———. 2008b. "IOC Chief Expects more Drugs Shame from Beijing." Agence France-Presse, 9 November 2008. http://afp.google.com/article/ALeqM5j89X-DQwfkqtT0M7RAksVyuWIvKpw. Accessed 24 November 2008.

———. 2008c. "Rogge Sees Long Battle against Drugs in Sport." Agence France-Presse, 26 November 2008. http://www.google.com/hostednews/afp/article/ALeqM5iFeba6tA3yRuLeXufCktJ5K6c6fQ. Accessed 27 November 2008.

———. 2008d. "WADA Chief Warns Sports to Beat Drugs or Face Irrelevance." Agence France-Presse, 7 August 2008. http://afp.google.com/article/ALeqM5hispSXtLzWuSeW6IVKIYQLUgzzfA. Accessed 19 August 2009.

Agencies. 2006. "Gold Medal Tainted by Drugs." *The Age*, 8 August 2006. http://www.theage.com.au/news/sport/gold-medal-tainted-by-drugs/2006/08/07/1154802822652.html. Accessed 8 August 2006.

AIC (Australian Institute of Criminology). 2009. "National Illicit Drug Strategy." Australian Institute of Criminology. http://www.aic.gov.au/crime_types/drugs_alcohol/illicit_drugs/strategy/illicit.html. Accessed 10 February 2015.

Aitken, C. 2002. "Lifting Your Game." *Meanjin (Melbourne)* 61 (2): 217–224.

Albergo, L. 2007. "Demetriou Defends Drug Code." *Australian Football Association of North America*, 1 April 2007. http://www.afana.com/drupal/node/43. Accessed 15 November 2007.

Allison, L. 1993. "The Changing Context of Sporting Life." In *The Changing Politics of Sport*, edited by Allison, L., 1–14. Manchester: Manchester University Press.

Altheide, D.L. 1997. "The News Media, the Problem Frame, and the Production of Fear." *Sociological Quarterly* 38 (4): 647–668.

Amies, N. 2007. "Soccer Powers to Increase Bundesliga Doping Controls." Deutsche Welle, 10 August 2007. http://www.dw-world.de/dw/article/0,2144,2733276,00.html. Accessed 14 August 2007.

Amis, J. 2005. "Beyond Sport: Imaging and Re-imaging a Transnational Brand." In *Sport and Corporate Nationalisms*, edited by Andrews, D.L., 143–165. Oxford: Berg.

Anderson, B. 1991. *Imagined Communities: Reflections on the Origin and Spread of Nationalism*. London: Verso.

Anderson, J. 2007. "Tom Harley Revved up over Drug Loopholes." *Herald Sun*, 22 November 2007. http://www.news.com.au/heraldsun/story/0,21985,22801005–11088,00.html. Accessed 28 December 2007.

Andrews, D.L., and Jackson, S.J. 2001. "Introduction—Sport Celebrities, Public Culture, and Private Experience." In *Sport Stars—The Cultural Politics of Sporting Celebrity*, edited by Andrews, D.L. and Jackson, S.J., 1–19. London: Routledge.

Andrews, I. 2000. "From a Club to a Corporate Game: The Changing Face of Australian Football 1960–1999." *International Journal of the History of Sport* 17 (2/3): 225–254.

Anshel, M.H. 1991. "A Survey of Elite Athletes on the Perceived Causes of Using Banned Drugs in Sport." *Journal of Sport Behavior* 14: 283–308.

Anshel, M.H., and Russell, K.G. 1997. "Examining Athletes' Attitudes Toward Using Anabolic Steroids and Their Knowledge of the Possible Effects." *Journal of Drug Education* 27 (2): 121–145.

AOC (Australian Olympic Committee). n/d. "Montreal 1976." Australian Olympic Committee. http://corporate.olympics.com.au/games/montreal-197. Accessed 19 February 2015.

AP (Associated Press). 2006. "Sports Losing the Battle against Doping Image and Credibility Taking a Hit." *The Winnipeg Sun*, 31 July 2006. http://winnipegsun.com/Sports/OtherSports/2006/07/31/1711477-sun.html. Accessed 1 August, 2006.

———. 2007a. "Acrobatic Gymnast Okulova Banned for Doping Offense." *International Herald Tribune*, 27 November 2007. http://www.iht.com/articles/ap/2007/11/27/sports/EU-SPT-GYM-Doping-Okulova.php. Accessed 29 November 2007.

———. 2007b. "Britain to Consider Criminalizing Doping in Sports." *International Herald Tribune*, 24 July 2007. http://www.iht.com/articles/ap/2007/07/24/sports/EU-SPT-OLY-Britain-Doping-Laws.php. Accessed 25 July 2007.

———. 2007c. "Court Case involving Fired Astana Rider will Challenge World Doping System." *International Herald Tribune*, 2 November 2007. http://www.iht.com/articles/ap/2007/11/02/sports/EU-SPT-CYC-Kashechkin-Doping.php. Accessed 19 December 2007.

———. 2007d. "Doping Conference Overshadowed by Uncertainty over Election of WADA President." *International Herald Tribune*, 15 November 2007. http://www.iht.com/articles/ap/2007/11/15/sports/EU-SPT-Doping-Conference.php. Accessed 12 December 2008.

———. 2007e. "FIFA Leads Team-Sport Criticism of WADA's New Anti-Doping Code." *International Herald Tribune*, 16 November 2007. http://www.iht.com/articles/ap/2007/11/16/sports/EU-SPT-Doping-WADA-Code.php. Accessed 11 December 2007.

———. 2007f. "IOC President says Marion Jones Doping Admission 'Good Thing' for Sport." *International Herald Tribune*, 15 October 2007. http://www.iht.com/articles/ap/2007/10/15/sports/EU-SPT-OLY-Rogge-Jones.php. Accessed 17 January 2008.

———. 2007g. "IOC: Recent Doping Busts at Tour de France Show Shift in Attitude Against Cheaters." 26 July 2007. http://www.winnipegfreepress.com/historic/32338974.html. Accessed 27 July 2007.

———. 2007h. "Marion Jones Pleads Guilty." Associated Press, 8 October 2007. http://ap.google.com/article/ALeqM5jUq0dOf2wXE-ySJWjMfV_pDxwfVQD8S3AB18. Accessed 10 October 2007.

———. 2007i. "WADA Chief Warns Lax Doping Rules could Cost Slot in Olympics." *International Herald Tribune*, 6 July 2007. http://www.iht.com/articles/ap/2007/07/06/sports/LA-SPT-OLY-IOC-Doping.php. Accessed 16 July 2007.

———. 2007j. "WADA Official: Gap Closing between New Drugs and Testing." *The Globe and Mail*, 1 June 2007.

———. 2008. "IOC: No Missing Test Results from Beijing." *International Herald Tribune*, 16 October 2008. http://www.iht.com/articles/ap/2008/10/16/sports/OLY-IOC-Beijing-Tests.php. Accessed 17 October 2008.

———. 2011. "WADA Drops Case vs. Mexico Players." ESPN, 12 October 2011. http://espn.go.com/sports/soccer/news/_/id/7091999/world-anti-doping-agency-drops-case-mexico-soccer-players. Accessed 13 April 2015.

———. 2013. "Lance Armstrong Says former UCI President Helped Cover up Doping." *USA Today*, 18 November 2013. http://www.usatoday.com/story/sports/cycling/2013/11/18/lance-armstrong-coverup-doping-uci-tour-de-france/3628059/. Accessed 14 June 2015.

———. 2014. "Italian Cycling President: Police must Act to Stop Michele Ferrari Influence." 19 *The Guardian*, December 2014. http://www.theguardian.com/sport/2014/dec/18/michele-ferrari-italy-police-must-act. Accessed 11 April 2015.

Armour, K., Jones, R., and Kerry, D. 2000. "Sport Sociology 2000." *Sociology of Sport Online*. http://physed.otago.ac.nz/sosol/v1i1/v1i1a7.htm. Accessed 30 May 2010.

ASC (Australian Sports Commission). 1999. "The Australian Sports Commission—Beyond 2000." Australian Sports Commission. http://www.ausport.gov.au/publications/ascbeyond_2000s.pdf. Accessed 15 November 2006.

———. 2007a. "Australian Sport Directory." Australian Sports Commission. http://www.ausport.gov.au/about/australian_sport_directory2/australian_sport_directory?sq_content_src=%2BdXJsPWh0dHAlM0ElMkYlMkZ3ZWJhdXNwb3J0JTJGbWF0cml4X3Nwb3J0ZGlyZWN0b3b3J5JTJTJGYXNj3RhdHVzLmFzcCZhbGw9MQ%3D%3D. Accessed 5 March 2008.

———. 2007b. "NSO 2006/07 Grants and AIS Allocations." Australian Government. http://www.ausport.gov.au/funding/NSO_funding_2006–2007.pdf. Accessed 6 September 2007.

ASDA (Australian Sports Drug Agency). 1999. 1998–99 Annual Report. Canberra: Commonwealth of Australia. https://secure.ausport.gov.au/__data/assets/pdf_file/0007/247858/ASDA_AR__1998–1999.pdf. Accessed 11 February 2015

———. 2001. Annual Report Australian Sports Drug Agency 00:01. Canberra.: Australian Sports Drug Agency. http://www.asada.gov.au/resources/reports/previous/ar01/asda_ar01.pdf. Accessed 20 November 2007

———. 2002. Australian Sports Drug Agency Annual Report 2001–02. Canberra.: Australian Sports Drug Agency. http://www.asada.gov.au/resources/reports/previous/ar02/index.htm. Accessed 20 November 2007

———. 2003. Australian Sports Drug Agency Annual Report 03:04. Canberra.: Australian Sports Drug Agency. http://www.asada.gov.au/resources/reports/previous/ar04/_docs/asda_ar04.pdf. Accessed 20 November 2007

Ashenden, M. 2002. "A Strategy to Deter Blood Doping in Sport." *Haematologica* 87 (3): 225–234.

AthletesCAN. 1999. "Athletes CAN supports OATH—Olympic Advocates Together Honorably." AthletesCAN The Association of Canada's National Team Athletes. http://www.athletescan.com/Content/News/News Archives/Archives 1999/990316OATH.asp. Accessed 20 February 2007.

The Australian. 2006. "Drugged AFL Men to Remain Unnamed." *The Australian*, 23 March 2006.

Australian Athletes Alliance. 2008. Submission to ASADA Regarding Amendments to National Anti-Doping (NAD) Scheme. Australian Athletes Association. http://www.athletesalliance.org.au/submissions.html. Accessed 25 June 2010.

———. 2010. "Welcome to Australian Athletes' Alliance." Australian Athletes Alliance. http://www.athletesalliance.org.au/. Accessed 8 August 2010.

Australian Athletes Association. 2007. "AAA Announces Policy Position on Illicit Drugs in Sport." Australian Athletes Association. http://www.pfa.net.au/index.php?id=103andaid=8. Accessed 21 September 2007.

Australian Government. 2007. *Illicit Drugs in Sport Policy—Tough on Drugs in Sport*. Australian Government. http://www.sport.gov.au/__data/assets/pdf_file/0003/74982/Illicit-Drugs-in-Sport-policy-Oct-07.pdf. Accessed 10 April 2008.

Backhouse, S.H., McKenna, J., Robinson, S., and Atkin, A. 2007. *International Literature Review: Attitudes, Behaviours, Knowledge and Education—Drugs in Sport: Past, Present and Future*. Carnegie Research Institute, Leeds Metropolitan University. http://www.wada-ama.org/rtecontent/document/Backhouse_et_al_Full_Report.pdf. Accessed 10 February 2009.

Baerveldt, C., Bunkers, H., de Winter, M., and Kooistra, J. 1998. "Assessing a Moral Panic Relating to Crime and Drugs Policy in the Netherlands: Towards a Testable Theory." *Crime, Law and Social Change* 29 (1): 31–47.

Balko, R. 2008. "Should We Allow Performance Enhancing Drugs in Sports?" Reason Online 23 January 2008. http://reason.com/news/show/124577.html. Accessed 24 December 2008.

Barney, R. K., Wenn, S. R., and Martyn, S. G. 2002. *Selling the Five Rings: The International Olympic Committee and the Rise of Olympic Commercialism*. Salt Lake City: The University of Utah Press.

Barrett, D., and Williams, R. 2007. "AFL Delay on Drugs Policy." *Fox Sports*, 17 December 2007. http://www.foxsports.com.au/story/0,8659,22935225-23211,00.html. Accessed 21 December 2007.

Battin, M. P., Luna, E., Lipman, A. G., Gahlinger, P.M., Rollins, D. E., Roberts, J. C., and Booher, T. L. 2008. *Drugs and Justice: Seeking a Consistent, Coherent, Comprehensive View*. Oxford: Oxford University Press.

Baum, G. 2007. "Sporting Heroes Carry Extra Burden in Drug Witch-Hunt." *Real Footy*, 7 September 2007. http://www.realfooty.com.au/news/news/sporting-heroes-carry-extra-burden-in-drug-witchhunt/2007/09/06/1188783414288.html?page=fullpage—contentSwap. Accessed 7 September 2007.

BBC. 2012. "Lance Armstrong Stripped of All Seven Tour de France Wins by UCI." BBC, 22 October 2012. http://www.bbc.com/sport/0/cycling/2000852. Accessed 27 March 2015.

BBC Berkshire. 2007. "Drugs Testing: Q and A." BBC Berkshire, 7 June 2007. http://www.bbc.co.uk/berkshire/content/articles/2007/05/10/speedway_wada_070510_feature.shtml. Accessed 7 June 2007.

BBC Sport. 2006. "Radcliffe Attacks Christie Role." *BBC Sport*, 13 August 2006. http://news.bbc.co.uk/sport2/hi/athletics/4788157.stm. Accessed 7 April 2011.

———. 2007. "The Fight Against Drugs in Sport." *BBC Sport*, 17 November 2007. http://news.bbc.co.uk/sport2/hi/other_sports/7099845.stm. Accessed 6 March 2008.

Beamish, R. 2009. "Steroids, Symbolism and Morality: The Construction of a Social Problem and its Unintended Consequences." In *Elite Sport, Doping and Public Health*, edited by Moller, V., McNamee, M. and Dimeo, P., 55–73. Odense: University of Southern Denmark.

Beamish, R., and Ritchie, I. 2005. "From Fixed Capacities to Performance-Enhancement: The Paradigm Shift in the Science of 'Training' and the Use of Performance-Enhancing Substances." *Sport in History* 25 (3): 412–413.

Beck, L. 2008. "Athletes Learn Risks, Rules at Anti-Doping Centre." *Reuters*, 10 August 2008. http://www.reuters.com/article/GCA-Olympics/idUSPEK24374 20080810?sp=true. Accessed 25 August 2009.

Becker, H. S. 1963. *Outsiders*. New York: The Free Press.

———. 1967. "Whose Side Are We On?" *Social Problems* 14: 239–247.

Beckett, A. H., and Cowan, D. A. 1978. "Misuse of Drugs in Sport." *British Journal of Sports Medicine* 12: 185–194.

Behlmer, G. K. 2003. "Grave Doubts: Victorian Medicine, Moral Panic, and the Signs of Death." *The Journal of British Studies* 42 (2): 206–235.

Ben-Yehuda, N. 1986. "The Sociology of Moral Panics: Toward a New Synthesis." *Sociological Quarterly* 27 (4): 495–513.

———. 2009. "Moral Panics—36 Years On." *British Journal of Criminology* 49: 1–3.

Benammar, E. 2013. "Stuart O'Grady, Lance Armstrong, Marco Pantani, Floyd Landis and Alberto Contador: Cycling's Doping Scandals." ABC News, 25 July 2013. http://www.abc.net.au/news/2013-07-25/cycling27s-infamous-doping-scandals/484206. Accessed 3 September 2014.

Berentsen, A. 2002. "The Economics of Doping." *European Journal of Political Economy* 18: 109–127.

Berg, C. 2008. "Politics, not Sport, is the Purpose of the Olympic Games." *Institute of Public Affairs* (July 2008): 14–18.

Bernstein, S. 2004. "IGHC Working Paper Series: The Elusive Basis of Legitimacy in Global Governance: Three Conceptions." In *Autonomy, Democracy, and Legitimacy in an Era of Globalization*, edited by W. D. Coleman. McMaster University,

Ontario: Institute on Globalization and the Human Condition. http://www.religiousstudies.mcmaster.ca/institute-on-globalization-and-the-human-condition/documents/IGHC-WPS_04-2_Bernstein.pdf. Accessed 1 March 2012

Best, J. 1990. *Threatened Children: Rhetoric and Concern about Child-Victims.* Chicago: University Press of Chicago.

———. 1999. *Random Violence: How We Talk about New Crimes and New Victims.* Berkeley: University of California Press.

———. 2002. "Monster Hype." *Education Next* Summer 2002: 51–55.

Bette, K., and Schimank, U. 2001. "Coping with Doping: Sport Associations under Organisational Stress." Proceedings from the Workshop Research on Doping in Sport, Oslo,, May 22, 2001. http://web.bi.no/forskning/isforg.nsf/62af2dc3 1b641632c12566f30039282c/c9d01468d7b9ebe8c125670100428c50/$FILE/proceedings—doping.PDF. Accessed 7 December 2009.

Bhandari, A., and Arce, L. 2011. "Five Mexico Stars Banned after Failing Drugs Test." CNN, 10 June 2011. http://edition.cnn.com/2011/SPORT/06/10/mexico.doping/. Accessed 24 April 2015.

Birchard, K. 2000. "Past, Present, and Future of Drug Abuse at the Olympics." *The Lancet* 356 (September 16 2000): 1008.

Bird, E. J., and Wagner, G. G. 1997. "Sport as a Common Property Resource—A Solution to the Dilemmas of Doping." *Journal of Conflict Resolution* 41 (6): 749–766.

Black, D. L. 2001. "Doping Control Testing Policies and Procedures." In *Doping in Elite Sport: The Politics of Drugs in the Olympic Movement*, edited by Wilson, W. and Derse, E., 29–42. Champaign, Il: Human Kinetics.

Blair, T. 2005. "Shame and Disgrace." *The Bulletin*, 18 May 2005. http://bulletin.ninemsn.com.au/bulletin/site/articleIDs/EE4EODCFFFF092D-0CA2570030011865B5. Accessed 7 March 2006.

Blumer, H. 1971. "Social Problems As Collective Behavior." *Social Problems* 18 (3): 298–306.

Bok, S. 1989. *Lying: Moral Choice in Public and Private Life.* New York: Vintage Books.

Bond, D. 2007. "Shake-Up in Fight against British Drug Cheats." *Telegraph*, 5 December 2007. http://www.telegraph.co.uk/sport/main.jhtml;jsessionid=F1EQ FKL0UXANHQFIQMFCFGGAVCBQYIV0?xml=/sport/2007/12/05/sofron105. xml. Accessed 12 December 2007.

Booth, D. 1995. "Sports Policy in Australia: Right, Just and Rational?" *The Australian Quarterly* 67 (1): 1–10.

Booth, D., and Tatz, C. 2000. *One Eyed: A view of Australian Sport.* St. Leonards, Australia: Allen and Unwin.

Bourdieu, P. 1998. *On Television and Journalism.* Translated by Priscilla Packhurst Ferguson. London: Pluto Press.

Bowen, K. 2007. "Mass Doping is Now the Order of the Day." Deutsche Welle, 24 May 2007. http://www.dw-world.de/dw/article/0,2144,2556989,00.html. Accessed 15 June 2007.

Bowers, L. D. 2002. "Abuse of Performance-Enhancing Drugs in Sport." *Therapeutic Drug Monitoring* 24: 178–181.

Boxill, I., and Unnithan, N. P. 1995. "Rhetoric and Policy Realities in Developing Countries: Community Councils in Jamaica, 1972–1980." *Journal of Applied Behavioral Science* 31 (1): 65–79.

Boyes, S. 2001. "The International Olympic Committee, Transnational Doping Policy and Globalisation." In *Drugs and Doping in Sport: Socio-Legal Perspectives*, edited by O'Leary, J., 167–179. London: Cavendish Publishing.

Breivik, G., Hanstad, D. V., and Loland, S. 2009. "Attitudes Towards use of Performance-Enhancing Substances and Body Modification Techniques. A Comparison between Elite Athletes and the General Population." *Sport in Society* 12 (6): 737–754.

Brennan, C. 2007. "A Call for Baseball to Toughen Drug Testing." *USA Today*, May 2007. http://www.usatoday.com/sports/columnist/brennan/2007–05–02-brennan-baseball-drug-testing_N.htm. Accessed 5 June 2007.

———. 2008. "Enough about the BCS; Why Aren't we Focusing on Doping?" *USA Today*, 21 November 2008. http://www.usatoday.com/sports/columnist/brennan/2008–11–19-Christine_N.htm. Accessed 24 November 2008.

Bright, R. 2007. "Doping Tests for Cycling to Increase." *Telegraph*, 23 October 2007. http://www.telegraph.co.uk/sport/main.jhtml?xml=/sport/2007/10/23/socycl123.xml. Accessed 4 December 2007.

Brissonneau, C. 2010. "An Interactionist Study of Phenomenon of Doping." Body Enhancement and (Il)legal Drugs in Sport—A Human and Social Science Perspective Conference, University of Copenhagen, 12 November 2010. http://www.newcyclingpathway.com/wp-content/uploads/2010/11/Intervention_Copenhague-09–11–10.pdf. accessed 1 February 2011.

British Medical Association. 2002. *Drugs in Sport: The Pressure to Perform*. London: BMJ Books.

Broadbent, R. 2007. "Britain's Drug Test Pioneer still Chasing Place on Front Line in War against Cheats." Times Online, 21 November 2007. http://www.timesonline.co.uk/tol/sport/more_sport/athletics/article2910302.ece. Accessed 27 December 2007.

———. 2008. "Maurice Greene Accused of Being Drugs Cheat." *Times Online*, 14 April 2008. http://www.timesonline.co.uk/tol/sport/more_sport/athletics/article3739937.ece. Accessed 14 April 2008.

Brohm, Jean-Marie. 1978. *Sport: A Prison of Measured Time*. London: Ink Links.

Brookes, J. 2011. "UK Athletics Sanction Drugs Cheat to Help Coach British Medal Hopeful Okoye." *Mail Online*, 31 July 2011. http://www.dailymail.co.uk/sport/othersports/article-2020585/UK-Athletics-sanction-drugs-cheat-help-coach-young-British-medal-hopeful-Okoye.html?ito=feeds-newsxml. Accessed 1 August 2011.

Brown, D.A. 2005. "The Olympic Games Experience: Origins and Early Challenges." In *Global Olympics: Historical and Sociological Studies of the Modern Games*, edited by Young, K. and Wamsley, K.B., 19–41. Amsterdam: Elsevier JAI.

Browne, A. 2013. "AFL to Boost Integrity Unit." Australian Football League. http://www.afl.com.au/news/2013–02–14/boost-for-integrity-unit. Accessed 29 June 2015.

Brunvand, J.H. 2001. *Encyclopedia of Urban Legends*. Santa Barbara, Calif.: Oxford.

Buchanan, A., and Keohane, R.O. 2006. "The Legitimacy of Global Governance Institutions." *Ethics and International Affairs* 4: 405–437.

Burnside, S. 2007. "Debate over NHL's Drug-Testing Policy Rages On." *ESPN*, 6 August 2007. http://sports.espn.go.com/nhl/columns/story?columnist=burnside_scottandid=296370. Accessed 8 August 2007.

Buti, A., and Fridman, S. 1994. "The Intersection of Law and Policy: Drug Testing in Sport." *Australian Journal of Public Administration* 53 (4): 489–507.

———. 2001. *Drugs, Sport and the Law*. Mudgeeraba, Queensland: Scribblers Publishing.

Cantelon, H. 2005. "Amateurism, High-Performance Sport, and the Olympics." In *Global Olympics: Historical and Sociological Studies of the Modern Games*, edited by Young, K. and Wamsley, K.B., 83–101. Amsterdam: Elsevier JAI.

Cantelon, H., and McDermott, L. 2001. "Charisma and the Rational-Legal Organisation: A Case Study of the Avery Brundage-Reginald Honey Correspondence Leading up to the South African Expulsion from the International Olympic Movement." *OlyMPIKA: The International Journal of Olympic Studies* X: 33–58.

Carroll, M.P. 1987. "'The Castrated Boy': Another Contribution to the Psychoanalytic Study of Urban Legends." *Folklore* 98 (2): 216–225.

Cashman, R. 1995. *Paradise of Sport: The Rise of Organised Sport in Australia.* Melbourne: Oxford University Press.

Cashmore, E. 1990. *Making Sense of Sport.* London: Routledge.

Cashore, B. 2002. "Legitimacy and the Privatization of Environmental Governance: How Non-State Market-Driven (NSMD) Governance Systems Gain Rule-Making Authority." *Governance: An International Journal of Policy, Administration, and Institutions* 15 (4): 503–529.

CBC News. 2007. "Pound Quits World Anti-Doping Agency." *CBC*, 18 September 2007. http://www.cbc.ca/canada/montreal/story/2007/09/18/qc-pound0918.html. Accessed 20 September 2007.

CBC Sports. 2007a. "WADA's Pound Calls for more Awareness on Public Health Problems Posed by Doping." *CBC*, 13 May 2007. http://www.cbc.ca/cp/sports/070513/s051347A.html. Accessed 25 May 2007.

———. 2007b. "World Anti-Doping Agency Boss Applauds U.S. Moves against Doping Underground." *CBC*, 12 March 2007. http://www.cbc.ca/cp/sports/070312/s031227A.html. Accessed 13 March 2007.

CBS News. 2012. "Lance Armstrong now Faces Justice Department in Lawsuit." CBS News, http://www.cbsnews.com/news/lance-armstrong-now-faces-justice-department-in-lawsuit/. Accessed 27 March 2015.

Chalkley-Rhoden, S. 2015a. "AFL Anti-Doping Tribunal to Hand Down Decision on Essendon Players over Supplements Program." *ABC News*, 31 March 2015. http://www.abc.net.au/news/2015–03–25/afl-anti-doping-tribunal-to-hand-down-essendon-decision/634772. Accessed 29 June 2015.

———. 2015b. "Essendon ASADA Invstigation: Players Not Guilty of Using Banned Peptide, AFL Anti-Doping Tribunal Finds." *ABC News*, 31 March 2015. http://www.abc.net.au/news/2015–03–31/essendon-supplements-afl-anti-doping-tribunal-decision/636100. Accessed 29 June 2015.

Chandrasekaran, R. 2000. "Sports Crazy: On the Fields, in the Stands and in the Betting Parlors, Australians may be the most Sports-Obsessed Nation on Earth." *The Washington Post*, 3 September 2000.

Chermak, S. 1997. "The Presentation of Drugs in the News Media: The News Sources Involved in the Construction of Social Problems." *Justice Quarterly* 14 (4): 687–718.

Chesterton, R. 2007. "Drugs Use in Sport is Out of Control." *The Daily Telegraph*, 3 October 2007. http://www.news.com.au/story/0,23599,22520718–2,00.html. Accessed 4 October 2007.

Christiansen, A. V. 2009. "Doping in Fitness and Strength Training Environments—Politics, Motives and Masculinity." In *Elite Sport, Doping and Public Health*, edited by Moller, V., McNamee, M. and Dimeo, P., 99–118. Odense: University Press of Southern Denmark.

Christie, J. 2006. "WADA May Move to Ban Oxygen Tents." Canadian Sport Centre. http://www.canadiansportcentre.com/Communications/SportPerformance-Weekly/SPW2006/05_15_06.html. Accessed 6 September 2006.

Clark, J., Harper, T., and Shackleton, S. 2013. "Ex-ASADA Chairman Richard Ings Says it's 'Blackest Day in Australian Sport' as Scandal Rocks Nation." *The Australian*, 7 February 2013. http://www.theaustralian.com.au/archive/news/ex-asada-chairman-richard-ings-says-its-blackest-day-in-australian-sport-as-scandal-rocks-nation/story-fncagcd8–122657270002. Accessed 29 June 2015.

Clarke, S. 2014a. "Germany Set to Introduce Jail Sentences for Doping Offences." *Cycling Weekly*, 12 November 2014. http://www.cyclingweekly.co.uk/news/latest-news/germany-set-introduce-jail-sentences-doping-offences-14404. Accessed 13 April 2015.

————. 2014b. "WADA President Denounces Jail Sentences for Doping Offenders." *Cycling Weekly*, 18 November 2014. http://www.cyclingweekly.co.uk/news/latest-news/wada-president-denounces-jail-sentences-doping-offenders-145219 — If4qPgZ72btyGwvM.9. Accessed 13 April 2015.

————. 2015. "Doping is Becoming a Public Health Issue, Says WADA Chief." *Cycling Weekly*, 28 January 2015. http://www.cyclingweekly.co.uk/news/latest-news/doping-becoming-public-health-issue-says-wada-chief-15466. Accessed 10 February 2015.

Coakley, Jay J. 2007. *Sports in Society: Issues and Controversies*. Boston: McGraw-Hill Higher Education.

CoE (Council of Europe). 2003. "Information Document Conclusions regarding WADA Part IV International Consultative Group on Anti-Doping in Sport (IIC-GADS)." Council of Europe. https://wcd.coe.int/ViewDoc.jsp?id=34911andSite=COE—P589_4228. Accessed 31 March 2015.

Cohen, S. 1967. "Mods, Rockers and the Rest: Community Reactions to Juvenile Delinquency." *The Howard Journal of Criminal Justice* 12 (2): 121–130.

————. 1972. *Folk Devils and Moral Panics: The Creation of the Mods and Rockers*. London: MacGibbon and Kee.

————. 2002. *Folk devils and moral panics: the creation of the Mods and Rockers* 3rd ed. Abingdon, Oxon, New York: Routledge.

Committee on the Judiciary, United States Senate. 1973. *Proper and Improper Use of Drugs by Athletes*. U.S. Government Printing Office, Washington D.C.: Subcommittee to Investigate Juvenile Deliquency.

Commonwealth of Australia. 2001a. *Backing Australia's Sporting Ability a More Active Australia*. Sport and Tourism. Commonwealth of Australia. http://www.dbcde.gov.au/__data/assets/pdf_file/0009/7677/BASA.pdf.

————. 2001b. *Game Plan 2006: Sport and Leisure Industry Strategic National Plan*. Department of Industry Science and Resources. Canberra: Commonwealth of Australia. http://fulltext.ausport.gov.au/fulltext/2001/feddep/gp2006.pdf. Accessed 15 November 2006.

Connor, J. 2009a. "Legitimacy and Decline: The Role of the Australian Democrats." Forum of Federations' Political Parties and Civil Society Roundtable, Australian Parliament House, Canberra, 2009. http://www.forumfed.org/en/events/event.php?id=457, accessed 9 September 2010.

————. 2009b. "Towards a Sociology of Drugs in Sport." *Sport in Society* 12 (3): 327–343.

Connor, J., and A. Kirby. 2011. "Sport and Global Governance: Foul Play Rewarded with Legitimacy." The annual conference of the International Sociological Association, Global Governance: Political Authority in Transition, Montreal, Quebec, Canada, 16–19 March, 2011. http://www.isanet.org/Conferences/Montreal-2011. Accessed 9 September 2011.

Cooper, A. 2006. "AFL Demanding Answers from Government over Drug Test Details." *AAP Sports News Wire*, 14 March 2006.

Cooper, A., and Fiamengo, M. 2006. "AFL: Identities Remain Secret, but Anger at System Continues." *AAP Sports New Wire*, 16 March 2001.

Cornwell, B., and Linders, A. 2002. "The Myth of 'Moral Panic': An Alternative Account of LSD Prohibition." *Deviant Behaviour* 23 (4): 307–330.

Critcher, C. 2002. "Media, Government and Moral Panic: The Politics of Paedophilia in Britain 2000–1." *Journalism Studies* 3 (4): 521–535.

Cromer, G. 1978. "Character Assassination in the Press." In *Deviance and Mass Media*, edited by Winick, C., 255–241. Beverley Hills, California: Sage Publications.

Crouse, K. 2010. "For Swimmer, Ban Ends, but Burden Could Last." *The New York Times*, 7 August 2010. http://www.nytimes.com/2010/08/08/sports/08hardy.html. Accessed 24 April 2015.

Crowther, N. 2002. "The Salt Lake City Scandals and the Ancient Olympic Games." *International Journal of the History of Sport* 19 (4): 169–178.

Davidson, D. 2014. "AFL Eyes as Much as $1.6bn for Television Rights Deal." *The Australian*, 27 October 2014. http://www.theaustralian.com. au/business/media/afl-eyes-as-much-as-16bn-for-television-rights-deal/ story-fna045gd-122710286382. Accessed 14 February 2015.

Davies, J. 2005. "White Line Fever." *The Bulletin*, 18 May 2005. http://bulletin. ninemsn.com.au/bulletin/site/articleIDs/7E2DAF12F1A64903CA25700200 72D07. Accessed 7 March 2006.

Dawson, A., and McNamee, M. 2009. "Doctors' Duties and Doping Dilemmas." In *Elite Sport, Doping and Public Health*, edited by Moller, V., McNamee, M. and Dimeo, P., 179–190. Odense: University Press of Southern Denmark.

DCITA (Dept. Communications Information Technology and the Arts). 2005. "New Anti-Doping Body Legislation Introduced" Media release. Department of Communications Information Technology and the Arts. http://www.minister.dcita.gov. au/kemp/media/media_releases/new_anti-doping_body_legislation_introduced. Accessed 6 March 2006.

Demetriou, A. 2005a. "The AFL and WADA: Room for Compromise." *AFL Record (Melbourne, Aust)* (8–10 July) : 6–8.

———. 2005b. "How the Final Decision was Made." *AFL Record (Melbourne, Aust)* (22–24 July 2005): 6.

———. 2007. "AFL Response to Behaviour." *AFL Record (Melbourne, Aust)* (May 4–6): 20–21.

Dept. of Health and Ageing. 2001. "Federal Health Minister Announces new Funding Commitments for *Tough on Drugs*." Commonwealth of Australia. http://www. ocs.gov.au/internet/main/publishing.nsf/Content/health-mediarel-yr2001-kp-kp01002.htm. Accessed 25 May 2011.

Deutsche Welle. 2007a. "German Cabinet Pushes New Anti-Doping Law." *Deutsche Welle*, 8 March 2007. http://www.dw-world.de/dw/article/0,2144,2377262,00. html. Accessed 9 March 2007.

———. 2007b. "German Government Probes Doping Scandal." *Deutsche Welle*, 30 May 2007. http://www.dw-world.de/dw/article/0,2144,2569575,00.html. Accessed 31 May 2007.

———. 2007c. "German Rider Admits to Doping From Notorious Spanish Doctor." *Deutsche Welle*, 30 June 2007. http://www.dw-world.de/dw/ article/0,2144,2652273,00.html. Accessed 5 July 2007.

Dillman, L. 2012. "Swimmer Jessica Hardy Gets Another Shot at the Olympics." *Los Angeles Times*, 25 April 2012. http://articles.latimes.com/2012/apr/25/ sports/la-sp-oly-jessica-hardy-2012042. Accessed 24 April 2015.

Dimeo, P. 2007. *A History of Drug Use in Sport 1876–1976: Beyond Good and Evil.* New York: Routledge.

———. 2009. "The Origins of Anti-Doping Policy Sports: From Public Health to Fair Play." In *Elite Sport, Doping and Public Health*, edited by Moller, V., McNamee, M. and Dimeo, P., 29–40. Odense: University Press of Southern Denmark.

Dingelstad, D., Gosden, R., Martin, B., and Vakas, N. 1996. "The Social Construction of Drug Debates." *Social Science and Medicine* 43 (12): 1829–1838.

Donnelly, P. 1996. "Prolympism: Sport Monoculture as Crisis and Opportunity." *Quest* 48 (1): 25–42.

Donohoe, T., and Johnson, N. 1986. *Foul Play: Drug Abuse in Sports.* Oxford: Blackwell.

Donovan, R.J., Egger, G., Kapernick, V., and Mendoza, J. 2002. "A Conceptual Framework for Achieving Performance Enhancing Drug Compliance in Sport." *Sports Medicine* 32 (4): 269–284.

Douglas, T. 2007. "Enhancement in Sport, and Enhancement outside Sport." *Studies in Ethics, Law, and Technology* 1 (1): 1–15.

DrugScope. 2004. "The Doping Scandal: A Question for Sport." DrugScope. http://www.drugscope.org.uk/about/project_hometemplate.asp?id=5. Accessed 12 September 2006

Duffield, M. 2002. "Koops is Absolved by Tribunal Football." *The Age*, 30 April 2002.

Dvorak, J., Graf-Baumann, T., D'Hooghe, M., Kirkendall, D., Taennler, H., and Saugy, M. 2006. "FIFA's Approach to Doping in Football." *British Journal of Sports Medicine* 40: 3–12.

Dwyer, B. 2008. "Olympic Drug Cheats still ahead of the Cops." *Los Angeles Times*, 1 August 2008. http://articles.latimes.com/2008/aug/01/sports/sp-olydwyredrugs. Accessed 14 August 2008.

Dyreson, M. 1998. *Making the American Team: Sport, Culture, and the Olympic Experience*. Urbana: University of Illinois Press.

Early, G. 1998. *Body Language: Writers on Sport*. Saint Paul: Graywolf Press.

Eber, N. 2008. "The Performance-Enhancing Drug Game Reconsidered A Fair Play Approach." *Journal of Sports Economics* 9 (3): 318–327.

Edmund, S., and Dunn, M. 2007. "Groups Split on AFL Drug Policy." *Herald Sun*, 18 October 2007. http://www.news.com.au/heraldsun/story/0,21985,22604881–662,00.html. Accessed 10 December 2007.

Eitzen, D. S., and Frey, J. H. 1991. "Sport and Society." *Annual Review of Sociology* 17: 503–522.

Entman, R. M. 2004. *Projections of Power: Framing News, Public Ppinion, and U.S. Foreign Policy*. Chicago: University of Chicago Press.

Ericson, R. V, Baranek, P.M., and Chan, J.B.L. 1987. *Visualizing Deviance: A Study of News Organisations*. Milton Keynes: Open University Press.

———. 1991. *Representing Order*. Toronto: University of Toronto Press.

Erikson, K.T. 1966. *Wayward Puritans: A Study in the Sociology of Deviance*. New York: John Wiley and Sons, Inc.

Espy, R. 1979. *The Politics of the Olympic Games*. Berkeley: University of California Press.

Essendon Football Club. 2011. "AFL Releases Illicit Drugs Policy Results." Essendon Football Club. http://www.essendonfc.com.au/news/2011–06–22/afl-releases-illicit-drugs-policy-results. Accessed 14 February 2015.

Fairchild, D. 1989. "Sport Abjection: Steroids and the Uglification of the Athlete." *Journal of the Philosophy of Sport* XVI: 74–88.

Farnen, R. F. 1990. "Decoding the Mass Media and Terrorism Connection: Militant Extremism as Systemic and Symbiotic Processes." In *Marginal Conventions: Popular Culture, Mass Media and Social Deviance*, edited by Sanders, C.R., 98–116. Bowling Green, Ohio: Bowling Green State University Popular Press.

Farquhar, G. 2008. "IOC Steps up War on Dopers." *BBC Sport*, 8 October 2008. http://www.bbc.co.uk/blogs/olympics/2008/10/ioc_steps_up_war_on_dopers.html. Accessed 10 October 2008.

Fife, G. 1999. *Tour de France: The History, the Legend, the Riders*. Edinburgh: Mainstream.

Fife, G. 2001. *Inside the Peloton: Riding, Winning and Losing the Tour de France*. Edinburgh: Mainstream.

Fine, G. A. 1985. "The Goliath Effect: Corporate Dominance and Mercantile Legends." *The Journal of American Folklore* 98 (387): 63–84.

Flick, U. 2002. *An Introduction to Qualitative Research*. London: Sage Publications.

Foster, K. 2001. "The Discourses of Doping: Law and Regulation in the War Against Drugs." In *Drugs and Doping in Sport: Socio-Legal Perspectives*, edited by O'Leary, J., 181–203. London: Cavenidsh Publishing.

Fotheringham, W. 2015. "Lance Armstrong and UCI 'Colluded to Bypass Doping Accusations.'" *The Guardian*, 9 March 2015. http://www.theguardian.com/sport/2015/mar/09/lance-armstrong-uci-colluded-circ-report-cycling. Accessed 14 June 2015.

Fotheringham, W. 2002. *Put Me Back on My Bike: In Search of Tom Simpson*. London Yellow Jersey.

Franke, W.W., and Berendonk, B. 1997. "Hormonal Doping and Androgenization of Athletes: A Secret Program of the German Democratic Republic Government." *Clinical Chemistry* 43 (7): 1262–1279.

Freidson, E. 1970. *Profession of Medicine: A Study of the Sociology of Applied Knowledge*. Chicago: The University of Chicago Press.

Fritz, N.J., and Altheide, D.L. 1987. "The Mass Media and the Social Construction of the Missing Children Problem." *Sociological Quarterly* 28 (4): 473–493.

Futterman, M. 2012. "Trials and Tribulations of the Angry Swimmer." *The Wall Street Journal*, 14 May 2012. http://www.wsj.com/articles/SB10001424052702304203604577396561119031937. Accessed 25 April 2015.

Gardini, A. 2010. "Keat No Drug Cheat." *Gold Coast Bulletin*, 13 February 2008. http://www.goldcoast.com.au/article/2008/02/13/7716_gold-coast-sport.html. Accessed 17 September 2010.

Garland, D. 2008. "On the Concept of Moral Panic." *Crime Media Culture* 4 (1) :9–31.

Ghareeb, E. 2000. "New Media and the Information Revolution in the Arab World: An Assessment." *Middle East Journal* 54 (3 The Information Revolution): 395–418.

Gilmour, R. 2009. "Andy Murray Awoken in New York Hotel Room by Early-Rising Drug-Testers." *The Telegraph*, 26 August 2009. http://www.telegraph.co.uk/sport/tennis/andymurray/6092431/Andy-Murray-awoken-in-New-York-hotel-room-by-early-rising-drug-testers.html. Accessed 27 March 2015.

Girginov, V. 2006. "Creating a Corporate Anti-doping Culture: The Role of Bulgarian Sports Governing Bodies." *Sport in Society* 9 (2): 252–268.

Giulianotti, R. 2005. *Sport: A Critical Sociology*. Cambridge: Polity Press.

Gleeson, M. 2006. "Footy Drugs Testing Finds 15 Under the Influence." *The Age*, 10 March 2006. http://www.theage.com.au/realfooty/articles/2006/03/09/1141701634085.html. Accessed 10 March 2006.

———. 2013. "AFL Considers 'Friends Register' for Player." *The Sydney Morning Herald*, 1 March 2013. http://www.smh.com.au/afl/afl-news/afl-considers-friends-register-for-players-20130228-2f98d.html?skin=text-only. Accessed 29 June 2015.

———. 2015. "WADA Wants Essendon Case Heard in Switzerland." *The Age*, 20 May 2015. http://www.theage.com.au/afl/afl-news/wada-wants-essendon-case-heard-in-switzerland-20150519-gh5ath.html. Accessed 29 June 2015.

Goffa, D. 2008. "Drug Questions Dog Dara." *Los Angeles Times*, 12 July 2008. http://latimesblogs.latimes.com/olympics_blog/2008/07/drug-questions.html. Accessed 30 September 2008.

Gonzenbach, W.J. 1992. "A Time-Series Analysis of the Drug Issue, 1985–1990: The Press, The President and Public Opinion." *International Journal of Public Opinion* 4 (2): 126–147.

Goode, E. 2012. "The Moral Panic: Dead or Alive?" Presentation at Seminar 1, *Moral Panics Seminar Series*, 23 November, Edinburgh: Edinburgh University.

Goode, E., and Ben-Yehuda, N. 1994a. *Moral Panics the Social Construction of Deviance*. Cambridge, Massachusetts: Blackwell Publishers.

———. 1994b. "Moral Panics: Culture, Politics and Social Construction." *Annual Review of Sociology* 20 (3): 149–171.

————. 2006. "Enter Moral Panics." In *Constructing Crime: Perspectives on Making News and Social Problems*, edited by Potter, G. W. and Kappeler, V. E., 21–28. Long Grove, IL: Waveland Press.

————. 2009. *Moral Panics: The Social Construction of Deviance*. Chichester, West Sussex: Wiley-Blackwell Publishing.

The Gold Coast Bulletin. 2006. "AFL and the Court just Don't Get It." *The Gold Coast Bulletin*, 1 September 2006.

Gordon, M. 2013. " 'This is the Blackest Day in Australian Sport.' " The *Sydney Morning Herald*, 8 February 2013. http://www.smh.com.au/national/this-is-the-blackest-day-in-australian-sport-20130207–2e1i3.html. Accessed 3 January 2015.

Grafstein, R. 1981. "The Failure of Weber's Conception of Legitimacy: Its Causes and Implications." *The Journal of Politics* 43 (2): 456–472.

Green, M. 2007. "Olympic Glory or Grassroots Development?: Sport Policy Priorities in Australia, Canada and the United Kingdom, 1960–2006." *The International Journal of the History of Sport* 24 (7): 921–953.

Green, M., and Houlihan, B. 2006. "Governmentality, Modernization, and the 'Disciplining' of National Sporting Organizations: Athletics in Australia and the United Kingdom." *Sociology of Sport Journal* 23: 47–71.

Grogan, S., Shepherd, S., Evans, R., Wright, S., and Hunter, G. 2006. "Experiences of Anabolic Steroid Use: In-depth Interviews with Men and Women Body Builders." *Journal of Health Psychology* 11 (6): 845–856.

The Guardian. 2009. "Murray Attacks 'Draconian' Anti-Doping Rules." *The Guardian*, 6 February 2009. http://www.theguardian.com/sport/2009/feb/06/tennis-andy-murray-anti-doping. Accessed 8 January 2015.

Gucciardi, D. F., Jalleh, G., and Donovan, R. 2010. "Does Social Desirability Influence the Relationship between Doping Attitudes and Doping Susceptibility in Athletes?" *Psychology of Sport and Exercise* 11 (6): 479–486.

————. 2011. "An Examination of the Sport Drug Control Model with Elite Australian Athletes." *Journal of Science and Medicine in Sport* 14 (6): 469–476.

Guinness, R. 2014. "Banned Australian Cyclist Michael Rogers Cleared to Ride Again." *The Sydney Morning Herald*, 23 April 2014. http://www.smh.com.au/sport/cycling/banned-australian-cyclist-michael-rogers-cleared-to-ride-again-20140423-zqybj.html. Accessed 1 April 2015.

Gusfield, J. R. 1955. "Social Structure and Moral Reform: A Study of the Woman's Christian Temperance Union." *American Journal of Sociology* 61 (3): 221–232.

————. 1963. *Symbolic Crusade, Status Politics and the American Temperance Movement*. Urbana: University of Illinois Press.

————. 1967. "Moral Passage: The Symbolic Process in Public Designations of Deviance." *Social Problems* 15: 175–188.

————. 1981. *The Culture of Public Problems: Drinking-Driving and the Symbolic Order*. Chicago: The University of Chicago Press.

Guttmann, A. 1984. *The Games Must Go On: Avery Brundage and The Olympic Movement*. New York: Columbia University Press.

————. 1988. *A Whole New Ballgame: An Interpretation of American Sports*. Chapel Hill: University of North Carolina Press.

————. 1992. *The Olympics: A History of the Modern Games*. Urbana: University of Illinois Press.

————. 2004. *From Ritual to Record: The Nature of Modern Sports*. New York: Columbia University Press.

Habermas, J. 1976. *Legitimation Crisis*. London: Heinemann Educational.

Hagdorn, K. 2001. "Hope on Koops." *Sunday Herald-Sun*, 6 May 2001.

Hall, S., Critcher, C., Jefferson, J., Clarke, J., and Roberts, B. 1978. *Policing the Crisis: Mugging, The State, and Law And Order*. London: The MacMillan Press Ltd.

Hanstad, D. V., and Loland, S. 2009. "Where on Earth is Michael Rasmussen?—Is an Elite Level Athlete's Duty to Provide Information on Whereabouts Justifiable Anti-Doping Work or an Indefensible Surveillance Regime?" In *Elite Sport, Doping and Public Health*, edited by Moller, V., McNamee, M. and Dimeo, P., 167–177. Odensa: University Press of Southern Denmark.

Hanstad, D. V., Smith, A., and Waddington, I. 2008. "The Establishment of the World Anti-Doping Agency: A Study of the Management of Organizational Change and Unplanned Outcomes." *International Review for the Sociology of Sport* 43 (3): 227–249.

Hanstad, D. V., Skille, E. Å., and Loland, S. 2010. "Harmonization of Anti-Doping Work: Myth or Reality?" *Sport in Society* 13 (2): 418–430.

Hardie, M., Shilbury, D., Ware, I., and Bozzi, C. 2010. *I wish I was Twenty One Now—Beyond Doping in the Australian Peloton*. Waurn Ponds, Victoria.: Deakin University Faculty of Business and Law. http://www.newcyclingpathway.com/wp-content/uploads/2010/09/21-NOW-FINAL-.pdf. Accessed 16 August 2011

Hargie, O., Mitchell, D. H., and Somerville, I. 2015. " 'People Have a Knack of Making you Feel Excluded if they Catch on to your Difference': Transgender Experiences of Exclusion in Sport." *International Review for Sociology of Sport*, 1–17. doi: 10.1177/1012690215583283.

Harvey, J., and Law, A. 2005. " 'Resisting' the Global Media Oligopoly? The Canada Inc. Response." In *Sport and Corporate Nationalisms*, edited by Andrews, D. L., 187–225. Oxford: Berg.

Haugen, K. K. 2004. "The Performance-Enhancing Drug Game." *Journal of Sports Economics* 5 (1): 67–86.

Hawdon, J. E. 2001. "The Role of Presidential Rhetoric in the Creation of a Moral Panic: Reagan, Bush and the War on Drugs." *Deviant Behaviour* 22 (5): 419–445.

Healey, D. J. 2003. *The History of Drug Use in Sport*. Balmain: The Spinney Press.

Hedge, M. 2006. "AFL Wins Drug Suppression Case." *Sunday Times*, 30 August 2006. http://www.news.com.au/perthnow/story/0,21598,20304037–5005361,00.html. Accessed 5 September 2006.

Hemphill, D. 1992. "Sport, Political Ideology and Freedom." *Journal of Sport and Social Issues* 16 (1): 15–33.

———. 2002. " 'Think It, Talk It, Work It': Violence, Injury and Australian Rules Football." *Sporting Traditions* 19 (1): 17–31.

———. 2008. "War on Drugs in Sport." *Bulletin of Sport and Culture* (29): 3–4.

Henne, K. 2015. *Testing for Athlete Citizenship: Regulating Doping and Sex in Sport*. New Brunswick, NJ: Rutgers University Press.

Henne, K. E., Koh, B., and McDermott, V. 2013. "Coherence of Drug Policy in Sports: Illicit Inclusions and Illegal Inconsistencies." *Performance Enhancement and Health* 2 (2): 48–55.

Henne, K. E., and McDermott, V. 2013. "Cruel Reality of Sport Business." 15 February 2013. http://www.canberratimes.com.au/comment/cruel-reality-of-sport-business-20130214–2efr0.html. Accessed 11 March 2015.

Herman, M. 2007. "IOC Calls on Britain to Criminalise Doping." *The Guardian*, 24 July 2007. http://sport.guardian.co.uk/breakingnews/feedstory/0,,-6801161,00.html. Accessed 26 July 2007.

Hier, S. 2008. "Thinking Beyond Moral Panic: Risk, Responsibility, and the Politics of Moralization." *Theoretical Criminology* 12 (2): 173–190.

Hier, S., Lett, D., Walby, K., and Smith, A. 2011. "Beyond Folk Devil Resistance: Linking Moral Panic and Moral Regulation." *Criminology and Criminal Justice* 11 (3): 259–276.

Hilgartner, S., and Bosk, C. L. 1988. "The Rise and Fall of Social Problems: A Public Arenas Model." *The American Journal of Sociology* 94 (1): 53–78.

Hill, C.R. 1992. *Olympic Politics*. Manchester, UK: Manchester University Press.
———. 1993. "The Politics of the Olympic Movement." In *The Changing Politics of Sport*, edited by Allison, L., 84–104. Manchester; New York: Manchester University Press.
Hiltzik, M.A. 2006. "Athletes' Unbeatable Foe." *Los Angeles Times*, 10 December 2006. http://articles.latimes.com/2006/dec/10/sports/sp-doping10/. Accessed 7 January 2015.
Himmer, A. 2007. "IAAF Wants Tougher Bans for doping." *Reuters Africa*, 23 August 2007. http://africa.reuters.com/sport/news/usnBAN331064.html. Accessed 6 September 2007.
Hoberman, J. 1986. *The Olympic Crisis: Sport, Politics and the Moral Order*. New Rochelle, New York: Aristide D. Caratzas.
———. 1992. *Mortal Engines: The Science of Performance and the Dehumanisation of Sport*. New Jersey: The Blackburn Press.
———. 2001. "How Drug Testing Fails: the Politics of Doping Control." In *Doping in Elite Sport: The Politics of Drugs in the Olympic Movement*, edited by Wilson, W. and Derse, E., 241–274. Champaign, Il: Human Kinetics.
———. 2005. "Olympic Drug Testing: An Interpretive History." In *Global Olympics: Historical and Sociological Studies of the Modern Games*, edited by Young, K. and Wamsley, K.B., 249–268. Amsterdam: Elsevier.
Hodgkinson, M. 2009. "US Open: Britain's Andy Murray Frustrated by 'Intrusive' Tennis Drug-Testing Protocol." *The Telegraph*, 28 August 2009. http://www.telegraph.co.uk/sport/tennis/andymurray/6106682/US-Open-Britains-Andy-Murray-frustrated-by-intrusive-tennis-drug-testing-protocol.html. Accessed 27 Marach 2015.
Hollands, R.G. 1984. "The Role of Cultural Studies and Social Criticism in the Sociological Study of Sport." *Quest* 36 (1): 66–79.
Holroyd, J. 2007. "AFL Flags Drug Code Review." *Real Footy*, 18 October 2007. http://realfooty.com.au/articles/2007/10/18/1192300914023.html. Accessed 8 November 2007.
Holton, R.J. 1987. "The Idea of Crisis in Modern Society." *The British Journal of Sociology* 38 (4): 502–520.
Horne, J. 2006. *Sport in Consumer Culture*. New York: Palgrave Macmillan.
Horvath, P. 2006. "Anti-Doping and Human Rights in Sport: The Case of the AFL and the *WADA Code*." *Monash University Law Review* 32 (2): 357–386.
Houlihan, B. 1994. *Sport and International Politics*. Hemel Hempstead: Harvester Wheatsheaf.
———. 1999. "Anti-Doping Policy in Sport: The Politics of International Policy Co-ordination." *Public Administration* 77 (2): 311–334.
———. 2001. "The World Anti-Doping Agency: Prospects for Success." In *Drugs and Doping in Sport: Socio-Legal Perspectives*, edited by O'Leary, J., 125–145. London: Cavendish Publishing Limited.
———. 2002. *Dying to Win*. Strasbourg Cedex: Council of Europe Publishing.
———. 2004. "Civil Rights, Doping Control and the World Anti-Doping Code." *Sport in Society* 7 (3): 420–437.
———. 2005. "International Politics and Olympic Governance." In *Global Olympics: Historical and Sociological Studies of the Modern Games*, edited by Young, K. and Wamsley, K.B., 127–142. Amsterdam: Elsevier JAI.
———. 2008. "Detection and Eduction in Anti-Doping Policy: A Review of Current Issues and an Assessment of Future Prospects." *Hitotsubashi Journal of Arts and Sciences* 49: 55–71.
———. 2009. "Doping, Public Health and the Generalisation of Interests." In *Elite Sport, Doping and Public Health*, edited by Moller, V., McNamee, M. and Dimeo, P., 41–54. Odense: University Press of Southern Denmark.

Howman, D. 2012. "Developing New Alliances to Tackle the Increasing Problem of Doping in Sport." Doping as a Public Health Issue Symposium, Stockholm, Sweden, 21–22 September 2012. https://wada-main-prod.s3.amazonaws.com/resources/files/ArneSymposium.pdf. Accessed 8 January 2015.

Hunt, A. 1999. *Governing Morals: A Social History of Moral Regulation.* Cambridge, U.K.: Cambridge University Press.

Hunt, T. M. 2007. "Sport, Drugs, and the Cold War: The Conundrum of Olympic Doping Policy, 1970–1979." *Olympika XVI:* 19–42.

Hurd, I. 1999. "Legitimacy and Authority in International Politics." *International Organisation* 53 (2): 379–408.

IICGADS (International Intergovernmental Consultative Group on Anti-Doping in Sport). 1999. *Sydney Communique.* International Intergovernmental Consultative Group on Anti-Doping in Sport. http://www.dcita.gov.au/drugsinsport/communique_17nov.doc. Accessed 26 September 2007.

———. 2003. *The Copenhagen Declaration.* World Anti-Doping Agency. http://www.wada-ama.org/rtecontent/document/copenhagen_en.pdf. Accessed 26 September 2007.

Innes, M. 2005. "A Short History of the Idea of Moral Panic." *Crime Media Culture* 1 (1): 106–111.

International Herald Tribune. 2007a. "Dutch Secretary of Health Advocates Removal of Recreational Drugs from Anti-Doping Code." *International Herald Tribune,* 12 February 2007. http://www.iht.com/articles/ap/2007/02/12/sports/EU-SPT-Netherlands-Anti-Doping-Code.php. Accessed 14 February 2007.

———. 2007b. "World Anti-Doping Head Sees Progress as Term Nears End." *International Herald Tribune,* 13 May 2007. http://www.iht.com/articles/ap/2007/05/14/sports/NA-SPT-WADA-Pound.php. Accessed 25 May 2007.

IOC (International Olympic Committee). 1980. "Olympic Charter." International Olympic Committee. http://www.olympic.org/Documents/Olympic Charter/Olympic_Charter_through_time/1980-Olympic_Charter.pdf. Accessed 24 June 2014.

———. 1991. "Olympic Charter." http://www.olympic.org/Documents/Olympic Charter/Olympic_Charter_through_time/1991-Olympic_Charter_June91.pdf.

———. 2000. "Olympic Movement Anti-Doping Code." In, 49. Lausanne: International Olympic Committee.

———. 2007. "Recognised Sports." International Olympic Committee. http://www.olympic.org/uk/sports/recognized/index_uk.asp. Accessed 27 April 2007.

———. 2009. "Olympic Movement Medical Code." International Olympic Committee. http://www.olympic.org/Documents/Fight_against_doping/Rules_and_regulations/OlympicMovementMedicalCode-EN_FR.pdf. Accessed 20 December 2010.

———. 2013. "Olympic Charter." International Olympic Committee. http://www.olympic.org/Documents/olympic_charter_en.pdf. Accessed 9 January 2015.

———. 2014a. "Olympic Charter." http://www.olympic.org/Documents/olympic_charter_en.pdf. Accessed 24 June 2015.

———. 2014b. "Professor Arne Ljungqvist." International Olympic Committee. http://www.olympic.org/professor-arne-ljungqvist. Accessed 31 January 2015.

ISM (International Sports Movement). 2007. "World Anti-Doping Agency WADA Executive Committee and Foundation Board Advance Closer to Final Revision of the World Anti-Doping Code." *Sports Features Communications,* 14 May 2007. http://www.sportsfeatures.com/index.php?section=ppandaction=showandid=3908. Accessed 24 May 2007.

ISR (Dept. of Industry Science and Resources). 1999a. "TODIS—Foreword." Commonwealth of Australia. http://www.dcita.gov.au/tough_on_drugs/p1.htm. Accessed 24 July 2008.

———. 1999b. "TODIS—Implementing International Best Practice in Drug Testing." Commonwealth of Australia. http://fulltext.ausport.gov.au/fulltext/1999/feddep/tough_on_drugs_in_sport/content.htm. Accessed 25 May 2011.

———. 1999c. "Tough on Drugs in Sport: Australia's Anti-Drugs in Sport Strategy 1999–2000 and Beyond." Commonwealth of Australia. http://fulltext.ausport.gov.au/fulltext/1999/feddep/tough_on_drugs_in_sport/content.htm. Accessed 25 May 2011.

Jacobs, J.B., and Samuels, B. 1995. "The Drug Testing Project in International Sports: Dilemmas in an Expanding Regulatory Regime." *Hastings International and Comparative Law Review* 18 (3): 557–589.

Jalleh, G., Donovan, R., and Jobling, I. 2014. "Predicting Attitude towards Performance Enhancing Substance Use: A Comprehensive Test of the Sport Drug Control Model with Elite Australian Athletes." *Journal of Science and Medicine in Sport* 17: 574–579.

Jeffery, N. 2008. "Performance Drug Fight Stepped Ip." *The Australian*, 3 May 2008. http://www.theaustralian.news.com.au/story/0,25197,23636365–5013449,00.html. Accessed 13 February 2009.

Jenkins, P. 1992. *Intimate Enemies: Moral Panics in Contemporary Great Britain.* New York: Aldine de Gruyter.

Jenkins, P., and Maier-Katkin, D. 1992. "Satanism: Myth and Reality in a Contemporary Moral Panic." *Crime, Law and Social Change* 17 (1): 53–75.

Jennings, A. 1996. *The New Lords of the Rings: Olympic Corruption and How to Buy Gold Medals.* London: Pocket Books.

Jensen, E.L., Gerber, J., and Babcock, G.M. 1991. "The New War on Drugs: Grass Roots Movement or Political Construction?" *Journal of Drug Issues* 21 (3): 641–667.

Johnson, L. 1997. "Charles Drug Hearing on Thursday." *The Age,* 2 September 1997.

———. 2005. "Drugs Impasse Costs AFL $1.5m." *The Age,* 1 July 2005.

Johnson, T.J., Wanta, W., Boudreau, T., Blank-Libra, J., Schaffer, K., and Turner, S. 1996. "Influence Dealers: A Path Analysis Model of Agenda Building during Richard Nixon's War on Drugs." *Journalism and Mass Communication Quarterly* 73 (1): 181–194.

Jones, B.J., McFalls, J.A., and Gallagher, B.J. 1989. "Toward a Unified Model for Social Problems." *Journal of the Theory of Social Behavior* 19 (3): 337–356.

Kayser, B. 2009. "Current Anti-Doping Policy: Harm Reduction or Harm Induction?" In *Elite Sport, Doping and Public Health,* edited by Moller, V., McNamee, M. and Dimeo, P., 155–166. Odense: University Press of Southern Denmark.

Kayser, B., Mauron, A., and Miah, A. 2007. "Current Anti-Doping Policy: A Critical Appraisal." *BMC Medical Ethics* 8 (2). doi:10.1186/1472-6939-8-2.

Kelly, J. 2008. "Fans Line up to Blast AFL's Drug Policy." *Herald Sun,* 22 January 2008. http://www.news.com.au/heraldsun/story/0,21985,23087790–2862,00.html. Accessed 22 January 2008.

Kelso, P. 2007. "Drug Taking is Rife in Golf, Claims Player." *The Guardian,* 19 July 2007. http://www.guardian.co.uk/frontpage/story/0,,2129777,00.html. Accessed 20 July 2007.

———. 2008. "War on Drugs will Never be Won, Says Anti-Doping Chief." *The Guardian,* 28 February 2008. http://www.guardian.co.uk/sport/2008/feb/28/athletics.sport. Accessed 17 April 2009.

Kennedy, M.C. 2000. "Newer Drugs Used to Enhance Sporting Performance." *Medical Journal of Australia* 173 (Special Olympic issue): 314–317.

Kidd, B., Edelman, R., and Brownell, S. 2001. "Comparative Analysis of Doping Scandals: Canada, Russia, and China." In *Doping in Elite Sport: The Politics of Drugs in the Olympic Movement,* edited by Wilson, W. and Derse, E., 153–188. Champgaign, IL.: Human Kinetics.

Killingbeck, D. 2006. "The Role of Television News in the Construction of School Violence as a 'Moral Panic.'" In *Constructing Crime: Perspectives on Making News and Social Problems*, edited by Potter, G. W. and Kappeler, V. E., 213–228. Long Grove, IL: Waveland Press.

Kimmage, P. 1998. *Rough Ride: Behind the Wheel with a Pro Cyclist*. London: Yellow Jersey Press.

Knight, T. 2008. "Drugs in Sport: Cheats Go to Great Lengths." *Telegraph*, 23 June 2008. http://www.telegraph.co.uk/sport/othersports/drugsinsport/2303890/Drugs-in-sport-Cheats-go-to-great-lengths.html. Accessed 19 February 2009.

Knopf, T. A. 1970. "Media Myths on Violence." *Columbia Journalism Review* 9 (1): 17–25.

Kogay, P., and Read, B. 2006. "Refusing to Name, Shame is Confusing." *The Australian*, 1 September 2006. http://www.theaustralian.news.com.au/story/0,20867,20319507-2722,00.html. Accessed 4 September 2006.

Koppell, J. 2005. "Pathologies of Accountability: ICANN and the Challenge of 'Multiple Accountabilities Disorder.'" *Public Administration Review* 65 (1 Jan-Feb 2005): 94–108.

———. 2007. "Structure of Global Governance: Explaining the Organizational Design of Global Rulemaking Institutions." Annual Meeting of the International Studies Association, Chicago, IL, 1 March 2007.

———. 2008. "Global Governance Organizations: Legitimacy and Authority in Conflict." *Journal of Public Administration Research and Theory* 18 (2): 177–203.

Krabel, H. 2008. "Meet Rebekah Keat." Slowtwitch.com. http://www.slowtwitch.com/Interview/Meet_Rebekah_Keat_415.html. Accessed 17 September 2010.

Kuriloff, A. 2007. "NFL, Players to Increase Drug Testing By 40 Percent." *Bloomberg.com*, 24 January 2007. http://www.bloomberg.com/apps/news?pid=20601079andsid=aYHjeRMj4cUcandrefer=home. Accessed 29 January 2007.

Kwak, H., Lee, C., Park, H., and Moon, S. 2010. "What is Twitter, a Social Network or a News Media?" World Wide Web Conference Committee, Raleigh, NC, 26–30 April, 2010. http://delivery.acm.org/10.1145/1780000/1772751/p591-kwak.pdf?ip=130.56.65.83andacc=ACTIVE SERVICEandCFID=88690867andCFTOKEN=27314921and__acm__=1331086236_6ea81063d9774287b98650b643da3e1. Accessed 7 March 2012.

Lalor, P. 2007. "Healthy Dose of Sense on Drug Row." *The Australian*, 15 September 2007. http://www.theaustralian.news.com.au/story/0,25197,22420227-5013576,00.html. Accessed 18 September 2007.

Lamont-Mills, A., and Christensen, S. 2008. "'I Have Never Taken Performance Enhancing Drugs and I Never Will': Drug Discourse in the Shane Warne Case." *Scandinavian Journal of Medicine and Science in Sports* 18 (2): 250–258.

Lane, S. 2005a. Canberra And AFL In A Clash Of The Codes. *The Sunday Age*. 12 June 2005, http://www.footballodds.com.au/football-odds-articles/2005/6/12/canberra-and-afl-in-a-clash-of-the-codes/. Accessed 29 January 2015

———. 2006a. "Brown Gacks Steroid Use." *The Age*, 13 August 2006. http://www.realfooty.theage.com.au/articles/2006/08/12/1154803147220.html. Accessed 14 August 2006.

———. 2006b. "Malthouse Takes Aim at AFL." *Sunday Age*, 12 March 2006.

———. 2013. "Bill Will Boost Powers of Anti-Doping Agency." *The Age*, 7 February 2013. http://www.theage.com.au/sport/bill-will-boost-powers-of-antidoping-agency-20130206-2dz2v.html—ixzz2KYVBv73s. Accessed 20 April2015.

Lane, T. 2005b. "AFL's Brave Drug Stand." *The Age*, 2 July 2005.

Laure, P. 2009. "In Praise of the Non-Dominant Sense of Doping Behaviour." In *Elite Sport, Doping and Public Health*, edited by Moller, V., McNamee, M. and Dimeo, P., 119–133. Odensa: University Press of Southern Denmark.

Leonard, J. 2001. "Doping in Elite Swimming: A Case Study of the Modern Era from 1970 Onward." In *Doping in Elite Sport The Politics of Drugs in the Olympic Movement*, edited by Wilson, J. and Derse, E., 225–239. Champaign, IL: Human Kinetics Publishers, Inc.

Lidz, C. W., and Walker, A. L. 1980. *Heroin, Deviance, and Morality*. Beverly Hills, Calif.: Sage Publications.

Linden, J. 2010. "WADA Loses Bid to Hike Suspension of Wwimmer Hardy." Reuters, 21 May 2010. http://www.reuters.com/article/2010/05/21/us-swimming-hardy-doping-idUSTRE64K49Y2010052. Accessed 25 April 2015.

Linnell, G. 1995. *Football Ltd: The Inside Story of the AFL*. Sydney: Pan Macmillan Australia Pty Limited.

Linnell, S. 1997. "Eagle Caught Out by Flu Medication." *The Age*, 1 September 1997.

———. 1998. "League Vows Swift Action on Drug Offences." *The Age*, 5 March 1998.

Lofquist, W. S. 1997. "Constructing 'Crime': Media Coverage of Individual and Organizational Wrongdoing." *Justice Quarterly* 14 (2): 243–263.

Lucas, J. A. 1992. *Future of the Olympic Games*. Champaign, IL: Human Kinetics Books.

Lull, J., and Hinerman, S. 1997. *Media Scandals: Morality and Desire in the Popular Culture Marketplace*. Cambridge, U.K.: Polity Press.

Lundy, Senator the Hon Kate, and The Hon Jason Clare MP. 2012. Media release: New partnership to tackle doping in sport. Australian Government http://www.asada.gov.au/publications/media/ministerial_media_releases/ministerial_release_121016_new_partnership_to_tackle_doping.pdf. Accessed 15 April 2015.

Lysaght, B. 2007. "Athlete Doping Incidents Are Rising, Enforcement Chief Says." *Bloomberg.com*, 1 November 2007. http://www.bloomberg.com/apps/news?pid=20601079andsid=a.CY1pwYDddgandrefer=home. Accessed 9 December 2008.

MacAloon, J. 1981. *This Great Symbol: Pierre de Coubertin and the Origins of the Modern Olympic Games*. Chicago: University of Chicago Press.

———. 1984. *Rite, Drama, Festival, Spectacle: Rehearsals toward a Theory of Cultural Performance*. Philadelphila: Institute for the Study of Human Issues.

———. 2001. "Doping and Moral Authority: Sport Organisations Today." In *Doping in Elite Sport: The Politics of Drugs in the Olympic Movement*, edited by Wilson, W. and Derse, E., 205–224. Champaign, IL: Human Kinetics.

———. 2006. "The Mighty Working of a Symbol: From Idea to Organization." *The International Journal of the History of Sport* 23 (3–4): 528–570.

Macintyre, S. 2011. "AFL Boss Andrew Demetriou: 'We are Trying to Control as much as we Can Control.'" *The Conversation*, 15 August 2011. http://theconversation.edu.au/afl-boss-andrew-demetriou-we-are-trying-to-control-as-much-as-we-can-control-281. Accessed 16 August 2011.

Macur, J. 2007. "Doping Officials Question Baseball's Policy on Drugs." *The New York Times*, 17 November 2007. http://www.nytimes.com/2007/11/17/sports/baseball/17madrid.html?ref=sports. Accessed 26 December 2007.

———. 2012. "Lance Armstrong Is Stripped of His 7 Tour de France Titles." *The New York Times*, 22 October 2012. http://www.nytimes.com/2012/10/23/sports/cycling/armstrong-stripped-of-his-7-tour-de-france-titles.html?_r=. Accessed 27 March 2015.

———. 2014. *Cycle of Lies: The Fall of Lance Armstrong*. London: William Collins.

Magdalinski, T. 2000. "The Reinvention of Australia for the Sydney 2000 Olympic Games." *The International Journal of the History of Sport* 17 (2–3): 305–322.

Magnay, J. 2006. "Government Gets Tough on AFL over Secrecy surrounding Drug-Testing Policy." *The Sydney Morning Herald*, 8 September 2006. http://www.smh.com.au/news/afl/government-gets-tough-on-afl-over-secrecy-surrounding-drug-testingpolicy/2006/09/07/1157222264974.html. Accessed 8 September 2006.

————. 2008a. "Baggaley Faces Drugs Charges in Two States." *The Sydney Morning Herald*, 2 May 2008. http://www.smh.com.au/news/sport/baggaley-faces-drugs-charges-in-two-states/2008/05/01/1209235055647.html. Accessed 13 February 2009.

————. 2008b. "Missing Test Results Turn Up but WADA Isn't Happy." *The Sydney Morning Herald*, 17 October 2008. http://www.smh.com.au/news/sport/missing-test-results-turn-up-but-wada-isnt-happy/2008/10/16/1223750232514.html. Accessed 17 October 2008.

Malloy, D.C., and Zakus, D.H. 2002. "Ethics of Drug Testing in Sport—An Invasion of Privacy Justified?" *Sport, Education and Society* 7 (2): 203–281.

Mark, D. 2015. "Stephen Dank Says AFL, ASADA 'Constructed' Story to Incriminate Him and Essendon Bombers in Supplements Saga." ABC News, http://www.abc.net.au/news/2015–02–05/afl-and-asada-constructed-story-to-incriminate-bombers-dank-says/607405. Accessed 15 February 2015.

Masters, R. 2004. "Drugs Chiefs Hold Secret Powwow over Latest Trends." *The Sydney Morning Herald*, 10 December 2004. http://www.smh.com.au/news/Sport/Drugs-chiefs-hold-secret-powwow-over-latest-trends/2004/12/09/1102182429497.html?oneclick=true. Accessed 19 February 2007.

————. 2007. "Party Drugs and Tootballers—The Cloud on the Horizon that Worries Kemp." *The Sydney Morning Herald*, 10 February 2007. http://www.smh.com.au/news/sport/party-drugs-and-footballers—the-cloud-on-the-horizon-that-worrieskemp/2007/02/09/1170524302699.html. Accessed 12 February 2007.

Matheson, C. 1987. "Weber and the Classification of Forms of Legitimacy." *The British Journal of Sociology* 38 (2): 199–215.

Mazanov, J., Huybers, T., and Connor, J. 2010. "Qualitative Evidence of a Primary Intervention Point for Elite Athlete Doping." *Journal of Science and Medicine in Sport* 14 (2011): 106–110.

McArdle, D. 2001. "'Say it Ain't So, Mo.' International Performers' Perceptions of Drug Use and the Diane Modahl Affair." In *Drugs and Doping in Sport: Socio-Legal Perspectives*, edited by O'Leary, J., 91–108. London: Cavendish Publishing Limited.

McAsey, J. 2007. "AFL Not Trying in Fight on Drugs." *The Australian*, 4 August 2007. http://www.theaustralian.news.com.au/story/0,25197,22185322–2722,00.html. Accessed 6 August 2007.

McCorkle, R.C., and Miethe, T.D. 1998. "The Political and Organizational Response to Gangs: An Examination of a 'Moral Panic' in Nevada." *Justice Quarterly* 15 (1): 41–64.

McDermott, V. 2012. "Legitimating the Fight against Drugs in Sport: The Australian Government and the Australian Football League." The annual conference of The Australian Sociological Association 2012, *Emerging and Enduring Inequalities*, The University of Queensland, 26–29 November 2012.

McGarry, A. 2015. "Essendon ASADA Investigation: Tribunal Decision to Reveal Guilt or Innocence for 34 Current and Former Bombers Players." *ABC News*, 31 March 2015. http://www.abc.net.au/news/2015–03–30/day-of-reckoning-arrives-for-essendon/636032. Accessed 29 June 2015.

McKay, J. 1986. "Hegemony, the State and Australian Sport." In *Power Play*, edited by Lawrence, G. and Rowe, D., 115–135. Sydney: Hale and Iremonger.

McKay, J., Hutchins, B., and Mikosza, J. 2000. "'Shame and Scandal in the Family': Australian Media Narratives of the IOC/SOCOG Scandal Matrix." Paper presented at the Bridging Three Centuries—Fifth International Symposium for Olympic Research, The University of Western Ontario, London, Ontario, Canada.

McKay, J., and Roderick, M. 2010. "'Lay Down Sally': Media Narratives of Failure in Australian Sport." *Journal of Australian Studies* 34 (3): 295–315.

McKay, S. 1996. "Famine Threatens a Footy Feast; Football's Boom Times." *The Age*, 9 September 1996.

McNicol, A. 2011. "Failed Drug Tests Down." *AFL.com.au*, 22 June 2011. http://www.afl.com.au/news/newsarticle/tabid/208/newsid/116819/default.aspx. Accessed 13 July 2011.

McRobbie, A. 1994. "Folk Devils Fight Back." *New Left Review* January-February: 107–116.

McRobbie, A., and Thornton, A.L. 1995. "Rethinking 'Moral Panic' for Multi-Mediated Social Worlds." *British Journal of Sociology* 46 (4): 559–574.

Mehlman, M.J. 2009. *The Price of Perfection: Individualism and Society in the Era of Biomedical Enhancement*. Maryland: The John Hopkins University Press.

Mendes, P. (2001) "Social Conservatism vs Harm Minimisation: John Howard on Illicit Drugs," *Journal of Economic and Social Policy* 6 (1), Article 2. Available at: http://epubs.scu.edu.au/jesp/vol6/iss1/2

Mendoza, J. 2002. "The War on Drugs in Sport: A Perspective from the Front-line." *Clinical Journal of Sport Medicine* 12: 254–258.

Miah, A. 2002. "Governance, Harmonisation, and Genetics: The World Anti-Doping Agency and its European Connections." *European Sport Management Quarterly* 2 (4): 350–369.

Mignon, P. 2003. "The Tour de France and the Doping Issue." *The International Journal of the History of Sport* 20 (2) : 227–245.

Millham, S., Bullock, R., and Cherrett, P.F. 1972. "Social Control in Organizations." *The British Journal of Sociology* 23 (4): 406–421.

Mills, C.W. 1973. *The Sociological Imagination*. Middlesex, England: Penguin Books.

Møller, V. 2005. "Knud Enemark Jensen's Death During the 1960 Rome Olympics: A Search for Truth?" *Sport in History* 25 (3): 452–471.

———. 2009. "Conceptual Confusion and the Anti-Doping Campaign in Denmark." In *Elite Sport, Doping and Public Health*, edited by Moller, V., McNamee, M. and Dimeo, P., 13–28. Odense: University Press of Southern Denmark.

———. 2010. *The Ethics of Doping and Anti-Doping: Redeming the Soul of Sport?* London: Routledge.

Monitoring the Future. 2015. "Monitoring the Future: A Continuing Study of American Youth." The Regents of the University of Michigan. http://monitoringthefuture.org/. Accessed 26 June 2015.

Moston, S.E., Engelberg, T., and Skinner, J. 2015. "Perceived Incidence of Drug Use in Australian Sport: A Survey of Athletes and Coaches." *Sport in Society: Cultures, Commerce, Media, Politics* 18 (1): 91–105.

Mugford, S., Mugford, J., and Donnelly, D. 1999. *Social Research Project: Athletes' Motivations for Using or Not Using Performance Enhancing Drugs*. Canberra: Australian Sports Drug Agency.

Munckton, S. 2010. "Fresh Hysteria on Drugs and Sport." *Green Left Weekly*: 851.

Murphy, P. 2006. "Drug Use at a Peak: AFL Star." *The Australian*, 31 March 2006.

Murphy, T. 1997. "Last week in the AFL. . . . AFL Round 22, Weekly Wrapup." Footy.com.au, 1 September 1997. http://www.footy.com.au/dags/97/wrapup/wrapup_r22.html. Accessed 30 January 2008.

Nadel, D. 1998a. "Colour, Corporations and Commissioners, 1976–1985." In *More Than A Game: An Unauthorised History of Australian Rules Football*, edited by Hess, R. and Stewart, B., 200–224. Melbourne: Melbourne University Press.

———. 1998b. "The League Goes National, 1986–1997." In *More Than a Game: An Unauthorised History of Australian Rules Football*, edited by Hess, R. and Stewart, B., 225–255. Carlton: Melbourne University Press.

Nafziger, J.A.R. 1992. "International Sports Law: A Reply of Characteristics and Trends." *American Journal of International Law* 86 (3): 489–518.

Nebehay, S. 2008. "Rogge Says IOC More Credible on Doping since Beijing." *Reuters*, 30 September 2008. http://www.reuters.com/article/sportsNews/idUS TRE48T4OE2008093. Accessed 24 October 2008.

Nicholson, M. 2006. "Moving the Goalposts: Change and Challenge in a Competitive Football Market." In *Football Fever: Moving the Goalposts*, edited by Nicholson, M., Stewart, B. and Hess, R., 1–10. Hawthorne, Vic: Maribyrnong Press.

Nixon, R. 1992. "Apartheid on the Run: The South African Sports Boycott." *Transition* 58: 68–88.

OATH. 1999a. "First Ever Olympic Athlete Sponsored Symposium on IOC Reform Convenes in New York." Olympic Advocates Together Honourably. http://www. prnewswire.com/cgi-bin/stories.pl?ACCT=104andSTORY=/www/story/06–11– 1999/0000961706andEDATE=. Accessed 20 July 2006.

———. 1999b. "Olympic Advocates Launch International organization to Renew Olympic Spirit." Olympic Athletes Together Honourably. http://www.prnews wire.co.uk/cgi/news/release?id=13026. Accessed 20 July 2006.

Opie, H. 2004. "Drugs in Sport and the Law—Moral Authority, Diversity and the Pursuit of Excellence." *Marquette Sports Law Review* 14: 267–77.

Ordway, C., and Rofe, S. 1998, November. "Drugs in Sport." *The Law Society of South Australia Bulletin*, 16–19.

Paccagnella, M., and Grove, R.J. 1997. "Drugs, Sex, and Crime in Sport: An Australian Perspective." *Journal of Sport and Social Issues* 21 (2): 179–188.

Page, C.H. 1973. "The World of Sport and its Study." In *Sport and Society: An Anthology*, edited by Talamini, J., and Page, C.H., 1–40. Boston: Brown Little.

Pakulski, J. 1986. "Legitimacy and Mass Compliance: Reflections on Max Weber and Soviet-Type Societies." *British Journal of Political Science* 16 (1): 35–56.

Palmer, C. 2000. "Spin Doctors and Sportsbrokers." *International Review for Sociology of Sport* 35 (3): 364–377.

———. 2001. "Outside the Imagined Community: Basque Terrorism, Political Activism, and the Tour de France." *Sociology of Sport Journal* 18: 143–161.

Parenti, M. 1986. *Inventing Reality*. New York: St. Martin's Press.

Parham, E. 2008. "Australia and the World Anti-Doping Code 1999–2008." World Anti-Doping Agency. http://www.wada-ama.org/rtecontent/document/Aus tralia_and_the_World_Anti_Doping_Code_1999_2008.pdf. Accessed 2 April 2009.

Parisotto, R. 2006. *Blood Sports: The Inside Dope on Drugs in Sport*. Prahran: Hardie Grant Books.

Pascoe, R. 1995. *The Winter Game: The Complete History of Australian Football*. Port Melbourne: Reed Books Australia.

———. 1997. "The AFL 1996 Centenary Celebrations." *Australian Historical Studies* 28 (108): 113–117.

Pearlman, J. 2013. " 'Darkest Day' Down Under as Australian Sport Rocked by Revelations of Drug Taking and Links to Organised Crime." *The Telegraph*, 7 February 2013. http://www.telegraph.co.uk/sport/othersports/drugsinsport/9854446/ Darkest-day-Down-Under-as-Australian-sport-rocked-by-revelations-of-drug-taking-and-links-to-organised-crime.html. Accessed 29 June 2015.

Pells, E. 2015. "Associating with Drug Cheats Forbidden in '15 Olympics code." *The China Post*, 4 January 2015. http://www.chinapost.com.tw/sports/other/2015/ 01/04/425592/Associating-with.htm. Accessed 7 April 2015.

Perez, A.J. 2008. "Poll: Doping Questions Cloud Americans' View of Games." *USA Today*, 31 July 2008. http://www.usatoday.com/sports/olympics/beijing/2008–0 7-31-poll-doping-cover_N.htm. Accessed 14 August 2009.

Petroczi, A. 2007. "Attitudes and doping: A Structural Equation Analysis of the Relationship between Athletes' Attitudes, Sport Orientation and Doping Behaviour." *Substance Abuse Treatment, Prevention, and Policy* 2: 34.

Petroczi, A., and Aidman, E. 2008. "Psychological Drivers in Doping: The Life-Cycle Model of Performance Enhancement." *Substance Abuse Treatment, Prevention, and Policy* 3 (7): published online 2008 March 2010. doi: 2010.1186/1747-2597X-2003-2007.

Phelan, J. 2008. "Illicit Drugs Policy Revamped." *Australian Football League*, 28 August 2008. http://afl.com.au/News/NEWSARTICLE/tabid/208/Default. aspx?newsId=6651. Accessed 29 August 2008.

Pierik, J. 2006. "Footy's Going to Pot: Rhys-Jones Says AFL a Drugs Playground." *The Mercury*, 5 April 2006.

———. 2015. "Swiss Court could 'Stike Down' Appeal against Essendon 34." *The Age*, 27 June 2015. http://www.theage.com.au/afl/afl-news/swiss-court-could-strike-down-appeal-against-essendon-34-20150627-ghz82k.html. Accessed 29 June 2015.

Pierre, J., and Røiseland, A. 2011. "Democratic Legitimacy by Performance? Exploring a Research Field." ECPR General Conference, Reykjavik, 25–27 August, 2011. http://www.ecprnet.eu/MyECPR/proposals/reykjavik/uploads/papers/1658.pdf. Accessed 15 July 2012.

Plummer, K. 2013. "Inspirations: The National Deviancy Conference." Ken Plummer. http://kenplummer.com/2013/02/08/inspirations-the-national-deviancy-conference/. Accessed 16 June 2013.

Pound, R. W. 2007. "Code Compliance: The Time is Now." *Play True: An Official Publication of the World Anti-Doping Agency* (2): 1–2.

Press Association. 2014. "Michael Rogers Cleared to Race as UCI Accepts Contaminated Meat Claim." *The Guardian*, 23 April 2014. http://www.theguardian.com/sport/2014/apr/23/michael-rogers-uci-contaminated-meat. Accessed 1 April 2015.

Pritchard, D., and Hughes, K. D. 1997. "Patterns of Deviance in Crime News." *Journal of Communication* 47 (3): 49–67.

Ralph, J. 2008. "AFL Clubs Happy with Drug Code Changes." *Herald Sun*, 29 August 2008. http://www.news.com.au/heraldsun/sport/afl/story/0,26576,24258903-19742,00.html. Accessed 2 September 2008.

Rasmussen, K. 2005. "The Quest for the Imaginary Evil: A Critique of Anti-Doping." *Sport in History* 25 (3): 515–535.

Reiner, R. 2007. "Media-Made Criminality: The Representation of Crime in the Mass Media." In *The Oxford Handbook of Criminology*, edited by Maguire, M., Morgan, R. and Reiner, R., 302–337. Oxford, UK: Oxford University Press.

Reuters. 2007a. "Ex-IOC Chief 'Not Interested in Doping.'" *The Sydney Morning Herald*, 25 October 2007. http://www.smh.com.au/news/Sport/ExIOC-chief-not-interested-in-doping/2007/10/25/1192941189806.html. Accessed 25 October 2007.

———. 2007b. "WADA Chief Pound Says Key Players Fear Doping Problem." *Reuters UK*, 22 July 2007. http://uk.reuters.com/article/UK_GOLF/idUKL2202024320070722?pageNumber=. Accessed 24 July 2007.

———. 2008. "FINA to Tackle Super Swim Suit Issue." *The Sydney Morning Herald*, 25 March 2008. http://news.smh.com.au/fina-to-tackle-super-swim-suit-issue/20080325-21bd.html. Accessed 25 March 2008.

Rielly, S. 1998. "Spectre of Another AFL Drug Scandal." *The Age*, 8 May 1998.

Riordan, J. 1993. "The Rise and Fall of Soviet Olympic Champions." *Olympika* 2: 25–44.

Roach, G. 2006. "So Certain Senior AFL Players Say they have No Confidence in the League's own Anti-Doping System." *The Advertiser*, 18 March 2006.

Robinson, M. 2014. "Essendon's Governance was Shoddy, but ASADA and AFL have Let us All Down." *Herald Sun*, 13 Aguust 2014. http://www.heraldsun.com.au/sport/afl/essendons-governance-was-shoddy-but-asada-and-afl-have-let-us-all-down-writes-mark-robinson/story-fni5f0at-1227023438691?nk=2f552dc2dd51 69d33ff17b73a46e4bcc. Accessed 17 August 2014.

Robinson, S. 2007. "Drugs in Sport: A Cure Worse than the Disease?" *International Journal of Sports Science and Coaching* 2 (4): 363–368.

Rohloff, A., and Wright, S. 2010. "Moral Panic and Social Theory: Beyond the Heuristic." *Current Sociology* 58 (3): 403–419.

Rommetvedt, H. 2005. "Norway: Resources Count, but Votes Decide? From neo-corporatist representation to neo-pluralist parliamentarism." *West European Politics* 28 (4): 740–763.

Rosen, D. M. 2008. *Dope: A History of Performance Enhancement in Sports from the Nineteenth Century to Today.* Westport, Conn.: Praeger.

Rothstein, B. 2009. "Creating Political Legitimacy: Electoral Democracy Versus Quality of Government." *American Behavioral Scientist* 53: 311–330.

Rowe, D. 1992. "Modes of Sports Writing." In *Journalism and Popular Culture*, edited by Dahlgren, P. and Sparks, C., 96–112. London: Sage.

Rushall, B. S., and Jones, M. 2007. "Drugs in Sport: A Cure Worse than the Disease?" *International Journal of Sports Science and Coaching* 2 (4): 335–358.

Ryan, R. 2015. "So Many Questions, So Few Answers." *The New Daily*, 30 January 2015. http://thenewdaily.com.au/sport/2015/01/30/asada-shambles-many-quest ions-answers/. Accessed 10 February 2015.

Sacco, V. F. 1995. "Media Constructions of Crime." *Annals of the American Academy of Political and Social Science* 539 :141–154.

Sanders, C. R. 1990. " 'A Lot of People Like It': The Relationship Between Deviance and Popular Culture." In *Marginal Conventions: Popular Culture, Mass Media and Social Deviance*, edited by Sanders, C. R., 3–13. Bowling Green, Ohio: Bowling Green State University Popular Press.

Saraceno, J. 2007. "For a Real Drug Deterrent, Start Naming Names." *USA Today*, 26 September 2007. http://www.usatoday.com/sports/columnist/saraceno/2007–09–25-drugs-feds_N.htm. Accessed 27 September 2007.

Savulescu, J., and Foddy, B. 2011. "Le Tour and Failure of Zero Tolerance: Time to Relax Doping Controls." In *Enhancing Human Capacities*, edited by Savulescu, J., Meulen, R. H. J. ter and Kahane, G., 304–312. Chichester, West Sussex, UK: Wiley-Blackwell.

Schlesinger, P., and Tumber, H. 1994. *Reporting Crime: The Media Politics of Criminal Justice.* Oxford: Clarendon Press.

Schneider, A. 2000a. "Olympic Reform, Are We There Yet?" Paper presented at the Bridging Three Centuries, Fifth International Symposium for Olympic Research, The University of Western Ontario, London, Ontario, Canada, September 2000.

———. 2004. "Privacy, Confidentiality and Human Rights in Sport." *Sport in Society* 7 (3): 438–456.

———. 2006. "Cultural Nuances: Doping, Cycling and the Tour de France." *Sport in Society* 9 (2): 212–226.

Schneider, J. W. 1985. "Social Problems Theory: The Constructionist View." *Annual Review of Sociology* 11: 209–229.

Schreiber, C., and Kassner, S. 2014. "Open Letter and Statement." German Athletes Commission. http://www.dosb.de/fileadmin/fm-dosb/arbeitsfelder/leistungssport/Antidoping/WADA_final_17122014__3_.pdf. Accessed 13 April 2015.

Schwartz, L., and Connolly, R. 1997. "New Claims of Steroid Use in AFL." *Sunday Age*, 31 August 1997.

Seib, P. 2008. *The Al Jazeera Effect: How the New Global Media are Reshaping World Politics*. Washington DC: Potomac Books, Inc.

Senate Standing Committee on Environment, Recreation and the Arts. 1989. *Drugs In Sport: Interim Report*. Canberra: Commonwealth of Australia. http://www.aph.gov.au/senate/committee/ecita_ctte/completed_inquiries/pre1996/drugs-int/report.pdf. Accessed 13 November 2007

———. 1990. *Drugs in Sport, Second Report* Canberra: Commonwealth of Australia.

Senator The Hon Kate Lundy. 2013. Media Release: Important New Anti-Doping Powers for ASADA Pass Through Parliament. Australian Government. http://www.asada.gov.au/media/ministerial.html. Accessed 15 April 2015.

Senator The Hon Rod Kemp. 2005. Media Release: AFL to Become WADA Code Compliant. Canberra: Australian Government. http://parlinfo.aph.gov.au/parlInfo/download/media/pressrel/8OPG6/upload_binary/8opg63.pdf;fileType=application%2Fpdf#search=%22kemp%20AFL%20pressrel%22. Accessed 4 February 2011.

Sheil, P. 1998. *Olympic Babylon: Sex, Scandal and Sportsmanship: The True Story of the Olympic Games*. Sydney: Pan Macmillan Australia.

Shermer, M. 2008. "The Doping Dilemma." *Scientific American*, 31 March 2008. http://www.sciam.com/article.cfm?id=the-doping-dilemma. Accessed 9 April 2008.

Siekmann, R.R.C., Soek, J., and Bellani, A. 1999. *Doping Rules of International Sports Organisations*. The Hague: T.M.C. Asser Press.

Silkstone, D. 2008. "Steroids Scourge Leaps from the Sports Field into the Community." *The Age*, 20 September 2008. http://www.theage.com.au/national/steroids-scourge-leaps-from-the-sports-field-into-the-community-20080919-4k8r.html?page=. Accessed 14 November 2008.

Silver, M.D. 2001. "Use of Ergogenic Aids by Athletes." *Journal of the American Academy of Orthopaedic Surgeons* 9: 61–70.

Silverman, D. 2001. *Interpreting Qualitative Data: Methods for Analysing Talk, Text and Interaction*. London: Sage.

Slater, M. 2008. "US Stars Lead Anti-Doping Battle." BBC Sport, 6 May 2008. http://news.bbc.co.uk/sport2/hi/olympics/athletics/7384365.stm. Accessed 11 May 2008.

Slattery, G. 2007. "The Drug Story you Haven't Read, Heard or Seen." *AFL Record* (Melbourne, Aust) (Aug 31 — Sept 2): 6–7.

Smith, Aaron C.T., and Stewart, B. 2008. "Drug Policy in Sport: Hidden Assumptions and Inherent Contradictions." *Drug and Alcohol Review* 27: 123–129.

Smith, P. 2006a. "AFL must Choose between Welfare of Player and Game." *The Australian*, 16 August 2006. http://www.theaustralian.news.com.au/story/0,20867,20142944–12270,00.html. Accessed 16 August 2006.

———. 2006b. "Appeasement Policy a Failure." *The Australian*, Tuesday July 25 2006.

———. 2008. "Contaminated by its own Drug Code." *The Australian*, 6 September 2008. http://www.theaustralian.news.com.au/story/0,25197,24301252–5013459,00.html. Accessed 11 September 2008.

———. 2010. "AFL Drugs Code must Protect the Sick." *The Australian*, 4 September 2010. http://www.theaustralian.com.au/news/sport/afl-drugs-code-must-protect-the-sick/story-e6frg7t6-122591403199. Accessed 15 February 2011.

Soek, J. 2003. "The WADA World Anti-Doping Code: The Road to Harmonisation." *The International Sports Law Journal* 2: 2–11.

Spaaij, R., Farquharson, K., and Marjoribanks, T. 2015. "Sport and Social Inequalities." *Social Compass* 9 (5): 400–411.

Spencer, M.E. 1970. "Weber on Legitimate Norms and Authority." *The British Journal of Sociology* 21 (2): 123–134.

Sportal.com.au. n/d. "AFL Beef Up Integrity Unit." *Sportal.com.au*, http://www.sportal.com.au/afl/news/afl-beef-up-integrity-unit/3yrn6ahkxwyh1g6vdsqx4b9sr. Accessed 29 June 2015.

Stevens, M. 2004. "Denial Led to Angwin Sacking." *The Daily Telegraph*, 8 April 2004.

Stevens, M., and Barrett, D. 2004. "Carlton Crisis Blue Bust: Carlton Board Investigates Norman, Angwin Breach." *Herald Sun*, 7 April 2004.

Stevens, M., Phillips, S., and Cunningham, M. 2004. "It's all Over for blackened Blue: Angwin Sacked over Drug Use." *The Mercury*, 8 April 2004.

Stewart, B. 2006. "The World Anti-Doping Agency and the Australian Football League: The Irresistible Force Bludgeons the Immoveable Object." In *Football Fever: Moving the Goalposts*, edited by Nicholson, M., Stewart, B. and Hess, R., 107–114. Hawthorne, Victoria: Maribyrnong Press.

———. 2007a. "Drugs in Australian Sport: A Brief History." *Sporting Traditions* 23 (2): 65–78.

———. 2007b. "The Political Economy of Football: Framing the Analysis." In *The Games Are Not the Same: The Political Economy of Football in Australia*, edited by Stewart, B., 3–22. Carlton, Vic.: Melbourne University Press.

Stewart, B., Dickson, G., and Smith, A. 2008. "Drug Use in the Australian Football League: A Critical Survey." *Sporting Traditions* 25 (1): 57–74.

Stewart, B., Nicholson, M., and Dickson, G. 2005. "The Australian Football Leagues' Recent Progress: A Study in Cartel Conduct and Monopoly Power." *Sport Management Review* (Melbourne, Aust) 8 (2): 95–117.

Stewart, B., Nicholson, M., Smith, A., and Westerbeek, H. 2004. *Australian Sport: Better by Design?: The Evolution of Australian Sport Policy.* London: Routledge.

Stewart, B., and Smith, A. C.T. 2008. "Drug Use in Sport Implications for Public Policy." *Journal of Sport and Social Issues* 32 (3): 278–298.

Stoddart, B. 1986. *Saturday Afternoon Fever: Sport in the Australian Culture.* London: Angus and Robertson.

Stokvis, R. 2003. "Moral Entrepreneurship and Doping Cultures in Sport." Amsterdam School for Social Science Research.

Strelan, P., and Boeckmann, R.J. 2003. "A New Model for Understanding Performance Enhancing Drug Use by Elite Athletes." *Journal of Applied Sport Psychology* 15: 176–183.

Strenk, A. 1980. "Diplomats in Tracksuits: The Role of Sport in the German Democratic Republic." *The Journal of Sport and Social Issues* 4 (1): 34–45.

Striegel, H., Vollkommer, G., and Dickhuth, H-H. 2002. "Combating Drug Use in Competitive Sports: An Analysis from the Athletes' Perspective." *Journal of Sports Medicine and Physical Fitness* 42 (3): 354–359.

Suchman, M.C. 1995. "Managing Legitimacy: Strategic and Institutional Approaches." *The Academy of Management Review* 20 (3): 571–610.

The Sunday Telegraph. 2014. "ASADA: Australia's Blackest Day in Sport was a Dark Day for Julia Gillard." *The Sunday Telegraph*, 10 August 2014. http://www.dailytelegraph.com.au/news/opinion/asada-australias-blackest-day-in-sport-was-a-dark-day-for-julia-gillard/story-fni0cwl5-1227018896179.

Sutherland, A. 2013. "Integrity Unit could Lose its Integrity." *The Roar*, 3 March 2013. http://www.theroar.com.au/2013/03/03/integrity-unit-could-lose-its-integrity/. Accessed 29 June 2015.

Swimming World. 2009. "Jessica Hardy Suspension Reduced to One Year, Supplement Ruled as Contaminated: USA Swimming Releases Statement: USADA Press Release; AdvoCare Disputes Findings—Updated." *Swimming World.* http://

www.swimmingworldmagazine.com/news/jessica-hardy-suspension-reduced-to-one-year-supplement-ruled-as-contaminated-usa-swimming-releases-statement-usada-press-release-advocare-disputes-findings-updated/. Accessed 24 April 2015.

Switkowski, Z. 2013. "Dr. Ziggy Switkowski Report." Essendon Football Club. http://www.essendonfc.com.au/news/2013–05–06/dr-ziggy-switkowski-report. Accessed 12 February 2015.

Teetzel, S. 2004. "The Road to Wada." Seventh International Symposium for Olympic Research, Windermere Manor, London, Ontario, 21–23 October 2004,. http://www.la84foundation.org/SportsLibrary/ISOR/ISOR2004t.pdf. Accessed 16 December 2010.

Thomas, J.J.R. 1984. "Weber and Direct Democracy." *The British Journal of Sociology* 35 (2): 216–240.

Thompson, B., and Greek, C. 2012. "Mods and Rockers, Drunken Debutants, and Sozzled Students: Moral Panic or the British Silly Season?" *Sage OPEN* 2 (3) (July–September 2012): 1–13. doi: 10.1177/2158244012455177.

Thompson, K. 1998. *Moral Panics.* London: Routledge.

Throgmorton, J.A. 1991. "The Rhetorics of Policy Analysis." *Policy Sciences* 24 (2): 153–179.

Timms, D. 2002. "Koops in Clear, Finally." *Herald Sun.* 30 April 2002.

Todd, J., and Todd, T. 2001. "Significant Events in the History of Drug Testing and the Olympic Movement." In *Doping in Elite Sport: The Politics of Drugs in the Olympic Movement*, edited by Wilson, W. and Derse, E., 65–128. Champaign, IL: Human Kinetics Publishers, Inc.

Tomlinson, A. 2005a. "The Commercialisation of the Olympics: Cities, Corporations, and the Olympic Commodity." In *Global Olympics: Historical and Sociological Studies of the Modern Games*, edited by Young, K. and Wamsley, K.B., 179–200. Amsterdam: Elsevier JAI.

———. 2005b. "The Making of the Global Sports Economy: ISL, Adidas and the Rise of the Corporate Player in World Sport." In *Sport and Corporate Nationalisms*, edited by Andrews, D.L., 35–65. Oxford: Berg.

Tonts, M., and Atherley, K. 2010. "Competitive Sport and the Construction of Place Identity in Rural Australia." *Sport in Society* 13 (3): 381–398.

Toohey, K. 2010. "Post-Sydney 2000 Australia: A Potential Clash of Aspirations Between Recreational and Elite Sport." *The International Journal of the History of Sport* 27 (16): 2766–2779.

Toohey, K., and Taylor, T. 2009. "Sport in Australia: 'Worth a Shout'." *Sport in Society* 12 (7): 837–841.

Toohey, K., and Veal, A.J. 2000. *The Olympic Games: A Social Science Perspective.* Wallingford: CABI Publishing.

Torres, C.R., and Dyreson, M. 2005. "The Cold War Games." In *Global Olympics: Historical and Sociological Studies of the Modern Games*, edited by Young, K. and Wamsley, K.B., 59–82. Amsterdam: Elsevier JAI.

Tucher, A. 1994. *Froth and Scum: Truth, Beauty, Goodness, and the Ax Murder in America's First Mass Medium.* Chapel Hill: University of North Carolina Press.

Turner, M., and McCrory, P. 2003. "Social Drug Policies for Sport." *British Journal of Sports Medicine* 37 (5): 378–379.

Turner, P.A. 1987. "Church's Fried Chicken and The Klan: A Rhetorical Analysis of Rumor on the Black Community." *Western Folklore* 4: 294–306.

UNESCO (United Nations Educational Scientific and Cultural Organization). 2014. "Background to the Convention." United Nations Educational Scientific and Cultural Organization. http://www.unesco.org/new/en/social-and-human-sciences/themes/anti-doping/international-convention-against-doping-in-sport/background/. Accessed 3 September 2014.

USADA (United States Anti-Doping Agency). 2012. "Members of the United States Postal Service Pro-Cycling Team Doping Conspiracy, Dr. Garcia Del Moral, Dr. Ferrari And Trainer Mart Receive Lifetime Bans for Doping Violations." USADA (United States Anti-Doping Agency). http://www.usada.org/members-of-the-united-states-postal-service-pro-cycling-team-doping-conspiracy-dr-garcia-del-moral-dr-ferrari-and-trainer-marti-receive-lifetime-bans-for-doping-violations/. Accessed 11 April 2015.

Vasciannie, S. 2006. "As Fast as a Drug." *Jamaica Gleaner*, 7 August 2006. http://www.jamaica-gleaner.com/gleaner/20060807/cleisure/cleisure2.html. Accessed 7 August 2006.

Verroken, M. 2000. "Drug Use and Abuse in Sport." *Bailliere's Clinical Endocrinology and Metabolism* 14 (1): 1023.

———. 2005. "Drug Use and Abuse in Sport." In *Drugs in Sport*, edited by Mottram, D.R., 29–63. New York, NY: Routledge.

Verroken, M., and Mottram, D.R. 2005. "Doping Control in Sport." In *Drugs in Sport*, edited by Mottram, D.R., 309–356. London: Routledge.

Victor, J.S. 1998. "Moral Panics and the Social Construction of Deviant Behavior: A Theory and Application to the Case of Ritual Child Abuse." *Sociological Perspectives* 41 (3): 541–565.

Voet, W. 2001. *Breaking the Chain: Drugs and Cycling: The True Story*. London: Yellow Jersey Press.

von Hoffman, N. 1985. "The Press: Pack of Fools. Killer Bees, Missing Kids, and Other Phoney Stories." *The New Republic* 3681: 9–11.

Voy, R. 1991. *Drugs, Sport and Politics*. Champaign, IL: Leisure Press.

WADA (World Anti-Doping Agency). 2005. "UNESCO International Convention against Doping in Sport—Overview." World Anti-Doping Agency. http://www.wada-ama.org/en/dynamic.ch2?pageCategory.id=39. Accessed 5 February 2007.

———. 2006a. "A Brief History of Anti-Doping." World Anti-Doping Agency. http://www.wada-ama.org/en/dynamic.ch2?pageCategory.id=31. Accessed 11 March 2006.

———. 2006b. "Chairman's Message." World Anti-Doping Agency. http://www.wada-ama.org/en/dynamic.ch2?pageCategory.id=25. Accessed 5 October 2006.

———. 2006c. "The Code and Sanctions." *Play True* 3: 7–8.

———. 2006d. "Letter of Ratification—UNESCO International Convention Against Doping in Sport." World Anti-Doping Agency. http://www.wada-ama.org/rte-content/document/WADA_Letter_Ratification_Convention_En.pdf. Accessed 5 February 2007.

———. 2006e. "Logo Story." World Anti-Doping Agency. http://www.wada-ama.org/en/dynamic.ch2?pageCategory.id=26. Accessed 9 January 2008.

———. 2006f. "The World Anti-Doping Code: A Guide." *Play True* 4 (3): 3–6.

———. 2007a. "Education." World Anti-Doping Agency. http://www.wada-ama.org/rtecontent/document/05_FS_Education_en.pdf. Accessed 2 February 2007.

———. 2007b. "QandA: The World Anti-Doping Agency." World Anti-Doping Agency. http://www.wada-ama.org/rtecontent/document/QA_The_World_Anti-Doping_Agency.pdf. Accessed 9 January 2008.

———. 2007c. "Science Honing in on Doping." *Play True* 5 (2): 5–8.

———. 2008a. "President's Welcome Message." World Anti-Doping Agency. http://www.wada-ama.org/en/dynamic.ch2?pageCategory.id=25. Accessed 9 January 2008.

———. 2008b. "WADA Advances Cooperation with Interpol, Athlete Passport Development." World Anti-Doping Agency. http://www.wada-ama.org/en/newsarticle.ch2?articleId=311574. Accessed 24 November 2008.

————. 2008 (July). "What is the Code—Introduction." World Anti-Doping Agency. http://www.wada-ama.org/en/dynamic.ch2?pageCategory.id=26. Accessed 14 July 2008.

————. 2009. "World Anti-Doping Program—Governments." World Anti-Doping Agency. http://www.wada-ama.org/en/World-Anti-Doping-Program/Governments/. Accessed 11 December 2009.

————. 2009 (January). "WADA History." World Anti-Doping Agency. June 2006. http://www.wada-ama.org/en/dynamic.ch2?pageCategory.id=31. Accessed 30 January 2009.

————. 2009 (October). "Programs—Education, Introduction." World Anti-Doping Agency. http://www.wada-ama.org/en/dynamic.ch2?pageCategory.id=26. Accessed 1 October 2009.

————. 2009, September. "Governance—List Working Committees." World Anti-Doping Agency. http://www.wada-ama.org/en/dynamic.ch2?pageCategory.id=31. Accessed 1 September 2009.

————. 2010a. "About WADA." World Anti-Doping Agency. http://www.wada-ama.org/en/About-WADA/. Accessed 12 August 2010.

————. 2010b. "Education and Awareness." World Anti-Doping Agency. http://www.wada-ama.org/en/Education-Awareness/. Accessed 2 January 2011.

————. 2010c. "WADA—Education and Awareness, Social Science Research." World Anti-Doping Agency. http://www.wada-ama.org/en/Education-Awareness/Social-Science/. Accessed 11 April 2010.

————. 2010d. "WADA—Education and Awareness, Social Science Research, Funded Research Projects." World Anti-Doping Agency. http://www.wada-ama.org/en/Education-Awareness/Social-Science/Funded-Projects/. Accessed 11 April 2010.

————. 2012a. "Code and International Standards (IS) Review." World Anti-Doping Agency. http://www.wada-ama.org/en/world-anti-doping-program/sports-and-anti-doping-organizations/the-code/code-review/. Accessed 7 December 2012.

————. 2012b. "The World Anti-Doping Code International Standard for Testing." World Anti-Doping Agency. https://wada-main-prod.s3.amazonaws.com/resources/files/WADA_IST_2012_EN.pdf. Accessed 3 September 2014.

————. 2013a. "2013 Anti-Doping Testing Figures—Sport Report." World Anti-Doping Agency. https://wada-main-prod.s3.amazonaws.com/resources/files/WADA-2013-Anti-Doping-Testing-Figures-SPORT-REPORT.pdf. Accessed 7 April 2015.

————. 2013b. "WADA Appoints Sir Craig Reedie as its new President." World Anti-Doping Agency. https://www.wada-ama.org/en/media/news/2013–11/wada-appoints-sir-craig-reedie-as-its-new-president. Accessed 31 January 2015.

————. 2014a. "Governance—Executive Committee." World Anti-Doping Agency. https://elb.wada-ama.org/en/who-we-are/governance/executive-committee. Accessed 3 September 2014.

————. 2014b. "Governance—Foundation Board." World Anti-Doping Agency. https://elb.wada-ama.org/en/who-we-are/governance/foundation-board. Accessed 3 September 2014.

————. 2014c. "International Standard for Testing and Investigations." https://wada-main-prod.s3.amazonaws.com/resources/files/WADA-2015-ISTI-Final-EN.pdf. Accessed 8 January 2015.

————. 2014d. "A Strong, Fair Set of Rules." *Play True* (2): 12–13.

————. 2014e. "What we Do—International Standards." World Anti-Doping Agency. https://elb.wada-ama.org/en/what-we-do/international-standards. Accessed 3 September 2014.

————. 2014f. "What we Do—The Code." World Anti-Doping Agency. https://www.wada-ama.org/en/what-we-do/the-code. Accessed 3 September 2014.

————. 2015a. "Anti-Doping Community." World Anti-Doping Agency. http://www.wada-ama.org/en/Anti-Doping-Community/. Accessed 19 March 2015.

————. 2015b. "Code Review Process." World Anti-Doping Agency. https://www.wada-ama.org/en/what-we-do/the-code/code-review-process. Accessed 18 March 2015.

————. 2015c. "Copenhagen Declaration—List of Signatories." World Anti-Doping Agency. https://www.wada-ama.org/en/who-we-are/anti-doping-community/governments/copenhagen-declaration-list-of-signatories. Accessed 18 March 2015.

————. 2015d. "Governments." World Anti-Doping Agency. https://www.wada-ama.org/en/who-we-are/anti-doping-community/governments. Accessed 19 March 2015.

————. 2015e. "International Standards." World Anti-Doping Agency. https://elb.wada-ama.org/en/what-we-do/international-standards. Accessed 31 March 2015.

————. 2015f. "Significant Changes Between the 2009 Code and the 2015 Code." World Anti-Doping Agency. https://www.wada-ama.org/en/resources/the-code/significant-changes-between-the-2009-code-and-the-2015-code. Accessed 24 April 2015.

————. 2015g. "World Anti-Doping Code 2015." https://wada-main-prod.s3.amazonaws.com/resources/files/wada-2015-world-anti-doping-code.pdf. Accessed 3 September 2014.

Waddington, I. 2000. *Sport, Health and Drugs: A Critical Sociological Perspective*. London: E and FN Spon.

————. 2005. "Changing Patterns of Drug Use in British Sport from the 1960s." *Sport in History* 25 (3): 472–496.

Wagner-Pacifici, R. E. 1986. *The Moro Morality Play: Terrorism as Social Drama*. Chicago: University of Chicago Press.

Walsh, D. 2007. *From Lance to Landis: Inside the American Doping Controversy at the Tour de France*. New York: Ballantine Books.

————. 2012. *Seven Deadly Sins: My Pursuit of Lance Armstrong*. London: Simon and Schuster.

Walter, B. 2007. "My 14 years of Drugs: Joey." *The Age, League HQ*, 31 August 2007. http://www.brisbanetimes.com.au/news/sport/my-14-years-of-drugs-joey/2007/08/30/1188067339383.html. Accessed 4 September 2014.

Wamsley, K. B., and Young, K. 2005. "Coubertin's Olympic Games: The Greatest Show on Earth." In *Global Olympics: Historical and Sociological Studies of the Modern Games*, edited by Young, K. and Wamsley, K. B., xiii-xxv. Amsterdam: Elsevier JAI.

Warner, M. 2011. "Six AFL Players Fail Illicit Drug Tests in 2010." *Herald Sun*, 22 June 2011. http://www.heraldsun.com.au/ipad/six-afl-players-fail-illicit-drug-tests-in-2010/story-fn6bfkm6–122607996800. Accessed 28 July 2011.

Weber, M. 1947. *The Theory of Social and Economic Organisation*. New York: Free Press.

————. 1954. *Max Weber on Law in Economy and Society*. Cambridge: Harvard University Press.

————. 1969. *Economy and Society, 2 vols*. Berkeley: University of California Press.

Weisman, L. 2007. "Anti-Doping Agency Assails NFL Policy, despite Changes." *USA Today*, 25 January 2007. http://www.usatoday.com/sports/football/nfl/2007-01-25-nfl-testing_x.htm. Accessed 5 February 2007.

Welch, M., Weber, L., and Edwards, W. 2000. "'All The News That's Fit to Print': A Content Analysis of the Correctional Debate in the *New York Times*." *The Prison Journal* 80 (3): 245–264.

Whannel, G. 2005. "The Five Rings and the Small Screen: Television, Sponsorship, and New Media in the Olympic Movement." In *Global Olympics: Historical and Sociological Studies of the Modern Games*, edited by Young, K. and Wamsley, K. B., 161–177. Amsterdam: Elsevier JAI.

Whateley, G. 2015. "Essendon Players the only ones Vindicated by AFL Tribunal Verdict, Gerard Whately Writes." *ABC News*, 1 April 2015. http://www.abc.net. au/news/2015–04–01/only-the-players-vindicated-by-verdict—whateley/636394. Accessed 29 June 2015.

Wheatcroft, G. 2003. *Le Tour: A History of the Tour de France*. London: Pocket Press.

Wheaton, B. 2015. "Assessing the Sociology of Sport: On Action Sport and the Politics of Identity." *International Review for Sociology of Sport* 50 (4): 634–639.

Whinnett, E. 2015. "'Darkest Day in Sport' now Looks more like a Political Stunt." *Herald Sun*, 1 April 2015. http://www.heraldsun.com.au/news/ victoria/darkest-day-in-sport-now-looks-more-like-a-political-stunt/ story-fni0fit3–122728719974. Accessed 29 June 2015.

White, R.J. 2015. "New Code Prohibits Olympic Athletes from Working with Drug Cheats." *CBS Sports.com*, 2 January 2015. http://www.cbssports.com/ general/eye-on-sports/24931946/new-code-prohibits-olympic-athletes-from-working-with-drug-cheats. Accessed 22 March 2015.

Whitham, J. 2010. "Failed Drugs Tests Falling." *AFL.com.au*, 13 May 2010. http://www.afl.com.au/news/newsarticle/tabid/208/newsid/94185/default.aspx. Accessed 13 July 2011.

———. 2011. "AFL's $1.25 billion Broadcast Deal." *Australian Football League*, 28 April 2011. http://www.afl.com.au/news/newsarticle/tabid/208/newsid/112560/ default.aspx. Accessed 16 August 2011.

Whittle, J. 2008. "The World Anti-Doping Agency's Diplomatic New Chief." *International Herald Tribune*, 29 February 2008. http://www.iht.com/articles/ 2008/02/29/sports/DRUGS.php. Accessed 13 April 2008.

Williams, A. 2006. "Football Folk Devils: Changes in Newspaper Representation of Sexual Assault Cases in the Australian Football League." In *Making Histories, Making Memories: The Construction of Australian Sporting Identities*, edited by Hess, R., 115–138. Melbourne: Australian Society for Sports History.

Williams, J.G.P. 1962. *Sports Medicine*. London: Edward Arnold.

———. 1975. "Drugs and Sport." *Medicine, Science and the Law* 15 (1): 9–15.

Wilson, J. 2006a. "Drugs Trio Fight to Stay Anonymous." *Herald Sun*, 22 May 2006.

———. 2006b. "Kennett Raises Heat on Drugs." *Herald Sun*, 4 April 2006.

———. 2006c. "Stop Protecting the Cheats: Gosper." *The Australian*, 1 September 2006. http://www.theaustralian.news.com.au/story/0,20867,20320923–23211,00. html. Accessed 4 September 2006.

Wilson, R. 2006d. "AFL Failing Everyone in War against Drugs." *The Advertiser*, 2 September 2006.

———. 2006e. "Name Names and End AFL Drug Farce." *The Advertiser*, 1 April 2006.

———. 2007. "A Sorry Situation." *The Daily Telegraph*, 20 October 2007. http:// www.news.com.au/dailytelegraph/story/0,22049,22614222–5006065,00.html. Accessed 31 December 2007.

Woodland, L. 1980. *Dope: The Use of Drugs in Sport*. Sydney: Reid.

Wright, R. 2000. "'I'd Sell You Suicide': Pop Music and Moral Panic in the Age of Marilyn Manson." *Popular Music* 19 (3): 365–385.

Wrynn, A. 2004. "The Human Factor: Science, Medicine and the International Olympic committee, 1900–70." *Sport in Society* 7 (2): 211–231.

Wuthnow, R., Hunter, J., Bergesen, A., and Kurzweil, E. 1984. *Cultural Analysis*. London: Routledge.

Xinhua. 2007. "WADA to Revise Anti-Doping Code." *China View*, 14 November 2007. http://news.xinhuanet.com/english/2007–11/15/content_7077921. htm. Accessed 26 December 2007.

Yesalis, C., and Bahrke, M.S. 2005. "Anabolic Steroid and Stimulant Use in North American Sport between 1850 and 1980." *Sport in History* 25 (3): 434–451.

Yesalis, C., and Cowart, V.S. 1998. *The Steroids Game*. Champaign, IL: Human Kinetics.

Young, J. 1971. "The Role of the Police as Amplifiers of Deviance, Negotiators of Reality and Translators of Fantasy." In *Images of Deviance*, edited by Cohen, S (27–61). Harmondsworth: Penguin.

———. 2009. "Moral Panic: Its Origins in Resistance, Ressentiment and the Translation of Fantasy into Reality." *British Journal of Criminology* 49: 4–16.

Zajdow, G. 2008. "Moral Panics: The Old and the New." *Deviant Behaviour* 29 (7): 640–664.

Zatz, M.S. 1987. "Chicano Youth Gangs and Crime: The Creation of a Moral Panic." *Contemporary Crises* 11 (2): 129–158.

Index

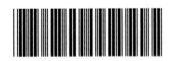